Acute Medicine

CLINICAL CASES UNCOVERED

For Tom and Matthew

Acute Medicine

CLINICAL CASES UNCOVERED

Chris Roseveare

BM FRCP

Consultant in Acute Medicine
Southampton University Hospitals NHS Trust
Southampton
UK

WILEY-BLACKWELL

A John Wiley & Sons, Ltd., Publication

This edition first published 2009, © 2009 by Chris Roseveare

Blackwell Publishing was acquired by John Wiley & Sons in February 2007. Blackwell's publishing programme has been merged with Wiley's global Scientific, Technical and Medical business to form Wiley-Blackwell.

Registered office: John Wiley & Sons Ltd, The Atrium, Southern Gate, Chichester, West Sussex, PO19 8SQ, UK

Editorial offices: 9600 Garsington Road, Oxford, OX4 2DQ, UK
      The Atrium, Southern Gate, Chichester, West Sussex, PO19 8SQ, UK
      111River Street, Hoboken, NJ 07030-5774, USA

For details of our global editorial offices, for customer services and for information about how to apply for permission to reuse the copyright material in this book please see our website at www.wiley.com/wiley-blackwell

Library of Congress Cataloging-in-Publication Data

Roseveare, Chris.
  Acute medicine / Chris Roseveare.
   p. ; cm. – (Clinical cases uncovered)
  Includes index.
  ISBN 978-1-4051-6883-0
  1. Critical care medicine. 2. Internal medicine. I. Title. II. Series.
  [DNLM: 1. Acute Disease–therapy–Case Reports. 2. Diagnosis, Differential–Case Reports. 3. Emergency Medicine–methods–Case Reports. 4. Emergency Treatment–Case Reports. WB 105 R817a 2009]
  RC86.7.R683 2009
  616.02′8–dc22

                    2008039514

ISBN: 978-1-4051-6883-0

A catalogue record for this book is available from the British Library.

Set in 9/12 pt Minion by SNP Best-set Typesetter Ltd., Hong Kong

Printed & bound in Singapore by Fabulous Printers Pte Ltd

1 2009

Contents

Colour plate section can be found facing p.148

Preface

One of the attractions of acute medicine is the enormous variety of conditions which may present on the medical 'take'. The nature with which these conditions can present is equally varied, although a large proportion of patients can be grouped into a much smaller number of common symptom 'categories'. The curriculum for training in acute medicine (*The Physicians of Tomorrow: Curriculum for General Internal Medicine (Acute Medicine)*. Federation of the Royal College of Physicians, London, 2006.) has identified 20 presenting symptoms which account for a large proportion of all emergency medical admissions (see Table I). Doctors undertaking training in hospital medicine are expected to attain competency in the management of all of these during their training.

The cases which are included in this book have been selected to illustrate the practical challenges which face clinicians involved with the initial management of acute medical patients. Most of the 'Top 20' presentations are included, with some minor modifications. Chest pain has been classified as 'cardiac-type' or 'pleuritic', since these two presentations usually require a different approach. Although patients do not usually use these terms when describing their symptoms, a referring clinician will often have categorised the patient's pain in this way. 'Breathlessness' has been divided to illustrate the differences in the initial management of suspected acute asthma, exacerbation of COPD and undiagnosed breathless elderly patients. Acute confusion presents different diagnostic challenges in an elderly patient compared to a younger patient with alcohol dependency. Abdominal and back pain more commonly present to surgical and orthopaedic teams, and have therefore been omitted to enable inclusion of diabetic ketoacidosis and acute renal failure.

Clearly it is impossible to base a book on symptoms without considerable overlap between the cases. In order to avoid duplication, the reader will find frequent cross-references to different chapters where a condition is described in more detail. Some symptoms will require a broad differential diagnosis, while other conditions may present in a variety of ways. Myocardial infarction, for example, most commonly presents with 'cardiac-type chest pain', but may result in pleuritic-type pain, breathlessness, syncope or acute confusion. So-called 'atypical' presentations of common conditions are more common

Table I 'Top 20 presentations' as defined in the *Curriculum for General Internal Medicine (Acute Medicine)*

Abdominal pain

Acute back pain

Blackout/collapse

Breathlessness

Chest pain

Confusion, acute

Cough

Diarrhoea

Falls

Fever

Fits/seizure

Haematemesis/melaena

Headache

Jaundice

Limb pain and swelling

Palpitations

Poisoning

Rash

Vomiting and nausea

Weakness and paralysis

in elderly patients, where it is particularly important for the clinician to keep an open mind. Attempts to categorise the patient's problem immediately on presentation may lead to the correct diagnosis being missed.

This book is designed to provide readers with a rationale with which to approach patients presenting on the acute medical take. It is not possible to cover every condition or possible outcome, and this should not be considered a comprehensive reference text. More detailed information about some of the conditions can be found in *Acute Medicine,* 4th edition by D. Sprigings and J.B.Chambers (Blackwell Publishing, 2008), which can be used as an accompaniment to this text. References to the relevant sections in this book are included at the end of some cases, along with other useful sources of further information.

All of the cases in this book are entirely fictitious, but are based on an amalgamation of real patients presenting with similar symptoms; hopefully this has resulted in realistic scenarios similar to those which readers will face in their clinical practice.

Chris Roseveare

Acknowledgements

Many people have assisted in the preparation of this manuscript and I will attempt to aknowledge all of these. Dr Ben Chadwick and Dr Stuart Henderson helped significantly in the writing of the chapters on the shocked and comatose patients; Dr Rebecca Strivens, Dr Nik Wennike, Dr Matt Todd, Dr Steven Hill and Dr Felicity Chastney also made very helpful contributions to the cases of chronic obstructive pulmonary disease, pyrexia, renal failure, seizure and the breathless elderly patient. I am also grateful to my colleagues, Dr Beata Brown, Dr Janet Butler, Dr Arthur Yue, Dr John Paisey, Professor Derek Bell and Dr Anindo Banerjee for reviewing some of the cases and for their helpful comments. I would also like to thank Dr Ivan Brown, Dr Harriet Joy and Dr Lynne Burgess in the radiology department at Southampton, for kindly providing radiographs for use in many of the cases.

Finally, I would like to thank my wife, Nicola, without whose patience and understanding I would not have been able to devote the necessary time to the production of this text.

How to use this book

Clinical Cases Uncovered (CCU) books are carefully designed to help supplement your clinical experience and assist with refreshing your memory when revising. Each book is divided into three sections: Part 1 Basics; Part 2 Cases; and Part 3 Self-assessment.

Part 1 gives you a quick reminder of the basic science, history and examination, and key diagnoses in the area. Part 2 contains many of the clinical presentations you would expect to see on the wards or in exams, with questions and answers leading you through each case. New information, such as test results, is revealed as events unfold and each case concludes with a handy case summary explaining the key points. Part 3 allows you to test your learning with several question styles (MCQs, EMQs and SAQs), each with a strong clinical focus.

Whether reading individually or working as part of a group, we hope you will enjoy using your CCU book. If you have any recommendations on how we could improve the series, please do let us know by contacting us at: medstudentuk@oxon.blackwellpublishing.com.

Disclaimer

CCU patients are designed to reflect real life, with their own reports of symptoms and concerns. Please note that all names used are entirely fictitious and any similarity to patients, alive or dead, is coincidental.

List of abbreviations

ABG	arterial blood gas
ACE	angiotensin-converting enzyme
ACS	acute coronary syndrome
AF	atrial fibrillation
ALP	alkaline phosphatase
ALT	alanine transaminase
ANA	anti-nuclear antibody
ANCA	anti-neutrophil cytoplasmic antibody
APTR	activated partial thromboplastin ratio
AST	aspartate transaminase
BBB	bundle branch block
BCT	broad complex tachycardia
BiPAP	biphasic positive airway pressure
CDU	clinical decision unit
COPD	chronic obstructive pulmonary disease
CPR	cardiopulmonary resucitation
CRP	C-reactive protein
CSF	cerebrospinal fluid
CT	computed tomography
CTPA	computed tomography pulmonary angiogram
CVP	central venous pressure
DIC	disseminated intravascular coagulation
DKA	diabetic ketoacidosis
DVT	deep vein thrombosis
EM	emergency medicine
ESR	erythrocyte sedimentation rate
EWS	early warning score
FBC	full blood count
FEV_1	forced expiratory volume in 1 second
FVC	forced vital capacity
GCS	Glasgow Coma Score
GI	gastrointestinal
GTN	glyceryl trinitrate
Hb	haemoglobin
HDU	high-dependency unit
HPC	history of presenting complaint
IBD	inflammatory bowel disease
INR	international normalized ratio
JVP	jugular venous pressure
LFT	liver function tests
LMN	lower motor neurone
LMWH	low molecular weight heparin
LP	lumbar puncture
MI	myocardial infarction
NSAIDs	non-steroidal anti-inflammatory drugs
NSTEMI	non-ST elevation myocardial infarction
OGD	oesophagogastroduodenoscopy
OSCE	objective structured clinical examination
PA	posteroanterior
PCI	percutaneous coronary intervention
PE	pulmonary embolism
PEA	pulseless electrical activity
PEFR	peak expiratory flow rate
PND	paroxysmal nocturnal dyspnoea
PPI	proton pump inhibitor
PT	prothrombin time
PTP	pretest probability
REM	rapid eye movement
SAH	subarachnoid haemorrhage
SLE	systemic lupus erythematosus
STEMI	ST elevation myocardial infarction
SVT	supraventricular tachycardia
TGA	transient global amnesia
TIMI	thrombolysis in myocardial infarction
U&E	urea and electrolytes
VF	ventricular fibrillation
VT	ventricular tachycardia
WCC	white cell count

Introduction and specialty overview

What is acute medicine?

The term *acute medicine* has been a relatively recent addition to the UK healthcare vocabulary. In its 2007 document *Acute medical care. The right person in the right setting – first time,* the Royal College of Physicians defines acute medicine as:

> that part of general (internal) medicine concerned with the immediate and early specialist management of adult patients suffering from a wide range of medical conditions who present to, or from within, hospitals requiring urgent or emergency care.

In short, acute medicine comprises the medical 'take' and its immediate aftermath.

Acute medicine: a brief history

Traditionally, responsibility for adult patients requiring admission to hospital, and whose care was deemed unlikely to require surgery ('medical patients'), fell within the remit of the 'general physician'. The increasing complexity of medicine over the last century led to the development of medical specialties, with specialty training programmes enabling physicians to acquire more detailed knowledge and skills in one area. However, most 'specialists' also maintained skills in *general medicine* (also termed *general (internal) medicine, or G(I)M*). This ensured that they were able to care for medical patients admitted to hospital as emergencies, or patients whose problem did not fall into a clear specialty category.

During the 1980s and 1990s, a number of challenges threatened to undermine traditional models of hospital care. A progressive increase in the number of medical patients admitted as emergencies was placing considera-

ble pressure on hospital resources. In some cases this led to the cancellation of surgical procedures because of overspill of medical patients into other parts of the hospital; in other cases, patients were forced to spend prolonged periods of time waiting in corridors for a bed to become available. Alongside this pressure was a need to reduce the excessive hours worked by junior hospital doctors. One approach to address these challenges was the development of acute admissions wards (also termed 'acute assessment wards', 'acute medical units', 'emergency admissions units', etc.). This concept enabled the concentration of medical staffing resources in one area of the hospital, thereby reducing the numbers of junior doctors required to manage the emergency service. In addition, processes could be developed within these units to streamline the care of patients admitted as emergencies, preventing unnecessary admissions or reducing their length of stay in hospital.

However, despite the advantages provided by acute admissions wards, challenges persisted. Without clear medical leadership, many admissions units became dysfunctional 'bottlenecks' in the hospital. Many physicians were under pressure to provide a greater level of service to their specialty and wished to opt out of on-call and G(I)M. Additionally, much of the care of patients admitted as emergencies continued to be delivered by doctors in training, whereas patients demanded a consultant-led service. The concept of a specialty of acute medicine was first proposed by the Royal Colleges in 1998, since when the expansion of the field has been dramatic. The Royal College of Physicians has recommended that all hospitals should aim to appoint consultants specialising in acute medicine. Many hospitals now employ several *specialist acute physicians*, and a training curriculum in this field has existed since 2002. Acute medicine is currently the most rapidly expanding hospital specialty in the UK, and this trend is likely to continue over the next decade.

Acute Medicine: Clinical Cases Uncovered. By C. Roseveare.
Published 2009 by Blackwell Publishing, ISBN: 978-1-4051-6883-0

Acute medicine and emergency medicine

The development of the specialty of acute medicine has addressed many of the challenges around delivering care to medical patients admitted as emergencies. However, the interface between this field and the existing specialty of *Emergency Medicine (EM)* (previously termed *Accident and Emergency*) remains a subject of considerable debate. Although most of the first consultants in EM were from surgical or orthopaedic backgrounds, many of the patients presenting directly to hospital emergency departments (EDs) have medical problems that require ongoing inpatient care. This is now reflected in the training curriculum for EM, and consultants in EM are now expected to be skilled in the initial management of medical patients. Given the overlap between these two fields, some have challenged whether both specialties can survive as separate entities in the longer term.

However, there remain significant differences between these two specialties (see Table 1). Patients presenting themselves to the ED are entirely 'unselected'. Emergency medicine consultants therefore have to be able to manage patients presenting to hospital with problems pertaining to any inpatient specialty, including paediatrics, obstetrics, surgery and trauma, as well as medicine. In addition, the main focus of the ED is usually the delivery of immediate care, identifying those patients who can be discharged and, for those requiring admission, ensuring stabilisation prior to referral to the appropriate specialty. By contrast, most of the patients seen by an acute medicine consultant will already have been seen by another clinician (either a GP or EM doctor) and deemed to have a 'medical' problem. Acute medicine specialists do not have the range of specialty knowledge of an EM specialist, although the depth of knowledge pertaining to patients

with medical problems would normally be greater. Furthermore, acute medicine places more emphasis on continuing care and follow-up for medical patients, particularly those who do not fall into a clear medical specialty category.

It is very likely that acute medicine and EM specialists will need to work in close collaboration in the future, to prevent unnecessary duplication of effort. Generic training programmes for acute specialties are already in existence and are likely to expand. The continued rise in the emergency workload will ensure that acute care of patients in hospital remains high on the UK healthcare agenda.

Models of care in acute medicine

Hospitals in the UK vary considerably in their size, structure and catchment population, resulting in a wide variation in the numbers of emergency medical admissions. This in turn will influence the model of acute medical service that is adopted by the hospital (see Table 2). Most larger hospitals will have an admissions ward, and many will have consultants with specific responsibility for this area. There will rarely be sufficient numbers of acute medicine consultants to provide a continuous service 24 hours a day, seven days per week; the service therefore usually relies on specialists with training in G(I)M to participate in an on-call rota. The Royal College of Physicians recommends that all patients are reviewed by a consultant within 24 hours of admission; in most cases this takes place during a 'post-take ward round'. Depending on the number of admissions this process may occur one or more times each day. In some cases, consultants in acute medicine may adopt a more hands-on approach, providing ongoing review of patients admitted during daytime hours. However, most medical patients admitted

Table 1 Differences between acute and emergency medicine

Emergency medicine	Acute medicine
Wide range of specialty skills including medicine, surgery, trauma, paediatrics	Medicine specific with greater depth of knowledge in this area
Patients self-present or brought by ambulance '999'	Patients usually referred by GPs or emergency medicine clinicians
Main focus is immediate care and management in first 4 h following presentation to hospital. A longer duration of stay may be feasible in some emergency departments with clinical decision units (CDU)	Greater focus on ongoing care and follow-up for medical patients, including ambulatory care

Table 2 Models of care in acute medicine

Model	Comments
On-call rota system	Traditional model where on-call consultant physician undertakes normal daytime commitments in their specialty followed by a 'post-take' ward round on the acute medicine unit at the end of this period
Physician of the day/week	Acute medicine service provided by physicians with other specialty interests, but specialty sessions are cancelled during their on-call day/week to enable provision of a more hands-on service
Acute medicine consultant	Specialist appointed specifically to provide part or all of the on-call service at consultant level. Large numbers are required to provide a comprehensive on-call rota so that a hybrid model with one of the other systems is usually adopted at present pending further expansion of specialist numbers

as emergencies will usually be 'clerked' by a more junior member of the on-call medical team shortly after their arrival in hospital.

The development of skills relating to the initial assessment and management of patients admitted to hospital as medical emergencies is an essential component of training for all junior doctors. Students should take every available opportunity to develop these skills during their clinical years. Some of the essential skills required to work in this field are described in the next section.

Admission avoidance and acute medicine

Patients with medical problems are usually admitted to hospital for one of the following reasons.
• They require treatment which can only be delivered in a hospital environment
• They require investigation to confirm or refute a serious diagnosis that cannot be provided in an outpatient setting
• They are not able to care for themselves in the community because of combinations of medical and social problems

There are many reasons for the increase in hospital admissions in recent years; some of the most common are summarised below.
• Increased medical technology: treatments are now available (and often considered mandatory) for conditions that might previously have been managed in the community (e.g. stroke, myocardial infarction)
• Increased fear of litigation: the need to exclude significant pathology often requires a period of hospital assess-

ment and investigation; conditions such as myocardial ischaemia, subarachnoid haemorrhage and meningitis may first present with relatively minor symptoms prior to life-threatening deterioration
• Increasing age of the population: older patients have greater medical and social needs, which can often not be met in the community

Much of the pressure to develop the specialty of acute medicine has centred around the need to prevent 'unnecessary' hospital admissions. Two of the strategies to deliver this are summarised below.

Risk stratification

Clinical features and targeted investigations can be used to produce a score that determines the likelihood of a condition or of an adverse outcome. Evidence-based risk scores for upper gastrointestinal bleeding (Rockall score, see Case 9), myocardial ischaemia (thrombolysis in myocardial infarction [TIMI] score, see Case 1) and pulmonary embolism (Wells score, see Case 2), are some of the best known.

It should be remembered that most scores continue to rely on a degree of subjective judgement, and should not be used in isolation. Senior clinical review is often required to support the use of this approach.

Ambulatory care

The term *ambulatory care* refers to the management of patients in an outpatient setting whose care would traditionally have required admission to a hospital bed. The service will often require a combination of rapid assessment, targeted investigation and treatment with regular review and follow-up. In many cases the setting for ambulatory care is within or adjacent to the acute medical unit, and specialist acute physicians are often responsible for the development and management of this service.

Examples of ambulatory care services include:

• Outpatient management of suspected and proven deep vein thrombosis, using daily injections of low molecular weight heparins (see Case 22)

• Daily provision of intravenous antibiotics for soft tissue infection (e.g. cellulitis)

• Supported early discharge of patients with chronic obstructive airways disease.

The precise model for such services may vary in different hospitals; however, access to the appropriate space, rapid diagnostic services and senior clinical review are essential components of ambulatory care.

Further reading

Department of Health. *Emergency care ten years on: reforming emergency care.* Professor Sir George Alberti. National Director of Emergency Access. DH, London, 2007

National Institute for Health and Clinical Excellence. *Acutely ill patients in hospital. Recognition of and response to acute illness in adults in hospital.* NICE clinical guideline 50. NICE, London, 2007

Royal College of Physicians. *The interface between accident and emergency medicine and acute medicine.* Report of a working party. RCP, London, 2002

Royal College of Physicians. *Acute medicine: making it work for patients. A blueprint for organisation and training.* Report of a working party. RCP, London, 2004

Royal College of Physicians. *Acute medical care. The right person in the right setting – first time.* Report of the Acute Medicine Task Force. RCP, London, 2007

Approach to the patient

Immediate assessment and resuscitation

The initial approach will need to be guided by the clinical needs of the patient. Patients who are admitted following cardiopulmonary arrest should be resuscitated according to the algorithms produced by the Resuscitation Council (see Fig. 1). Fortunately, this represents only a tiny minority of cases. However, the ability to recognise an acutely unwell adult is a vital skill for clinicians working in acute medicine. Many hospitals use an 'early warning score' as an aid for the recognition of acute illness and deterioration in a patient's condition (see Table 3). It should be remembered that these scores are not infallible and should not be used in isolation.

In some cases immediate treatment may be required before a more detailed assessment is possible. Many of the cases described in this book illustrate this, and the precise approach will depend on the clinical scenario. However, for any acutely unwell patient a generic ABCDE approach is the appropriate starting point, as described here.

A Airway

A patent airway is required to deliver oxygen to the lungs. Untreated, this will rapidly lead to cardiopulmonary arrest. Airway obstruction requires immediate treatment; senior or anaesthetic assistance is likely to be required.

Consider the questions below.

Is the airway obstructed?

• Listen (without a stethoscope) to the breath sounds: complete obstruction will result in the absence of breath sounds at the mouth or nose; partial obstruction results in harsh or gurgling inspiratory sounds

• Look at the chest/abdominal wall – complete obstruction may result in paradoxical 'see-saw' movements of the chest and abdomen

Why is the airway obstructed?

• There may be fluid (e.g. vomit) or solid matter (e.g. food) in the mouth or upper airway

• The tongue may have slipped posteriorly in cases of reduced conscious level

How can the obstruction be relieved?

• Suction or a 'finger sweep' should enable removal of liquid or solid material from the mouth and throat

• Positioning of the patient with a reduced conscious level on their side or in the 'recovery position' (unless there is a concern about possible neck injury)

• Use airway adjuncts such as a nasopharyngeal or Guedel airway

• Use endotracheal intubation if these measures fail

B Breathing

Adequate breathing is required to deliver oxygen to the circulation.

Is the patient breathing effectively?

• Look at the patient's breathing pattern; determine whether they are using accessory muscles of respiration and whether they appear to be struggling with inspiration or expiration

• Measure the respiratory rate: a fast rate (>20 breaths/min) suggests difficulty in maintaining oxygenation; a slow rate (<12 breaths/min) may imply reduced central respiratory drive

• Auscultate the chest: quiet breath sounds often suggest inadequate breathing

• Measure oxygen saturation: either use pulse oximetry or obtain an arterial blood gas; hypoxaemia implies inadequate oxygenation of the blood

Acute Medicine: Clinical Cases Uncovered. By C. Roseveare.
Published 2009 by Blackwell Publishing, ISBN: 978-1-4051-6883-0

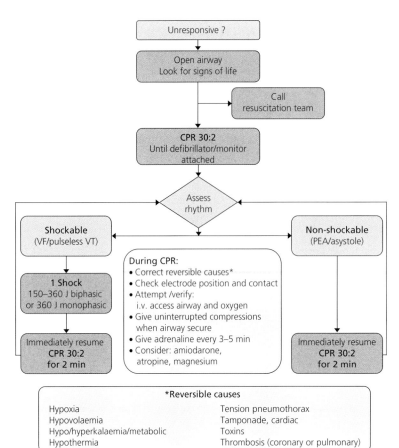

Figure 1 Advanced life support algorithm. CPR, cardiopulmonary resuscitation; PEA, pulseless electrical activity; VF, ventricular fibrillation; VT, ventricular tachycardia. Reproduced with permission from the Resuscitation Council, UK.

Table 3 Typical early warning score

Score	3	2	1	0	1	2	3
Respiratory rate	<8	<8–10		11–14	15–20	21–30	>30
Urine output	<10 mL/h	10–30 mL/h		>30 mL/h			
Heart rate		<40	41–50	51–100	101–110	111–130	>130
Systolic blood pressure	<70	71–80	81–100	101–179	180–199	200–220	>220
Temperature		<35	35.1–36	361–38	38.1–38.5	>38.5	
Neurological status			New confusion	Alert	Responds to voice	Responds to pain	Unresponsive

A score of 4 or more usually suggests that the patient requires immediate assessment (many variations of this are used in hospitals across the UK, with different trigger points for escalation of care – refer to local guidelines if in doubt).

Why is the patient's breathing ineffective?
• Look at the patient: a reduced conscious level may lead to reduced respiratory drive; exhaustion may result in respiratory muscle fatigue

• Auscultate carefully: harsh inspiratory sounds imply large airway narrowing (e.g. tracheitis, epiglottitis, obstructing tumours) whereas musical expiratory sounds suggest small airway narrowing (e.g. asthma, broncho-

spasm); coarse bilateral crackles suggest pulmonary oedema or fibrosis whereas focal crackles may imply infection
• Percuss the lung fields: dull percussion may suggest failed lung expansion because of pleural fluid accumulation; hyperresonance may imply deflation of a lung due to pneumothorax

What should be done?
• Deliver oxygen: in most cases where breathing is inadequate a high oxygen concentration should be delivered using a mask with a reservoir and a flow rate of >10 L/min. Patients with chronic obstructive airways disease and chronic hypoxaemia may require a controlled oxygen flow rate (see Case 6)
• Treat the cause, if this can be identified: bronchodilators for asthma (see Case 5), pleural drainage for effusions and pneumothorax or diuretics for pulmonary oedema
• Consider mechanical ventilatory support if oxygenation cannot be improved with the above measures or if inadequate respiratory drive or fatigue is the likely cause

C Circulation
An effective circulation is required to deliver the oxygenated blood to the vital organs. The effectiveness of the circulation will be determined by the cardiac output, the circulating volume of fluid and the capacity of the vascular system.

Is the circulation effective?
• Feel the pulse volume and skin temperature and measure capillary refill time (usually <2 s)
• Assess the pulse rate: a fast or slow pulse rate may be a *cause* or *effect* of inadequate circulation. Tachycardia may be the only sign of inadequate circulation in young patients whose compensatory mechanisms are highly effective. As a general rule of thumb a pulse rate greater than the systolic blood pressure reading often implies inadequate circulation
• Measure the blood pressure: generally a blood pressure of >90 systolic is required to perfuse major organs, although absolute figures are often difficult to interpret in isolation; changes in blood pressure measured over a series of readings will give a better indication of their significance

Why is the circulation ineffective?
• Look for 'obvious' causes: haemorrhage, fluid loss, cardiac arrest

• Check for cardiac causes: assess the rate and rhythm on a cardiac monitor (see p. 14) and 12-lead ECG and exclude obvious ST elevation myocardial infarction (STEMI) (see Case 1 and pp. 20–23)
• If the patient is cool, pale and sweaty with a weak, thready pulse consider hypovolaemia to be the most likely cause
• If the patient is warm with a large volume pulse and low diastolic pressure consider sepsis (see Case 8)

What should be done?
• Insert one (or preferably two) large bore cannulae
• Consider the likely underlying cause: if hypovolaemia or sepsis is likely, administer a rapid fluid challenge (e.g. 250–500 mL of 0.9% saline over 10–15 min) and assess response
• Attempt to correct cardiac arrhythmias (see Cases 2 & 3)
• Insert a urinary catheter to enable hourly measurement of urine output: this will give a good guide to the effectiveness of the circulation
• Ensure regular repeat measurements of blood pressure and pulse to assess response to treatment
• Obtain senior help and consider the insertion of a central venous cannula to enable the measurement of right atrial pressure: this will help to guide fluid requirements

D Disability
In this context, assessment of 'disability' implies the assessment of *conscious level*.

How can the conscious level be assessed?
• The AVPU score will enable a rapid initial assessment of the patient's level of alertness: **A**lert – responds to **V**oice – responds to **P**ain (but not voice) – **U**nresponsive (to pain or voice)
• The Glasgow Coma Scale (GCS, see p. 127) enables a more detailed assessment of conscious level and should be used for any patient who scores 'V' or worse on the AVPU score

What is the significance of reduced conscious level in the acute setting?
• Reduced conscious level may result in impairment of the natural protective reflexes for the airway (coughing/choking) and therefore requires medical measures to prevent aspiration of secretions or vomit into the lung. It is generally considered that this is more likely when the GCS is <8

• Reduced conscious level may reduce the effectiveness of breathing

• The cause of the reduced consciousness may be relevant to the underlying process leading to the patient's admission.

What should be done if the conscious level is reduced?

• If the GCS is <8 or there are other concerns about the airway, obtain immediate senior assistance and consider intubation

• Look for external signs of head injury

• Examine the pupils: bilateral pinpoint pupils suggest opiate drug use; inequality or lack of light response may imply intracranial pathology

• Move the patient into the lateral or recovery position if there is no risk of neck injury

• Measure capillary blood glucose; administer glucose if this is low: NB. If there is a possibility of alcohol abuse or chronic malnutrition administer intravenous vitamin B simultaneously (see Case 16)

E Exposure

This final stage requires a more general assessment of the patient; a full external examination will often be necessary, although this may take place as part of a more structured clinical examination provided the patient's condition has been stabilised and a working diagnosis has been reached.

History and examination

In the setting of the acute medical 'take' the ability to assess patients in a timely fashion is an important skill. As most patients will not require immediate resuscitation, the process of assessment will usually begin with the history. Challenges which face the admitting clinician when trying to obtain a history may include:

• Time pressures: the volume of work may tempt clinicians to cut corners by abbreviating the history

• Frequent interruptions: a succinct history is difficult if your train of thought is constantly interrupted by your pager

• Incomplete information: confused, uncooperative or unconscious patients may not be able to give a complete history; other sources of information may need to be sought

The importance of a clear and accurate history cannot be overstated.

The history represents your best opportunity to discover what is wrong with the patient, and subsequently to determine your treatment plan.

The history of presenting complaint (HPC)

This is the most important aspect of the history for any patient presenting acutely; the importance of this should be reflected in the time spent concentrating on this area. Virtually all of the diagnostic information will be gleaned by concentrating on the patient's presenting symptoms; if a differential diagnosis is not apparent in the mind of the assessing clinician on completion of this section of the history it is unlikely that the remainder of the history or examination will make it any clearer. It is crucial to know how to approach this area.

1 Preparation. Before approaching the patient, ensure that you have equipped yourself with all the available information.

• Read any accompanying letter from the patient's general practitioner

• If the patient has been seen already in the accident and emergency department, read the notes made regarding any initial assessment

• If a nurse or therapist has already assessed the patient, read their notes; some acute medical units use a multidisciplinary care record to reduce the need for duplication of notes and improve communication between healthcare professionals

• Look at observation recordings (pulse, blood pressure, etc.)

• For patients arriving at the hospital by ambulance, read the ambulance transfer information: this will give useful information about what happened prior to arrival in hospital

2 Opening lines. Establishing a good rapport with the patient will make an enormous difference to the remainder of your encounter with them. Patients will frequently have told their story to other clinicians before they see you, and may find it irritating to have to repeat this. However, it remains important to hear the symptoms directly from the patient. A useful way around this is to use the following opening line:

'I am aware that you have probably gone over this several times before, and I have read your GP's letter, but it is always very helpful to hear it in your own words'.
followed by:

'tell me about the problem which has brought you to hospital today'.

The use of this open question at the outset gives the patient the opportunity to describe the principal symptom, which they believe resulted in their referral to hospital. In some cases this may be very different from that described by the GP; it is important to remember that a GP consultation is generally considerably shorter than a hospital 'clerking'; if discrepancies are apparent there may be a need to take a step further back and ask the patient to describe specifically the reason they went to see their doctor that day.

3 Onset of symptoms. The nature of the onset of symptoms is frequently helpful in determining their cause.

Sudden onset
• Patients will often use the term 'sudden', when describing onset of symptoms, but it is vital to clarify this. Very few conditions are truly of sudden (i.e. 'explosive') onset; it is important to establish whether this is what the patient means. The following questions can be helpful.

  ○ *'When you say the (e.g. pain) started suddenly, do you mean that it built up quite quickly or was it truly sudden like this?' (then clap your hands)*
  ○ *'What were you doing when the (symptom) started?'*
  ○ *'Was the symptom worst at onset or did it worsen or change with time?'*

If any symptom was truly of sudden onset the patient will usually remember precisely what they were doing at the time; if the patient is unsure or vague about this, then it is likely that the symptom built up in a less dramatic fashion. This does not necessarily mean that the problem is any less severe, but it may help to refine your differential diagnosis (see Table 4).

Sometimes a practical issue arises when a patient's symptoms are present on waking. It may be hard to determine whether the patient was woken by the pain (implying an abrupt onset) or woke with pain (which may have developed more gradually). If the patient awoke unusually early this may suggest the former, but in practice it is wise to assume the worst case scenario and investigate accordingly.

Precipitating and relieving factors
• Identifying what the patient was doing immediately before the onset of the symptoms may provide useful information. If the symptom was brought on by exertion, change of posture, eating, sudden movement or trauma, this may help to define the cause.

Ask specifically 'What do you think may have caused the (symptom)?'

In some cases asking *'What made it go away?'* may be as helpful as establishing what brought it on. Relief following rest may reinforce the likelihood of the

Table 4 Conditions associated with symptoms of truly 'sudden' onset

Symptom	Causes of sudden onset	Comments
Cardiac-type chest pain	Aortic dissecting aneurysm	Often described as 'tearing' or 'ripping'; usually radiates to the back 'Cardiac' chest pain from myocardial infarction or angina usually builds over a few minutes
Pleuritic chest pain	Pneumothorax Nerve entrapment/muscular strain	Pleuritic chest pain caused by pulmonary embolism usually starts more gradually
Breathlessness	Pulmonary embolism Pneumothorax Bronchospasm Airway obstruction Hyperventilation Cardiac arrhythmia	
Headache	Subarachnoid haemorrhage 'Thunderclap' migraine	
Unilateral weakness	Stroke	Usually worst at onset – symptoms can evolve over a few hours

cause being exertional; specific drug remedies such as an antacid in the case of gastro-oesophageal reflux or glyceryl trinitrate in the case of angina may also help to define a cause.

Table 5 illustrates how questioning around this area can be helpful in the case of a patient with cardiac-type chest pain.

4 What happened next. There are many routes by which a patient may end up in hospital.

- They may have self-presented to the accident and emergency department or called for the ambulance that brought them
- They may have contacted a GP who arranged for admission
- A concerned relative or friend may have arranged for the ambulance or GP assessment
- They may have telephoned NHS Direct for advice and been advised to attend hospital

Establishing the sequence of events which led to the patient's arrival in hospital may give useful clues to the cause and severity of the problem.

Consider the two scenarios below.

Scenario 1

A 45-year-old man is awoken by chest pain. He takes an antacid but is still uncomfortable after 30 min. His wife suggests he contact NHS Direct. The telephone operator arranges a blue-light ambulance to bring the patient to hospital. By the time the ambulance arrives the pain has resolved, but the patient reluctantly agrees to being brought to hospital. On arrival in the accident and emergency

department he appears well with a normal ECG. Close questioning reveals a long history of similar symptoms that have been investigated in the past and attributed to gastro-oesophageal reflux.

Scenario 2

A 45-year-old man is awoken by chest pain. He asks his wife to call for an ambulance. The pain subsides spontaneously within 30 min and he appears well on arrival in hospital with a normal ECG. He tells you he feels a fraud and asks if he can go home. Subsequent investigation reveals an elevated troponin level and he is diagnosed with a non-ST elevation myocardial infarction.

In both of these cases the patient may have cardiac chest pain; however, the patient's actions at the time of the symptoms give a clue to the severity of the problem. Both patients may warrant further inpatient investigation, particularly if there are risk factors for ischaemic heart disease (see Case 1). However, the actions of the patient in Scenario 2 should ring loud alarm bells in the mind of the clinician.

Be wary of the patient who insists there is nothing wrong with him or her, despite having previously called an ambulance – a symptom that was severe at the time of onset always requires careful evaluation.

Examining the patient
By the end of the history it should be possible to summarise the key problem areas. Although physical examination of the areas relevant to the presenting complaint should be particularly thorough, most patients will

Table 5 Precipitating and relieving factors and likely causes of cardiac-type chest pain

Precipitating/exacerbating factor	Relieving factor	Likely cause
Exertion such as walking	Rest/GTN spray	Ischaemic heart disease
Lying flat or leaning forward	Sitting upright	Pericarditis/gastro-oesophageal reflux
Sudden movement/rotation of upper thorax	Sitting still, simple analgesia	Musculoskeletal (e.g. referred from thoracic spine, intercostal muscle strain, etc.)
Eating/drinking	Antacid	Gastro-oesophageal reflux
Chest wall trauma (e.g. car accident while wearing seatbelt)/local pressure over chest wall	Rest, simple analgesia	Chest wall bruising

GTN, glyceryl trinitrate.

require a comprehensive examination of all systems at the time of their initial presentation.

Before conducting any examination always consider the following.

• Always remember to ask the patient's permission prior to examination and to take a chaperone wherever possible (particularly when conducting intimate examination in members of the opposite sex)

• The presence of a family member may be helpful in some cases, but you must confirm that the patient is happy for them to remain present during the examination

• Explain clearly what you are going to do, and confirm that an area of the body is not painful or tender before palpation or percussion

• Disinfect your hands (and stethoscope) before and after examining any patient

• Watches and jewellery should be removed from your wrists, sleeves rolled up, and neck ties firmly secured or removed

Unexpected findings should be documented, allowing careful consideration of their relevance to the presenting complaint, or the need for future investigation if incidental. It should also be remembered that normal physical examination does not preclude serious pathology.

A summary of the procedure for patient examination is given in the objective structured clinical examination (OSCE) checklist below.

Objective structured clinical examination (OSCE) checklist
1 General inspection
• Always take a few minutes to step back and take in as much information as possible about the patient and their surroundings

• Establish whether the patient appears comfortable or distressed

• Establish whether the patient appears pale, flushed, cyanotic, jaundiced, etc.

• Look for clues to the nature of the patient's illness (e.g. inhalers/glyceryl trinitrate (GTN) spray on the bedside table, sputum pot, temperature chart, etc.)

2 The hands
• Feel the temperature

• Examine finger nails for 'clubbing' (see Plate 1), splinter haemorrhages, etc.

• Inspect the palmar surfaces for evidence of erythema (chronic liver disease) or pallor (anaemia)

• Feel the pulse: rate, rhythm and character

3 The neck/face
• Examine the jugular venous pulsations in the neck

• Check the colour of the conjunctival membranes (pale in anaemia)

• Check sclera for evidence of jaundice

• Examine the buccal mucosa and inside the lower lip for evidence of central cyanosis

4 The precordium
• Feel for parasternal heaves and for the apex beat

• Listen carefully to the heart sounds over the apex (mitral area), left lower sternal edge (tricuspid area) and left and right upper sternal edge (pulmonary and aortic areas)

• Any murmur should be characterised as systolic or diastolic, preferably with some indication about the likely valvular lesion (site, radiation and quality, e.g. pansystolic or ejection systolic)

• Establish whether a murmur is louder during inspiration (probably a right-sided valvular lesion, e.g. tricuspid/pulmonary valves) or expiration (mitral or aortic valve lesions)

5 The chest
• Percuss anteriorly and posteriorly over the chest wall, checking for areas of dullness

• Auscultate both anteriorly and posteriorly, asking the patient to breathe slowly through their mouth

• If crackles are heard, ask the patient to cough and then re-auscultate to see whether the crackles are reduced (when caused by secretions within the airways) or unchanged (suggestive of interstitial fibrosis, consolidation or pulmonary oedema)

6 The abdomen
• Inspect for scars and obvious abnormalities

• Check that the patient has no areas of tenderness (if so approach these with caution, asking the patient to tell you if you inflict significant discomfort)

• Palpate gently over all quadrants of the abdomen, then more deeply to feel for masses

• Next palpate specifically for the liver, pressing initially in the right lower quadrant and asking the patient to breathe in, while slowly moving the hand towards the chest

- The spleen is palpated similarly, moving the hand from the right lower quadrant to the left upper quadrant as the patient breathes
- Enlargements of kidneys may be apparent by pressing deeply in the flanks with one hand while using the other hand to press from behind (balloting the kidney)
- Percuss in the flanks for evidence of dullness: if present, rotate the patient away from you to see if it 'shifts' (ascites)
- External genitalia should normally be inspected
- Rectal examination should be considered for most patients, although this is not always indicated

7 Neurological system
- Check tone, power, coordination and all reflexes
- Check sensation in each dermatomal area (usually light touch only, unless symptoms suggest a problem that may need to be assessed in more detail)
- Examine cranial nerves (including papillary responses)
- Examine fundi using ophthalmoscope

8 Legs, feet and locomotor system
- Ensure that the patient's legs have been uncovered and inspected for evidence of erythema, warmth, tenderness and swelling
- Check for asymmetry (measure calf circumference if any doubt)
- Check for ulcers or pressure sores
- Check for peripheral oedema around ankles and sacral area
- Check peripheral pulses (dorsalis pedis and posterior tibial – if not palpable always feel for popliteal and femoral pulses)
- Carefully inspect any joints which the patient has described as painful, or which appear swollen or deformed: look, feel and move, taking care not to cause pain if the joint is inflamed or appears abnormal

9 Remember urinalysis
- Bedside analysis of urine should be considered part of any clinical examination

Blood tests: which, when and why?
It is likely that most patients admitted to hospital will need some form of venous blood testing. Increasingly, the pressure to accelerate decision making in the Emergency Department has led to the development of 'protocol-driven' blood sampling. In such cases, selection of investigations is determined by the presenting symptom, often before detailed clinical assessment has been undertaken.

There is no doubt that this approach is helpful in some cases, speeding up discharge for patients with minor illness, or enabling more rapid intervention. It is also helpful to take blood at the time of venous cannulation, to save the patient undergoing additional venipuncture. However, there may also be drawbacks.

- In some cases unnecessary investigation may prove costly
- Patients may require additional venous sampling after more detailed clinical assessment
- Abnormal test results may cloud the clinician's judgement or lead to inappropriate investigation (see Box 1)

Wherever possible the following approach to investigation should be adopted.
- Start with the history and examination
- Formulate a differential diagnosis
- Select investigations that enable confirmation/elimination of these

In addition, it is important to consider the following.
- Has the test been undertaken recently, and if so is it likely to have changed?
  - most hospitals now have computerised laboratory services enabling the results of recent tests to be accessed rapidly
  - tests such as lipids, thyroid function and autoimmune or tumour markers are relatively expensive and will usually not have changed unless specific therapy has been instituted
- Should the test be delayed to enable appropriate interpretation?
  - cardiac troponin continues to rise for 10–12 h after an ischaemic event; if measured too early a repeat test may be required
  - the paracetamol level should be delayed for 4 h following overdose to enable accurate interpretation
  - overnight sampling may not always be required: the costs associated with out-of-hours testing are often significant; if the result will not affect the patient's immediate management it may be appropriate to delay the test until the following morning
- Will the results of the test influence the patient's treatment?
  - if a decision has already been taken not to treat a patient who is terminally ill, blood testing is probably unnecessary

---

Box 1 Abnormal troponin: a cautionary tale

A 30-year-old woman who worked in the hospital mentioned to one of the junior doctors working with her that she had been experiencing chest pains intermittently during the past few weeks. These were not severe and had not required any alteration in her busy lifestyle. The junior doctor completed a blood form for some investigations, including troponin I, and suggested that she attend the pathology laboratory for these to be taken.

Two hours later the junior doctor was paged by a concerned laboratory technician to inform him that the troponin level was markedly elevated at 11.9 ng/mL (normal range <0.15; a level >1.5 is usually considered diagnostic of myocardial infarction). The staff member was found and admitted to the coronary care unit, where a more detailed history was obtained. She reiterated that the pain was mild and usually occurred after eating; it was not in any way related to exertion and there were no risk factors for coronary artery disease. Her ECG was entirely normal. Considering a laboratory error to be likely the cardiology senior house officer repeated the sample, which again was markedly elevated (12.2 ng/mL). Two further samples produced similar results.

She was reviewed by a consultant cardiologist and underwent a series of further investigations including echocardiography, coronary angiography, cardiac MRI scan and myocardial biopsy, all of which were entirely normal. She was discharged from hospital after 1 week on a combination of aspirin, clopidogrel, bisoprolol, ramipril and simvastatin, in line with the normal protocol following suspected myocardial infarction.

Two weeks later the patient was readmitted to hospital after an upper gastrointestinal bleed relating to the aspirin and clopidogrel. The repeat troponin was again noted to be markedly raised (12.4 ng/mL), although she had not experienced any chest pain since discharge. The laboratory was contacted and asked to re-examine this sample. The clinical biochemist noted that she had a monoclonal antibody in her blood that may have cross-reacted with the system used for the troponin assay. The antibody was filtered out of her blood and the troponin assay was repeated, using the same sample, and produced a value of <0.15 ng/mL. All her medication was stopped and she has remained well ever since.

○ if a diagnosis has already been confirmed, e.g. pulmonary embolism confirmed by computed tomography pulmonary angiogram (CTPA); there is usually no need to undertake a second diagnostic test (e.g. D-dimer)

Before taking any blood sample ask yourself the following questions.
- What will I do if the test is abnormal?
- What will I do if the test is normal?

If the answer is the same for both questions, reconsider whether the test is necessary.

Interpreting the results of blood tests

When interpreting the results of blood tests it is important to remember the following.
- No normal blood test will ever completely exclude any condition (i.e. no test is 100% *sensitive*)
- No abnormal blood test is ever completely diagnostic of one condition (i.e. no test is 100% *specific*)

Knowledge of the sensitivity and specificity of certain tests will help the clinician to determine the likelihood of a particular condition. However, a blood test result should always be interpreted in the context of the clinical presentation. If the result appears to contradict a strong clinical suspicion, you should always consider whether further investigation is required (see Box 1).

'Near patient' testing

Many acute units have access to equipment that enables rapid analysis of blood samples without the need for specimens to be sent to the laboratory (see Fig. 2). Provided these analysers are appropriately quality controlled and appropriately used, the results are usually as accurate as those provided by the laboratory.

Common tests available using 'near patient' analysers include:
- Arterial blood gases (see p. 24)
- Sodium, potassium, calcium, glucose
- Lactate
- Troponin (and other cardiac enzymes)
- D-dimer

Costs associated with maintenance, quality control and reagents used mean that use of these systems is often more expensive than the equivalent laboratory service; in addition there is a danger that the ease of access increases the number of unnecessary investigations undertaken. However, provided they are used in accordance with a clear departmental policy the costs are usually offset by the benefits in relation to speed of diagnosis, treatment and discharge.

An acute physician's guide to the ECG

Interpretation of the ECG is one of the key skills required of a clinician working in acute medicine. There are many causes of an abnormal ECG and the many abnormalities that can be identified can help in establishing a diagnosis. Some of these are covered in the relevant cases and there are numerous textbooks on this subject. The intention here is to concentrate on two key areas of relevance to the acute physician.

These can be summarised in the form of two questions.
• Is there an abnormality of rate or rhythm?
• Is there evidence of myocardial ischaemia or infarction?

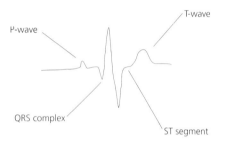

P-wave

T-wave

QRS complex

ST segment

Figure 2 Components of the ECG.

A brief revision of the key components of the ECG is shown in Fig. 2.

First steps
• Take a deep breath – and don't panic!
• Confirm that the name on the ECG relates to the patient being assessed
• Take note of the date and time that the ECG was taken
• Confirm the 'print rate' of the ECG (usually 25 mm/second) – see Fig. 3
• Note any comments written on the ECG, e.g. 'complaining of chest pain', 'short of breath', 'after treatment', etc.

Is there an abnormality of rate or rhythm?
Information about heart rate and rhythm can be obtained from a number of sources.
• A 12-lead ECG (usually includes a 'rhythm strip' at the bottom of the page)
• A single lead 'rhythm strip' printout
• By observing a cardiac monitor connected to the patient
• By palpating the patient's pulse
• By auscultating the heart or palpating the apex beat

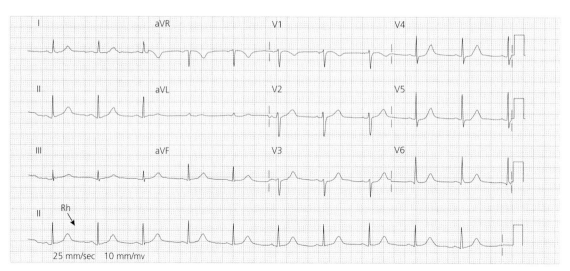

Figure 3 Standard 12-lead ECG. The date and time should appear at the top of the sheet. The patient's name would normally also appear here, along with information about the patient's condition at the time of the recording (in pain, breathless, etc.). The recording rate is indicated at the foot of the page (in this case 25 mm, the usual default setting). The voltage settings are also usually standardised at 10 mm/mv.

The 'rhythm strip' (Rh) at the bottom of the recording can be used to calculate the heart rate: in this case there are almost exactly four big squares between the QRS complexes, giving a rate of 75 beats/min (300/4). There are P-waves before each QRS complex indicating sinus rhythm. This ECG is otherwise normal.

Although this section deals predominantly with the interpretation of the ECG in isolation, it should never be forgotten that findings should always be confirmed by clinical assessment.

What is the heart rate?

The ECG paper comprises squares of 1 mm diameter ('small squares') and 5 mm diameter ('big squares').

Assuming a print rate of 25 mm/s (five big squares per second), each small square represents 0.04 s, whereas a big square represents 0.2 s.

In order to calculate the heart rate where the rhythm is regular:
- Count how many 'big squares' there are between the top of two R-waves
- Divide this figure into 300 to give you the heart rate in beats per minute

See Fig. 3.

The heart rate calculation can be more difficult when the rhythm is irregular. In this case:
- Count out 30 big squares (equivalent to 6 s of ECG time)
- Count the number of R-waves within this period
- Multiply by 10 to give the rate per minute

See Fig. 4.

Is the rhythm regular or irregular?

Identifying whether the rhythm is regular or irregular will help to identify the cause of any rhythm disturbance.
- In some cases it may be clear that the rhythm is irregular simply from brief inspection of the ECG
- If the rate is very fast or slow this may be more difficult
- **If in doubt: map it out:**
  - lay a piece of paper alongside the 'rhythm strip' at the bottom of the ECG
  - make a mark on this next to four consecutive R-waves
  - move the paper along and see if the marks still correspond to the next four R-waves: if not the rhythm is irregular

Irregular tachycardia

If the rhythm is fast and irregular it is likely that the rhythm represents one of the two following abnormalities.
- Fast atrial fibrillation
- Multiple ectopic beats

Table 6 shows how these may be distinguished.

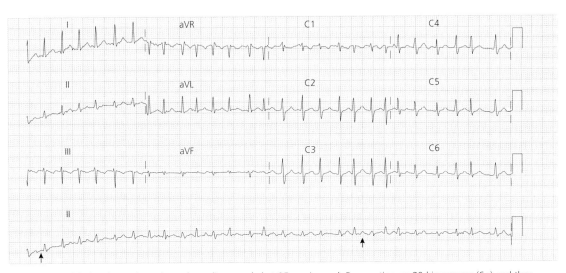

Figure 4 An ECG showing an irregular tachycardia, recorded at 25 mm/second. By counting up 30 big squares (6 s) and then counting the number of QRS complexes in this time period, the heart rate can be calculated: in this case the rate is 190 beats/min. There are no discernible P-waves and the QRS complexes are all of similar morphology, with an irregularly irregular rhythm. These features indicate that the rhythm is *fast atrial fibrillation*.

Table 6 Distinguishing between fast atrial fibrillation and multiple ectopic beats

Atrial fibrillation (Fig. 4)	Multiple ectopic beats (Fig. 5)
All complexes appear similar	Some complexes appear bizarre/broad/larger than others
No P-waves (irregular baseline)	P-waves before some QRS complexes
Rhythm completely 'random' – irregularly irregular	Some areas of regularity with 'ectopic' beats occurring within this pattern

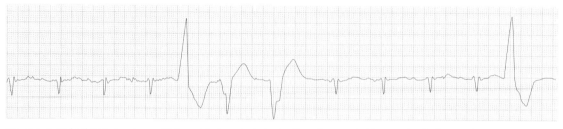

Figure 5 A 12-lead ECG showing multiple ventricular ectopic beats. There is an underlying regular rhythm produced by the narrow complex beats. The irregularity results from ventricular ectopics, which appear broad and very different in configuration. These ectopics also differ from each other, indicating that they arise from different foci within the ventricular wall.

Box 2 Atrial flutter

This is a common tachyarrhythmia in which the normal coordinated atrial activity is lost and replaced by rapid depolarisation at a rate of 300 beats/min. In most cases the atrioventricular (AV) node prevents transmission of some of these into the ventricle. The ventricular rate is therefore determined by the degree of 'block' at the AV node.

- If alternate beats are conducted the rate is 150 beats/min (2:1 block) – the most common scenario.
- If every third beat is conducted the rate is 100 beats/min (3:1 block), and so on.

In some cases the block may be variable (2:1 in some areas, 3 or 4:1 in others), resulting in an irregular rhythm.

When the degree of block is 3 or 4:1, the flutter waves (F-waves) are usually visible between the QRS complexes with a jagged saw-tooth appearance, one occurring in each big square (300 beats/min) (Fig. 6).

Atrial flutter with 2:1 block is often more difficult to distinguish from other tachyarrhythmias as the F-waves are often hidden within the QRS complex and T-wave (see Fig. 7). Where doubt exists, use of an AV nodal blocking agent such as adenosine can reveal the F-waves by increasing the degree of block (temporarily changing the rhythm from 2:1 to 4 or 5:1 block) (see p. 59).

Regular tachycardia

If the rhythm is **fast and regular** there are four common causes.

- Sinus tachycardia
- Atrial flutter with 2:1 block (see Box 2)
- Supraventricular tachycardia
- Ventricular tachycardia

When distinguishing these abnormalities (see Table 7), consider the following questions.

- Are there clearly defined P-waves before each QRS complex?

  Probably sinus tachycardia (see Fig. 8)

- Is the heart rate at (or very close to) 150 beats/min?

  Probably atrial flutter with 2:1 atrioventricular block

- Are the QRS complexes 'narrow' (<0.12 s or 3 mm) and very rapid, with no discernible P-waves?

  Probably supraventricular tachycardia (see Fig. 9)

- Are the QRS complexes 'broad' (>0.12 s or 3 mm)? – Fig. 10

  Either ventricular tachycardia or supraventricular tachycardia with associated bundle branch block (BBB) (see Case 4)

Bradycardias

There are two common causes of bradycardia.

- Sinus bradycardia

Table 7 Key features of different rhythm abnormalities in regular tachycardia

	Sinus tachycardia	Atrial flutter with 2:1 block	Supraventricular tachycardia	Ventricular tachycardia
Rate	Rarely >150 beats/min Usually some variation – often improves with treatment of underlying cause	Usually very close to 150 beats/min Very regular	Often very fast (>160 beats/min) Very regular	Rarely >180 beats/min Slight irregularity may be seen
P-waves	Present before each QRS complex	'Saw-tooth' flutter wave – may mimic P- or T-waves	Usually not visible; may be inverted	If visible will be dissociated from QRS complex
QRS complex	<0.12 s (unless bundle branch block)	<0.12 s (unless bundle branch block)	<0.12 s (unless bundle branch block)	>0.12 s (broad complex tachycardia)

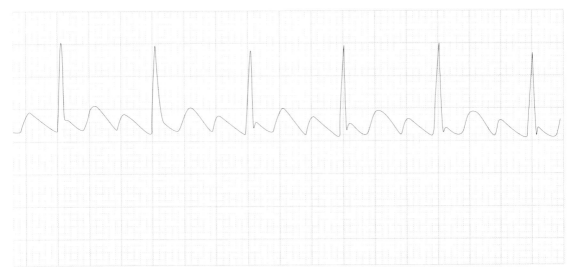

Figure 6 Atrial flutter with 3:1 block. The flutter waves are clearly visible between the QRS complexes with a ventricular rate of 100 beats/min.

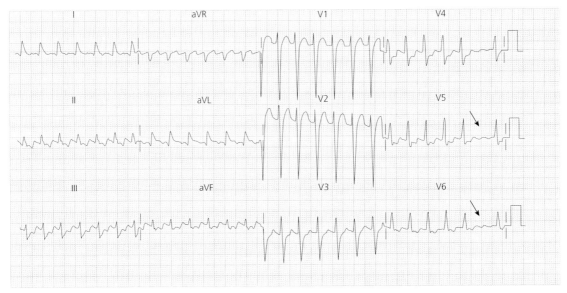

Figure 7 Atrial flutter with 2:1 block. Flutter waves are not clearly visible in any of the leads, but the rate is 150 beats/min. At the end of the tracing the level of 'block' increases to 3:1 (arrow), revealing the flutter waves (seen in leads V4–V6).

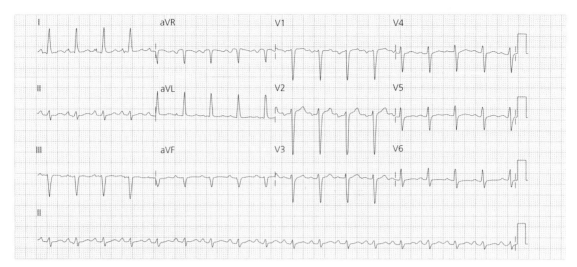

Figure 8 Sinus tachycardia. There are P-waves before each QRS complex and the rate is 120 beats/min.

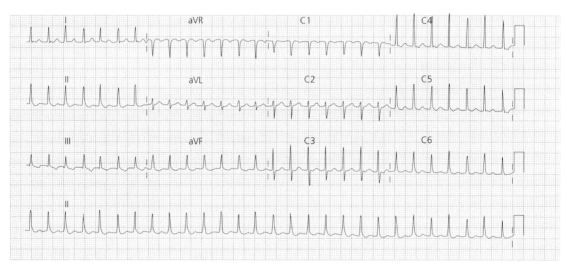

Figure 9 Supraventricular tachycardia. The complexes are narrow, and at a regular rate of around 180 beats/min with no P-waves visible.

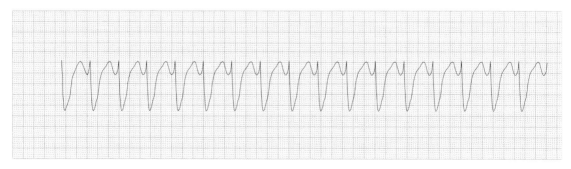

Figure 10 Rhythm strip showing broad complex tachycardia at a rate of 120 beats/min.

- Heart block (usually second or third degree – see Table 8)

Ask the following questions.

- Are there P-waves before every QRS complex?
  Sinus bradycardia
- Is the PR interval >5 mm (0.2 s) but constant?
  First-degree heart block
- Are there some P-waves *not* followed by QRS complexes?

Second-degree heart block – if progressive lengthening of PR interval this is Mobitz type 1 (Fig. 11); otherwise it is Mobitz type 2 (Fig. 12).

- Is there complete dissociation between P-waves and QRS complexes?
  Third-degree (complete) heart block

Evidence of myocardial ischaemia or infarction

Although interpretation of the rate and rhythm can be

Table 8 Some of the key features of rhythm disturbances in bradycardia

Rhythm	Key features
Sinus bradycardia	P-wave before each QRS complex Heart rate <60 beats/min
First-degree heart block	P-wave before each QRS complex PR interval >0.2 s (5 mm)
Second-degree heart block	Not all P-waves followed by QRS complex Mobitz type 1: progressive lengthening of PR interval over 2 or 3 beats followed by P-wave without subsequent QRS complex (Fig. 11) Mobitz type 2: all other cases of second-degree heart block (Fig. 12)
Third-degree heart block	Complete dissociation of P-waves and QRS complexes (Fig. 13) Ventricular beats are produced because of an 'escape' rhythm, arising either in the AV node ('nodal escape') or in the ventricular wall ('ventricular escape')

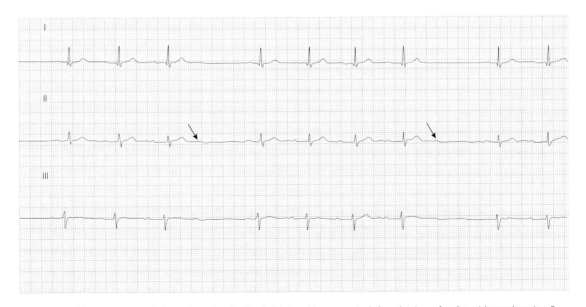

Figure 11 Mobitz type 1 second-degree heart block. The P–R interval is progressively lengthening; after 3 or 4 beats there is a P-waves (arrow) without a QRS complex, after which the P–R interval reverts to normal and the cycle repeats.

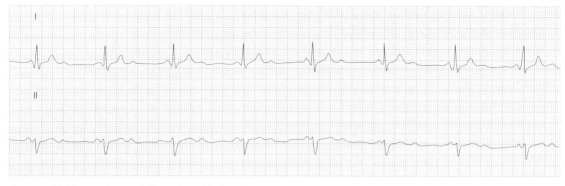

Figure 12 Mobitz type 2 second-degree heart block. In this example, alternate P-waves are followed by QRS complexes.

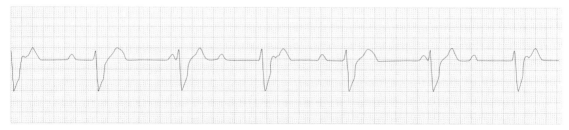

Figure 13 Complete heart block. The P-waves are completely dissociated from the QRS complexes.

made from a single ECG lead or inspection of the patient's heart monitor, information about the myocardium can only be accurately interpreted by looking at the 12-lead ECG as a whole.

To understand which area of the heart is affected by a particular abnormality it is necessary to consider the ECG leads in groups. Each group of leads gives information about a different region of heart muscle, as shown in Fig. 14.

The major regions can be summarised as follows.
- Inferior myocardium: leads II, III, AVF
- Anterior myocardium: leads V2–V4
- Lateral myocardium: leads V5, V6, I, II and AVL

Leads AVR and V1 offer some information about the right side of the heart, but rarely add to the diagnostic use of the ECG in the context of suspected myocardial ischaemia.

Sometimes more than one area can be affected simultaneously (inferolateral or anterolateral)

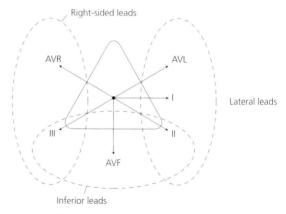

Figure 14 Diagramatic representation of the heart, showing regions represented by the limb leads.

Acute myocardial ischaemia/infarction

Evidence of acute myocardial ischaemia/infarction is usually identified by looking at the following areas (see Fig. 2).

- The ST segment
- The T-wave

ST segment abnormalities

ST segment abnormalities are usually considered significant if they affect two or more leads in one ECG 'region'.

ST segment abnormality takes two forms.

- ST elevation: the key feature of STEMI – see Fig. 15
- ST segment depression: often indicative of myocardial ischaemia or non-ST elevation myocardial infarction (NSTEMI) – see Fig. 16

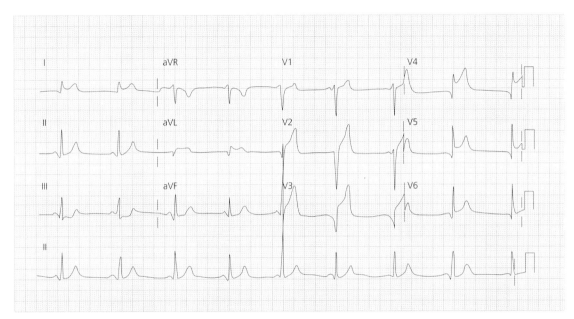

Figure 15 A 12-lead ECG showing ST segment elevation in leads V2–V6, I and AVL, indicating anterolateral ST elevation myocardial infarction.

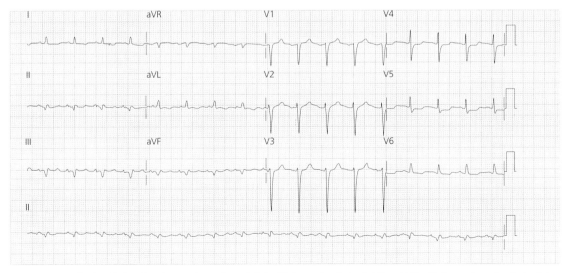

Figure 16 A 12-lead ECG showing sinus tachycardia and slight ST depression in leads V4 and V5 with T-wave inversion in leads I, AVL, V5 and V6. This suggests lateral ischaemia.

T-wave abnormalities

The T-wave usually adopts one of three shapes.

- Upward deflection
- Flattened
- Inverted

It can be normal for the T-waves to be inverted in leads AVR and V1 (see Fig. 3) and as an isolated finding in lead III (see Fig. 4).

Inverted or flattened T-waves in other leads may be indicative of myocardial ischaemia (see Fig. 16), NSTEMI or evolving STEMI.

Sometimes T-waves may adopt a 'biphasic' appearance – half up and half down; this may be a result of 'evolving' myocardial ischaemia. Serial ECGs are often required to clarify this.

Previous myocardial infarction

It is sometimes useful to establish evidence of a previous myocardial infarction. Full-thickness damage to the myocardium may leave ECG evidence in the form of:

- Q-waves:
  - a Q-wave is defined as a downward deflection before any upward deflection of the QRS complex
  - to be considered significant a Q-wave should be at least 2 mm deep or 25% of the height of the subsequent R-wave

- Small R-waves:
  - particularly significant in the anterior leads
  - R-waves should progressively enlarge from V2 to V6
  - Lack of 'R-wave progression' may indicate previous anterior infarction (see Fig. 17).

Bundle branch blocks

The left and right bundles of His carry the electrical wave of depolarisation through the interventricular septum after its passage through the atrioventricular node. Abnormalities of conduction through these bundles may result in ECG changes, characterised as left or right bundle branch blocks (LBBB and RBBB). Recognition of these abnormalities is important for a number of reasons.

- Bundle branch blocks (particularly LBBB) may be the presenting ECG abnormality of a myocardial infarction. When this occurs it is associated with a high mortality rate
- The presence of LBBB may make interpretation of ST segment and T-wave abnormalities extremely difficult. LBBB in the context of symptoms suggestive of myocardial infarction should be treated in the same way as STEMI (see Case 1)
- Although RBBB may be a normal variant, LBBB almost always implies underlying heart disease.

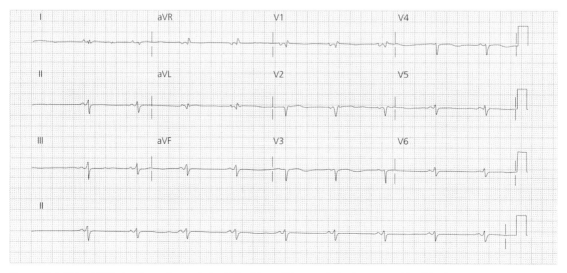

Figure 17 A 12-lead ECG showing a Q-wave in lead V2 with small R-waves in leads V2–V6 with minimal R-wave progression. This patient had experienced a previous anterolateral myocardial infarction but was asymptomatic at the time of this ECG.

ECG abnormalities in bundle branch blocks

Bundle branch block results in two abnormalities.
• Widening of the QRS complex because of slowed conduction through the abnormal bundle, which delays depolarisation of the ventricle
• Abnormal 'notched' QRS complex
The pattern of the notched QRS in different leads will usually give a clue to the nature of the block. When considering this pattern, imagine that you are facing the patient – the right-sided ECG leads (AVR, III, V1) will be on your left, whereas the left-sided ECG leads (I, II, V5, V6) will be on your right.

Left bundle branch block (see Figs 18 and 19)
The 'notch' in the right-sided leads will often resemble a 'W'.
   The 'notch' in the left-sided leads will often resemble an 'M'.
   As an *aide-memoire* remember the name 'WiLLiaM'.
• With the patient facing you, the 'W' is on their right
• The 'M' is on their left
• The 'LL' in the middle of the word defines the BBB as 'left'

Right bundle branch block (see Figs 18 and 20)
The 'notch' in the right-sided leads will often resemble an 'M'.
   The 'notch' in the left-sided leads will often resemble a 'W'.
   This time remember the word 'MaRRoW'.
• The 'M' is on the patient's right
• The 'W' is on the patient's left
• The 'RR' in the middle defines the BBB as 'right'

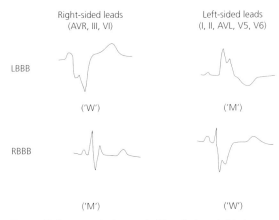

Figure 18 Assessment of suspected bundle branch block (BBB).

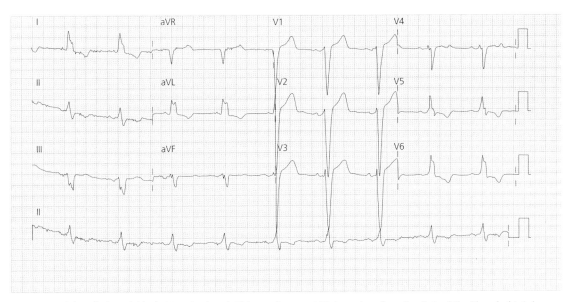

Figure 19 Left bundle branch block. Note the broad QRS complexes and W-shaped configuration in lead III, although this is less noticeable in leads V1 and AVR. The M configuration is seen in leads I, AVL, V5 and V6.

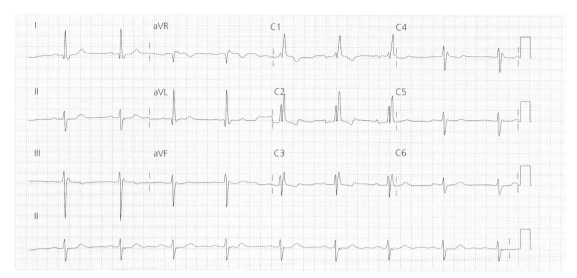

Figure 20 Right bundle branch block. The M-shaped QRS complexes are clearly evident in the right-sided leads (particularly V1 and V2). The W configuration is less obvious and can only be seen in leads I and AVL. This ECG also shows prolongation of the PR interval (first-degree heart block). More advanced readers may also note the left axis deviation. The combination of left axis deviation with first-degree heart block and right bundle branch block is termed trifascicular block.

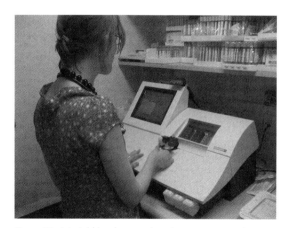

Figure 21 Arterial blood gas analyser in use on an acute medical unit.

This section on ECG interpretation has been deliberately simplified and should not be considered as a comprehensive summary. However, it is intended to highlight some of the most significant practical challenges that will be encountered on the acute medical unit. Other aspects of ECG interpretation cannot be ignored in medical school exams or OSCE stations and students are advised to seek out one of the more comprehensive textbooks on this subject to gain a more detailed insight into ECG interpretation in other settings.

Arterial blood gas interpretation on the acute medical unit

Most acute medical units have access to an arterial blood gas analyser (see Fig. 21), which can be invaluable in providing rapid diagnostic information for patients admitted as emergencies. Junior doctors will usually be trained to operate the machine, which gives a result within approximately 2 min. Interpretation of the result is an essential skill for any junior doctor working in this environment.

What information does an arterial blood gas provide?

The information provided by an arterial sample can be summarised as follows.
• Information about the patient's respiratory status
• Information about the patient's acid–base and metabolic status

In addition many analysers will provide other information, including:

- Electrolyte, calcium and glucose level
- Serum lactate
- Haemoglobin

It should be remembered that proper interpretation of an arterial blood gas result always requires:

- Information about the inspired oxygen concentration (FiO_2)
- Clinical information about the patient's condition

If presented with an arterial blood gas sample in an OSCE examination or on a ward round, a student should always ask for this additional information before attempting interpretation.

Information about the patient's respiratory status

This will be obtained by looking at the following.

The pO_2 level (normal range 12–16 kPa)

- **Low pO_2** is termed hypoxia (or hypoxaemia) and implies either inadequate gas exchange at the alveolar level or inadequate ventilation

Low pO_2 sometimes reflects inadvertent venous, rather than arterial, blood sampling; if the result is lower than anticipated from the clinical scenario, look at the oxygen saturation level: if the value on the blood sample is significantly lower than that obtained by pulse oximetry it is likely that the sample was venous and should be repeated

- **Raised pO_2** usually implies that the patient is breathing oxygen via a mask

The pCO_2 level (normal range 4.7–6.3 kPa)

- **Low pCO_2** (hypocapnia) implies that the patient is hyperventilating – i.e. they are 'blowing off' more CO_2 than normal due to a high respiratory rate (see 'respiratory alkalosis', below)
- **Raised pCO_2** (hypercapnia) implies that the patient is either hypoventilating, because of impaired respiratory drive, or inadequately ventilating their alveoli (see 'respiratory acidosis', below)

Information about the patient's acid–base and metabolic status

This will be obtained by looking at:

- **The pH** (normal range 7.35–7.45):
  - low pH is termed acidaemia
  - raised pH is termed alkalaemia
- **The base excess** (normal range −2 to +2) and **standard bicarbonate** (normal range 22–24):
  - low (i.e. negative) base excess, and low standard bicarbonate indicates a metabolic acidosis
  - high (i.e. positive) base excess and high bicarbonate indicates a metabolic alkalosis
- **The pCO_2** (again):
  - low pCO_2 indicates a respiratory alkalosis
  - high pCO_2 indicates a respiratory acidosis

The body will always attempt to correct an acid–base disturbance in order to restore the pH to normal.

- **In a primary metabolic acidosis** the patient's respiratory rate will usually increase resulting in a fall in the pCO_2 and consequent compensatory respiratory alkalosis
- **In a primary metabolic alkalosis** the patient's respiratory rate will fall resulting in compensatory respiratory acidosis
- **In a primary respiratory acidosis** the patient will retain bicarbonate resulting in compensatory metabolic acidosis
- **In a primary respiratory alkalosis** the patient will lose bicarbonate resulting in compensatory metabolic alkalosis

It should be noted that although respiratory compensation for a metabolic acidosis/alkalosis usually occurs very rapidly (often within minutes), metabolic compensation is much slower (24–48 h). This may give a clue to the acuity of the acid–base disturbance – i.e. if metabolic compensation has already occurred the problem is likely to have been ongoing for >24 h.

What is the 'dominant' metabolic disturbance?

As indicated above it is common to find a combination of acidosis and alkalosis on the same sample because of respiratory or metabolic compensation. In this situation, it is important to try to establish the dominant or primary metabolic disturbance.

It should be remembered that the body will not usually overcompensate for an acidosis or alkalosis; in other words:

- If the pH is high, the dominant disturbance is likely to be the alkalosis
- If the pH is low, the dominant disturbance is likely to be the acidosis

If the pH is normal (i.e. full compensation), the dominant disturbance may be more difficult to establish; in this situation, the clinical information will usually be invaluable (see the examples below).

Example 1

A 25-year-old female is brought into hospital drowsy and dehydrated. She is noted to be breathing rapidly.

Her arterial blood gas sample (while breathing room air) is as follows:

pH 7.19

pCO_2 2.1

pO_2 15.9

base excess −16

standard bicarbonate 12

oxygen saturation 99%

She has a high normal pO_2 with a low pCO_2 (respiratory alkalosis), negative base excess and low bicarbonate (metabolic acidosis). Given that the pH is low it is likely that the metabolic acidosis is the dominant abnormality, with compensatory respiratory alkalosis attempting to correct the pH.

Further investigation revealed raised blood glucose and ketonuria indicative of diabetic ketoacidosis (see Case 18).

Example 2

A 75-year-old man is brought into accident and emergency by ambulance. He has a history of chronic obstructive pulmonary disease and has been more breathless today. He was markedly hypoxic on arrival of the ambulance crew and was given high-flow oxygen during his transit to hospital. On arrival he appears drowsy, with laboured breathing. His arterial blood gases while breathing 40% oxygen are as follows:

pH 7.22

pCO_2 10.9

pO_2 10.4

base excess +7

standard bicarbonate 33

oxygen saturation 96%

He is slightly hypoxic with a raised PCO_2 (respiratory acidosis) and raised base excess/bicarbonate (metabolic alkalosis). His pH is low, which implies that the acidosis is the dominant lesion; given that the bicarbonate level is raised it is likely that there is an element of chronic compensated acidosis, which predates the recent deterioration, given that metabolic compensation takes 24–48 h to take effect. However, the low pH implies an acute uncompensated element, which may have coincided with the onset of drowsiness.

The patient was deemed to have CO_2 narcosis caused by uncontrolled oxygen delivery (see Case 6). The oxygen flow rate was reduced to 28% and the patient was treated with biphasic positive airway pressure (BiPAP), which resulted in improvement of his conscious level.

Example 3

Blood gases for the above patient were repeated after 1 h of BiPAP with the patient breathing 28% oxygen and revealed the following:

pH 7.31

pCO_2 7.2

pO_2 8.5

base excess +7

standard bicarbonate 31

saturation 93%

His pO_2 has fallen and his pCO_2 remains high. However, the pCO_2 has fallen compared with the previous result and the pH has nearly normalised as a result of more effective alveolar ventilation. The base excess and bicarbonate are largely unchanged. The features indicate compensated respiratory acidosis, and may be close to his normal metabolic status.

Arterial blood gas interpretation in practice

The following checklist should aid blood gas interpretation in the clinical setting or OSCE station.

1 Check the FiO_2 and *ask* for clinical information (if not provided).

2 Look at the pO_2: if this is low, is the CO_2 raised (Type II respiratory failure) or low (Type I respiratory failure)?

3 Look at the pH: is the patient acidaemic or alkalaemic?

4 If the pH is *low*, is there evidence of respiratory acidosis (high pCO_2) or metabolic acidosis (low bicarbonate or negative base excess)? Is there evidence of 'partial compensation' – respiratory acidosis plus high bicarbonate or metabolic acidosis plus low pCO_2?

5 If the pH is *high*, is there evidence of respiratory alkalosis (low pCO_2) or metabolic alkalosis (high bicarbonate or positive base excess)? Is there evidence of 'partial compensation' – respiratory alkalosis plus low bicarbonate or metabolic alkalosis plus raised pCO_2?

6 If the pH is *normal*, is there evidence of respiratory or metabolic compensation (low pCO_2 with low bicarbonate/base excess or high pCO_2 with raised bicarbonate/base excess)? If so consider the history to determine the 'dominant' disturbance.

7 Look at the haemoglobin, sodium, potassium, glucose and lactate (if provided).

Further reading

Cooper N, Forrest K, Cramp, P. *Essential guide to generic skills.* Blackwell Publishing, Oxford, 2006

Cooper N, Forrest K, Cramp, P. *Essential guide to acute care*, 2nd edition. Blackwell Publishing, Oxford, 2006

Resuscitation Guidelines. Resuscitation Council UK, London, 2005 (http://www. resus.org.uk)

Singer M, Webb AR. *Oxford handbook of critical care*, 2nd edition. Oxford University Press, Oxford, 2005

Sprigings D, Chambers JB. *Acute medicine: a practical guide to the management of medical emergencies*, 4th edition. Blackwell Publishing, Oxford, 2008

PART 1: BASICS

Case 1 A 45-year-old man with 'cardiac-type' chest pain

You receive a call from a general practitioner about a 45-year-old man he has seen in his surgery this morning. Mr John Porter had attended for a routine blood pressure check, but while in the waiting room he experienced severe central chest pain. The GP said that Mr Porter appeared pale and sweaty. An ambulance was called and arrived within 10 min, at which time Mr Porter was still in pain. Mr Porter is already en route to the hospital.

What challenges will this patient present?

• Chest pain is the commonest symptom resulting in referral to hospital for acute medical admission
• In many cases the reason for referral is either to confirm or refute the diagnosis of a 'cardiac' cause of the pain
• The term 'cardiac chest pain' is usually used to describe a pain resulting from either ischaemia of the cardiac muscle (myocardium) as a result of insufficient blood flow through a coronary artery or infarction as a result of blockage of an artery. Some common terminology is summarised in Table 9
• Rapid diagnosis or exclusion of myocardial infarction (MI) will be necessary to enable appropriate therapy to be given quickly
• A variety of other conditions can present with chest pain that may mimic the symptoms of ischaemic heart disease (see Table 10)

The ambulance has arrived at the Accident and Emergency department and you are 'fast bleeped' to attend. The ambulance crew report that Mr Porter has continued to experience pain during the trip to hospital. Mr Porter is responsive, breathing spontaneously and has a blood pressure of 120/50. The ambulance crew have inserted an intravenous cannula and applied oxygen via a mask. They have also administered two doses of glyceryl trinitrate (GTN) sublingually. The GP has enclosed a letter that details Mr Porter's past medical history. This includes high blood pressure, for which Mr Porter takes the angiotensin-converting enzyme (ACE) inhibitor ramipril. There is no prior history of angina or other cardiac disease.

What immediate management is required?

• Introduce yourself to Mr Porter and establish whether he is still in pain; if so reassure Mr Porter that you will be able to relieve it very quickly
• Confirm that Mr Porter is receiving 'high-flow' oxygen by mask (e.g. facemask with reservoir bag and 10–15 L/min flow rate): any degree of hypoxia will worsen the effects of myocardial ischaemia
• Recheck the blood pressure and heart rate
• Connect Mr Porter to a cardiac monitor and pulse oximeter
• Confirm that the cannula is patent and (if Mr Porter is still in pain) administer intravenous opiate analgesia, along with an anti-emetic drug (e.g. 5–10 mg of morphine sulphate with 50 mg of cyclizine)
• Obtain an ECG
• Take blood for a full blood count, urea and electrolytes, and lipids
• Administer 300 mg of aspirin and 300 mg of clopidogrel orally (see Box 3 – use 600 mg of clopidogrel if percutaneous coronary intervention is likely to be undertaken)

Mr Porter is given 300 mg of aspirin, 300 mg of clopidogrel and 5 mg of morphine sulphate intravenously along with 50 mg of cyclizine. Mr Porter is now pain free. He continues to look pale with cool perpiherae: oxygen saturation is 100% while breathing high-flow oxygen. Mr Porter's cardiac monitor reveals sinus rhythm, and his blood pressure is 110/60. An ECG is currently being recorded.

Acute Medicine: Clinical Cases Uncovered. By C. Roseveare.
Published 2009 by Blackwell Publishing, ISBN: 978-1-4051-6883-0

Table 9 Terminology used in the context of 'cardiac-type chest pain'

Term	Explanation
ST segment elevation myocardial infarction (STEMI)	Myocardial infarction (MI) characterised by the presence of ST segment elevation on ECG in one or more regions of the heart
Non-ST segment elevation myocardial infarction	MI without ST segment elevation – the ECG is normal or there may be ST segment depression or T-wave changes; the diagnosis is confirmed by measurement of biochemical markers (e.g. troponin)
Unstable angina	Ischaemic chest pain occurring at rest or with minimal exertion, usually implying critical narrowing of a coronary artery; ECG may be normal or show ST segment depression/T-wave changes; troponins are normal or marginally elevated
Crescendo angina	Ischaemic-type chest pain occurring on exertion, when the amount of exertion required to produce pain reduces progressively with time
Acute coronary syndrome (ACS)	An 'umbrella' term encompassing all of the above, recognising that ischaemia and infarction represent a continuum rather than distinct entities
Stable angina	Pain originating from ischaemic myocardium that is induced by exertion and relieved by rest and/or glyceryl trinitrate spray. Not usually considered part of the ACS spectrum, but may still require urgent investigation
Non-cardiac chest pain	Chest pain, which may be of 'cardiac type' but where myocardial ischaemia has been excluded
'Atypical' chest pain	A term which is frequently used but best avoided – usually implies a non-cardiac cause or diagnostic uncertainty

PART 2: CASES

Box 3 Why give aspirin and clopidogrel?

Aspirin has antiplatelet effects and has been shown to provide significant benefits when given to patients with ischaemic heart disease, particularly following myocardial infarction. Aspirin will often have been given by the ambulance crew or GP prior to arrival in hospital; if not, the patient should be given 300 mg of aspirin as soon as possible, unless the patient describes a previous severe allergy to the drug.

Clopidogrel is another antiplatelet agent that has additional benefits when given with aspirin. Patients with severe aspirin allergy should be given clopidogrel alone.

Following ST segment elevation myocardial infarction (STEMI) aspirin (75 mg daily) should be continued for life. Current evidence supports the use of clopidogrel 75 mg daily for 1 month following STEMI. If the patient undergoes percutaneous coronary intervention (PCI) and insertion of a coronary artery stent, the patient should take 75 mg of clopidogrel and 150 mg of aspirin daily for 1 year. After 1 year the clopidogrel can usually be stopped and the aspirin dose may be lowered to 75 mg daily. Following non-ST segment elevation myocardial infarction, clopidogrel should also be continued for 1 year.

Remember that severe allergy to aspirin is unusual. Much more commonly patients may have chosen or been told to avoid the drug because of previous peptic ulcer. It is generally considered that the benefits of aspirin in reducing mortality following myocardial infarction outweigh the small risk of precipitating gastrointestinal ulceration from a single dose of 300 mg. The decision on whether to continue aspirin treatment will be determined by the results of subsequent investigations and the nature/severity of the previous intolerance. Protection of the stomach with a proton pump inhibitor (e.g. omeprazole 20 mg daily) to reduce acid secretion may also be considered in this situation.

Table 10 'Non-cardiac' causes of 'cardiac-type' chest pain

Organ type	Specific examples	Comments
Cardiovascular	Dissection of thoracic aorta	Usually abrupt onset, radiating to back; may produce ECG changes mimicking ST segment elevation myocardial infarction (STEMI); discrepancy in upper limb blood pressures and widened mediastinum on chest radiograph may provide the clue to the diagnosis. Diagnosis is almost always made predominantly on the history
	Pericarditis	Patient often feels 'fluey'/unwell. Pain usually worse on lying flat and when leaning forward. The pain is also worsened by inspiration. Widespread ST elevation on ECG may cause confusion with STEMI
Musculoskeletal	Costochondritis	Pain results from inflammation of costal cartilage. It is often viral in origin – patient feels generally unwell. Usually exquisite localised tenderness ('reproduces the pain precisely') over the affected area
	Referred pain from neck or thoracic spine	Common in golfers or following heavy lifting. A careful history of recent activity may reveal a precipitant. Try rotating the thorax to see if this reproduces the pain
Gastro-oesophageal	Reflux disease	Usually described as 'burning' with relation to food. However, cardiac pain can often mimic this. Rapid relief with antacid may be suggestive
	Oesophageal spasm	Often indistinguishable from cardiac pain – usually a diagnosis of exclusion; may be eased by glyceryl trinitrate, but usually non-exertional; patients may have had repeated attacks over a long period
Neurogenic	Shingles	Pain of shingles follows a dermatome and may precede onset of the rash by 24 h. Often described as a 'shooting' pain, and always unilateral; carefully inspect the skin for vesicles
Abdominal	Pancreatitis/biliary colic/ peptic ulcer disease	Pain may originate from below the diaphragm; epigastric tenderness suggests an intra-abdominal cause; however, remember that myocardial infarction can also present with abdominal symptoms

Is the pain likely to be cardiac in origin?

As will be discussed below, it is crucial to act quickly. A detailed history may waste valuable minutes if this delays treatment. However, it is important to establish whether the symptoms are compatible with a cardiac origin for the pain, as this will help to guide subsequent treatment. Focused questioning should enable this information to be obtained in a matter of minutes. You should establish:

• The time of onset of symptoms
• The nature and severity of the pain, and associated symptoms (see Table 11)
• Any prior cardiac history
• Risk factors for coronary artery disease (see Table 12)

Mr Porter says that the pain built up rapidly, approximately 45 min earlier. He says this started centrally and then radiated across the chest as a 'tight band'. His left arm also felt 'heavy'. The pain became severe – probably the worst pain Mr Porter has experienced. He felt anxious and light headed and became sweaty. Mr Porter has had no previous episodes like this; however, he had experienced some intermittent central chest pains over the past few weeks that he had attributed to indigestion. In hindsight, Mr Porter now thought that these tended to come on with exertion rather than eating and they did not respond to treatment with an antacid. Mr Porter had not consulted a doctor about these pains. He has been treated for high blood pressure for the past five years with ramipril. Mr Porter smokes 20 cigarettes per day and his father died of a heart attack at the age of 55 years.

The ECG is now available (see Fig. 22).

Table 11 Clinical features of 'typical' cardiac pain (classified according to the 'Socrates' mnemonic)

		Comments
Site	Retrosternal area – often quite diffuse	Often radiates right across chest; very localised pain is unusual
Onset	Usually rapid (over 5–10 min)	Very abrupt onset is suspicious for dissecting thoracic aortic aneurysm
Character	Heavy, tight, band-like	Sometimes sharp or burning – do not assume the latter always implies an oesophageal source
Radiation	To neck, jaw, left shoulder and arm	Sometimes pain may be confined to arm or shoulder
Associated symptoms	Sweating, anxiety, pallor	These symptoms result from adrenaline release and may be found in any patient with severe pain
Time course	Myocardial infarction usually results in pain lasting >30 min; angina may result in briefer episodes	Very short-lived pain (seconds only) usually suggests non-cardiac cause
Exacerbating/relieving factors	Angina usually exacerbated by exertion, relieved by rest or GTN; myocardial infarct pain usually only relieved by opiate analgesia	If GTN is taken in the form of a sublingual spray the onset of action is very rapid (within 1–2 min). If a patient says that the pain disappeared after GTN check how long this took – a pain that took >10 min to disappear was probably relieved spontaneously, rather than by the GTN
Severity	Myocardial infarction pain is usually very severe – if the patient is asked to grade this on a scale of 1 to 10 it is usually described as 8–10 (or 'worst ever' pain). Patients who experience repeated attacks of angina-type chest pain may be able to give an indication of how this episode compares to previous pains	Remember that some patients may 'play down' the significance of their pain, particularly if this has been eased by the time you see them and they are keen to avoid a hospital stay. If the pain was severe enough to require them to call an ambulance and they do not normally visit a doctor it is likely that this was severe at the time of onset

GTN, glyceryl trinitrate.

Table 12 Risk factors for coronary artery disease

Hypertension

Diabetes mellitus

Obesity

Family history of ischaemic heart disease

Hyperlipidaemia

Smoking

Alcohol

PART 2: CASES

Does Mr Porter require immediate therapy to unblock a coronary artery?

The following can now be noted.

• Mr Porter is describing symptoms that are consistent with an ischaemic/cardiac origin of pain (see Table 11)

• The onset of symptoms was 45 min prior to Mr Porter's arrival in hospital

• Mr Porter has a number of risk factors for coronary artery disease (smoking, previous hypertension, family history) (see Table 12)

• The ECG shows evidence of ST segment elevation in leads II, III, AVF, V5 and V6. This is diagnostic of an inferolateral ST segment elevation myocardial infarction (STEMI) (see Part 1, p. 21)

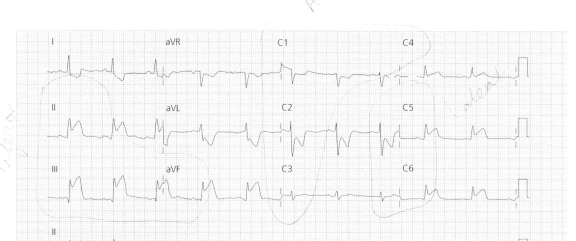

Figure 22 ECG showing marked ST elevation in leads II, III, AVF, V5 and V6 indicative of inferolateral ST elevation myocardial infarction. The ST depression and T-wave inversion seen in lead I, AVL and V2 is an electrical phenomenon termed 'reciprocal depression', commonly seen in patients with ST segment elevation myocardial infarction.

The theory behind therapies designed to unblock coronary arteries is summarised in Box 4. In this case, Mr Porter appears to fulfil the criteria for thrombolytic therapy or percutaneous coronary intervention (PCI), as listed in Box 5. The following actions are now required as quickly as possible.

• If local facilities exist for PCI, contact the on-call cardiology team immediately and follow the local protocol
• If PCI is not feasible, confirm that Mr Porter has no contraindications to thrombolysis (Box 5 – this may require you to take some further history if you have not asked these questions earlier)
• Ensure that the clinical features do *not* suggest thoracic aortic dissection as a cause for the symptoms/ECG changes (see Table 10). Abrupt onset of pain radiating to the back or discrepancy in upper limb blood pressure should lead to consideration of thoracic computed tomography before thrombolysis
• Explain the benefits and potential risks of thrombolysis to the patient
• Prescribe (and if necessary draw up and administer) the appropriate thrombolytic drug according to local guidelines (see Table 13)
• Arrange a bed in the coronary care unit

Mr Porter is given 40 mg of tenecteplase by a single bolus (based on an approximate weight of 75 kg) followed by intravenous heparin (bolus dose of 4000 units followed by infusion of 900 units/h). Arrangements are being made for transfer to the coronary care unit.

What further actions are required after thrombolysis?

• Ensure continuous cardiac monitoring, pulse oximetry, regular recording of blood pressure (every 5–10 min). Mr Porter should remain on oxygen
• Ensure that a full history and examination has been documented – this may not have been done earlier. Listen carefully to the heart sounds and document any heart murmurs.
• Review the results of blood tests – particularly the serum potassium level: if this is <4 mg/dL this should be supplemented in an intravenous infusion, taking care not to overload Mr Porter with fluid
• Arrange a chest radiograph
• Measure cardiac troponin (I or T) 12 h after onset of symptoms

Mr Porter's condition is now stable enough for transfer to the coronary care unit. The nurses have asked whether a drug chart has been completed.

What drugs should be prescribed for Mr Porter's stay in hospital?

Following MI most patients should be prescribed the following:

Box 4 Thrombolysis or percutaneous coronary intervention?

During the 1980s a number of large-scale clinical trials demonstrated that early treatment with drugs designed to dissolve a thrombus (thrombolytic drugs) reduced mortality following myocardial infarction where the ECG demonstrated ST segment elevation. The earlier such drugs were administered, the greater the degree of benefit. These benefits offset the risks of bleeding, provided the drugs were administered within 12 h of the onset of pain.

More recently, there has been considerable interest in an alternative approach to the opening of blocked arteries using percutaneous coronary intervention (PCI). This technique involves the insertion of metal stents through blocked arteries to re-establish blood flow. Recent studies indicate that PCI is likely to be superior to thrombolysis in many cases. However, such techniques require considerable expertise from doctors, nurses and theatre technicians, as well as equipment that is only available in a limited number of centres at present. Even in larger centres this may not be available outside normal working hours. It is therefore likely that many patients will continue to receive thrombolytic drugs in this situation.

Factors which favour the use of PCI rather than thrombolysis include:

- the ability to perform PCI within 90 min from presentation to hospital
- the presence of Q-waves on initial ECG

- time to presentation >3 h
- cardiogenic shock
- severe heart failure and/or pulmonary oedema
- contraindications to thrombolysis (see Box 5)
- doubt about diagnosis of ST segment elevation myocardial infarction (STEMI)

Whichever technique is employed to open a coronary artery, the key is that it should be undertaken rapidly. In 2000 the British government published the National Service Framework for Coronary Artery Disease, in which it set targets for the delivery of thrombolytic drugs. The time from the arrival of the patient in hospital to the time of administration of the drug ('door to needle time') should be <30 min, and the time from the onset of symptoms ('pain to needle time') should not exceed 1 h. These targets resulted in dramatic changes in the early management of STEMI: in some areas paramedics have been trained to administer the thrombolytic prior to arrival in hospital (pre-hospital thrombolysis). Many hospitals trained specialist nurses to ensure the early administration of these drugs. Local guidelines and care pathways exist in most hospitals to ensure that this process happens as quickly as possible. The staff in the emergency department will usually be familiar with the local practice and should be able to guide you where necessary.

Box 5 Indications for thrombolysis

History compatible with the diagnosis of myocardial infarction in the past 12 h associated with the following ECG changes:
ST segment elevation >2 mm in two contiguous chest leads
ST segment elevation >1 mm in two limb leads
Bundle branch block

Contraindications
Absolute
Haemorrhagic stroke (or other spontaneous intracerebral bleed) at any time in the past
Ischaemic stroke in the preceding 3 months
Central nervous system neoplasm
Major trauma/surgery/head injury within the preceding 3 months
Gastrointestinal bleeding within the past 1 month
Known bleeding disorder
Aortic dissection

Relative
Transient ischaemic attack in preceding 6 months
Oral anticoagulant therapy (e.g. warfarin – risk is greater with higher international normalised ratio)
Pregnancy or within 1 week post partum
Non-compressible puncture wound (e.g. failed subclavian central venous cannula insertion)
Prolonged/traumatic cardiopulmonary resuscitation
Refractory hypertension (systolic BP >180 mmHg despite treatment)
Advanced liver disease
Infective endocarditis
Active peptic ulcer disease

Table 13 Fibrinolytic regimens

Drug	Dose (all intravenous)	Heparin requirement?	Comment
Streptokinase	1.5 million units in 100 mL of normal saline over 30 min	None (prescribe prophylactic heparin for deep vein thrombosis prevention)	Least expensive, but high incidence of allergy and hypotension following infusion
Alteplase	15 mg bolus Then 0.75 mg/kg over 30 min Then 0.5 mg/kg over 60 min (Total dose not >100 mg)	Bolus 60 units/kg (maximum 4000 units) Infusion 12 units/kg/h (max 1000 units/h) for 24 h Check APTT at 3, 6, 12, 24 h and adjust dose, aiming for APTT of 50–70 s	
Reteplase	10 unit bolus Further 10 units at 30 min	As for alteplase	
Tenecteplase	Single bolus according to weight: <60 kg – 30 mg 60–69 kg – 35 mg 70–79 kg – 40 mg 80–89 kg – 45 mg >90 kg – 50 mg	As for alteplase	Simple dosing regimen makes this the most appropriate thrombolytic for pre-hospital use

APTT, activated partial thromboplastin time.

- Aspirin 75 mg daily (unless previous severe allergy or high risk of peptic ulceration)
- Clopidogrel 75 mg daily
- Beta-blocker (e.g. atenolol 25–50 mg daily), unless contraindicated (e.g. patients with asthma)
- HMGCoA reductase inhibitor ('statin') (e.g. simvastatin 40 mg daily)
- ACE inhibitor (e.g. ramipril) – a starting dose of 2.5 mg daily (or 1.25 mg in older patients) for patients not already taking the drug will reduce the likelihood of hypotension on starting this drug; the dose should be slowly titrated up to 10 mg per day if Mr Porter will tolerate this
- Deep vein thrombosis (DVT) prevention (e.g. enoxaparin 40 mg subcutaneously – start after completion of heparin infusion)
- Opiate analgesia as required (e.g. morphine sulphate 5–10 mg i.v.)
- Antiemetic as required (e.g. cyclizine 50 mg, 8 hourly)
- GTN sublingually as required

It may also be worth considering adding paracetamol 1 g qds as required, night sedation and an antacid to cover other possible eventualities during his hospital stay.

Mr Porter is transferred to the coronary care unit where he is observed on a cardiac monitor for 24 h, after which he mobilises uneventfully. Mr Porter's cardiac troponin I was elevated at 12.5 ng/mL (normal <0.15 ng/mL), confirming the diagnosis of MI. Mr Porter is discharged from hospital on day 5, with arrangements made for coronary angiography to be carried out as an outpatient within four weeks of discharge.

CASE REVIEW

A 45-year-old man is admitted with a history of recent-onset cardiac-type chest pain. Mr John Porter has a number of risk factors for coronary artery disease, and an ECG confirms the diagnosis of STEMI. Local facilities for PCI are not available and there are no contraindications to thrombolysis, so Mr Porter is administered tenecteplase within 30 min of arrival in hospital. Mr Porter is transferred to the coronary care unit and spends five days in hospital making an uneventful recovery.

Although this case illustrates a very important scenario, it should be noted that STEMI is diagnosed in only a small proportion (around 5–10%) of patients presenting to hospital with 'suspected cardiac' chest pain. It is far more common that the pain is 'consistent' with a cardiac cause but the ECG is either normal or non-diagnostic. In this situation there are three possibilities:

• the patient has some other form of 'acute coronary syndrome' (see Table 9)
• the pain is cardiac in origin but the patient is at low risk
• the pain is non-cardiac in origin (see Table 10).

Scarcity of hospital beds will often result in pressure to discharge patients in the last two groups as early as possible. However, it is important to identify patients in the first group who may be at high risk of more serious cardiac complications or death. The approach to these patients should include:

• a careful history – true cardiac pain does not always present in a 'typical' way, and non-cardiac causes may produce the classic symptoms described in Table 9

• there may be other factors which point towards an alternative explanation (see Table 10)
• careful evaluation of the risk factors for cardiac disease – sometimes a formal risk score, such as the thrombolysis in myocardial infarction (TIMI) risk score, may be helpful (see Table 14)
• measurement of biochemical markers of cardiac muscle damage, particularly troponin I or troponin T.

It is important to remember that cardiac troponins will rise for up to 24 h from the onset of damage (although the peak is usually at 12 h). A 'normal' value can only be confirmed if measurement is delayed until 12 h from the patient's most severe pain. Furthermore, although a normal value does help to guide prognosis, it does not exclude a cardiac cause for the patient's symptoms. This must be taken in the context of the patient's symptoms and risk factors. Many patients will still require further cardiac investigation, although this may often be arranged after discharge from hospital.

Finally, remember that a discharge diagnosis of 'non-cardiac chest pain' may do little to satisfy the patient's anxiety about their symptoms. Where possible a 'positive' explanation for a patient's symptoms should always be sought; if this is not possible then this should be discussed carefully with the patient, paying particular attention to the plan of action if the symptoms should recur. Non-cardiac pain from a musculoskeletal or gastro-oesophageal source is frequently recurrent, and a telephone call to NHS Direct describing the chest pain may result in re-admission to hospital.

KEY POINTS

• Immediate resuscitation, oxygen and analgesia is the first priority for all patients presenting to hospital with chest pain.
• If a cardiac cause is suspected, an ECG should be obtained at the earliest opportunity.
• Confirmation of ST segment elevation on ECG should result in immediate consideration of thrombolysis or percutaneous coronary intervention: *time is muscle!*
• Patients should be observed closely for complications such as arrhythmias and heart failure, which should be treated promptly.

• If the ECG is normal or non-diagnostic, carefully evaluate the risk of acute coronary syndrome by clinical assessment and measurement of cardiac troponins.
• If a cardiac cause is thought to have been excluded always try to make a positive diagnosis before discharge and communicate carefully with the patient to prevent unnecessary re-admission.

Variable	Score
Age >65	1
History of hypertension	1
History of diabetes	1
Current smoker	1
Hypercholesterolaemia	1
Family history of coronary artery disease	1
Prior angiographic stenosis >50%	1
≥2 episodes of rest pain in past 24 h	1
Use of aspirin in past 7 days	1
Elevated troponin or creatinine kinase MB isoenzyme	1
Horizontal ST depression or transient ST elevation ≥1 mm	1
Total	
Event likelihood:	
score 0/1	4.7%
score 2	8.3%
score 3	13.2%
score 4	19.9%
score 5	26.2%
score 6/7	40.9%

Table 14 Thrombolysis in myocardial infarction (TIMI) risk score for unstable angina/non-ST segment elevation myocardial infarction

Further reading

Antman EM, Cohen M, Peter J et al. The TIMI risk score for unstable angina/non-ST elevation MI: a method for prognostication and therapeutic decision making. *JAMA* 2000; **284**: 835–42

Bassand JP, Hamm CW, Ardissino D et al. Guidelines for the diagnosis and treatment of non-ST-segment elevation acute coronary syndromes. *Eur Heart J* 2007; **28**: 1598–660

European Society of Cardiology. Guidelines for the management of patients with ST elevation myocardial infarction (2003). http://www.escardio.org/guidelines-surveys/esc-guidelines/Pages/acs-st-segment-elevation.aspx

Keeley EC, Hillis LD. Primary PCI for myocardial infarction with ST-segment elevation. *N Engl J Med* 2007; **356**: 47–54

Case 2 A 35-year-old woman with 'pleuritic' chest pain

You are contacted by a general practitioner regarding Mrs Sarah Williams, a 35-year-old woman he has seen in his surgery this morning. Mrs Williams woke this morning with left-sided chest pain, which is sharp and increased with inspiration. She also describes mild shortness of breath on exertion. Mrs Williams is a non-smoker and takes the combined oral contraceptive pill but no other medication. She is normally fit and well. Mrs Williams had an eight-hour journey by aeroplane two weeks ago, but has not had any symptoms suggestive of deep vein (DVT) thrombosis. The GP explains that he is concerned about the possibility of pulmonary embolism (PE) and would be grateful if you could exclude this.

What challenges will this patient present?

• When chest pain is described as 'sharp' and increased by inspiration or coughing the pain is termed 'pleuritic'
• Pleuritic pain usually results from inflammation of the parietal pleura, which contains an abundance of nerve cells
• The range of conditions that commonly present with pleuritic chest pain is considerable (see Table 15)
• In addition, pain originating in the chest wall, frequently termed 'musculoskeletal' chest pain, may mimic pleuritic chest pain
• Frequently, the referring clinician's main concern is to exclude PE as the cause of the patient's symptoms
• It should be remembered that many of the conditions listed in Table 15 may be serious enough to justify hospital treatment; furthermore, establishing an alternative diagnosis may help in the exclusion of PE

On arrival Mrs Williams is experiencing significant ongoing chest pain. Respiratory rate is 24 breaths/min and pulse

oximetry reveals a saturation of 91% while breathing room air. Pulse is 110 beats/min with a blood pressure of 100/50.

What immediate management is required?

• High-flow oxygen should be applied via a re-breathe/reservoir mask; if feasible, obtain an arterial blood gas sample immediately before applying the oxygen, with the patient breathing room air
• Connect the patient to a cardiac monitor
• Administer analgesia, according to the patient's needs; if the pain is severe an intravenous opiate may be required (e.g. morphine sulphate 5–10 mg)
• Site an intravenous cannula
• Take a venous blood sample for full blood count (FBC), urea and electrolytes (U&E), liver function tests (LFT), clotting and D-dimer (see below)
• Obtain an ECG and request an urgent chest radiograph *Fibrin degredation prod (from clot break down ... ie resolving thrombosis*

Mrs Williams is now more comfortable after administration of 5 mg of morphine sulphate intravenously. Respiratory rate has slowed to 18 breaths/min and saturation is reading 100% while breathing high flow oxygen.

The ECG shows a sinus tachycardia but no other abnormalities.

*Arterial blood gases taken **prior** to the administration of oxygen revealed the following: pH 7.56, pCO$_2$ 3.25, pO$_2$ 8.56, base excess −1.8, standard bicarbonate 22.*

What do the arterial blood gas results indicate?

• Arterial blood gases taken with the patient breathing room air show an acute respiratory alkalosis (see p. 25) and significant hypoxaemia
• Given that she apparently has no prior history of pulmonary disease, this degree of hypoxaemia is highly significant

Acute Medicine: Clinical Cases Uncovered. By C. Roseveare.
Published 2009 by Blackwell Publishing, ISBN: 978-1-4051-6883-0

Table 15 Differential diagnosis of 'pleuritic' type chest pain

Classification	Specific examples	Comments
Respiratory	Pulmonary embolism	See text and Table 16
	Viral infection with pleurisy	Symptoms of recent or ongoing viral illness
	Pneumonia	Infective symptoms and cough productive of purulent sputum; evidence of pulmonary consolidation on examination and chest radiograph
Pleural diseases	Pleural tumours (e.g. mesothelioma)	Ask about asbestos exposure; usually long history with gradual onset
	Connective tissue diseases – e.g. SLE, rheumatoid	Usually a past history of rheumatological disease is apparent
Cardiac	Pericarditis	Pain worsened by lying flat and leaning forward; ECG shows widespread concave ST segment elevation. Usually viral origin – patient feels unwell
	Myocardial infarction	Pain not typically pleuritic, but occasionally patient describes pain worsened by breathing – listen carefully to the history and check the ECG
Musculoskeletal	Costochondritis (Tietze's syndrome, Bornholm disease)	Usually viral in origin; patient describes localised pain over costochondral junction with point tenderness
	Referred pain from thoracic spine	Often band-like, radiating to back and worsened by rotation of thorax. Often abrupt onset. May be history of preceding injury/heavy lifting/golf, etc.)
	Chest wall injury (bruising, rib fracture)	History of prior trauma (e.g. seatbelt injury in car accident). Marked local tenderness
	Shingles	Sharp 'shooting' pain; unilateral; pain may precede onset of rash. Look closely for vesicles in the distribution of the pain
Abdominal	Cholecystitis	May cause referred pain to right shoulder blade, exacerbated by inspiration; examine carefully for abdominal (right upper quadrant) tenderness

SLE, systemic lupus erythematosus.

• The low pCO_2 and raised pH suggest that she is attempting to compensate for the hypoxia by hyperventilating (type 1 respiratory failure)

• The normal bicarbonate and base excess suggest that this problem is of acute onset, since metabolic compensation has not yet occurred. This corresponds with the history

• Although it is reassuring to note that the oxygen saturation has risen to 100% on high-flow oxygen, this should ideally be confirmed by repeating the arterial blood gas

Repeat arterial blood gases with Mrs Williams breathing high flow oxygen reveal a pCO_2 of 4.1 and pO_2 12.5.

Mrs Williams' condition is now stabilised. It is now important to consider the clinical likelihood of PE and differential diagnosis; this requires a detailed history and examination.

Mrs Williams describes having felt breathless for the two weeks prior to the onset of pain. For the past 24 hours she has felt generally unwell with a fever and general malaise. She has noted a slight dry cough but without sputum production. During the night Mrs Williams was aware of left-sided chest pain, which started in the axillary area and radiated anteriorly. This pain has become more intense this morning and is notably worsened by inspiration and by coughing, as well as by certain movements. As a result Mrs

Williams feels that she can only take shallow breaths. This morning when walking to the GP's surgery she felt very breathless and became light-headed.

In the past Mrs Williams has been well, with no significant medical history, specifically no prior history of DVT or PE, and no recent surgery. She is a non-smoker and takes no regular medication apart from the combined (oestrogen and progesterone) oral contraceptive pill. Mrs Williams recently returned from a two-week holiday in the USA during which she undertook several internal air flights. During the flight home Mrs Williams noticed that both ankles swelled up, but there was no redness or calf tenderness.

On examination Mrs Williams has a mild pyrexia (37.5°C) and persistent tachycardia 100 beats/min. Cardiovascular and respiratory examination is otherwise unremarkable and there is no evidence of DVT on examination of her legs. Mrs Williams' chest wall is mildly tender over the site of the pain, which is also worsened by rotation of the thorax.

Are the symptoms/signs compatible with a diagnosis of pulmonary embolism?

• Symptoms and signs of pulmonary embolism are summarised in Table 16.
• Breathlessness, pleuritic chest pain and light-headedness in combination with a fast respiratory rate and tachycardia are all suggestive of pulmonary embolism

• Breathlessness often precedes the onset of pleuritic chest pain in the context of pulmonary embolism
• Significant breathlessness with hypoxia and a clear chest on examination are strong indicators of pulmonary embolism

Are there any features that point to an alternative diagnosis?

The differential diagnosis for pleuritic chest pain is summarised in detail in Table 15.
• The prior history of cough, fever and malaise might suggest respiratory infection as a possible cause, although there are physical examination findings to suggest pneumonia and Mrs Williams has not expectorated discoloured sputum
• The presence of chest wall tenderness and increased pain on rotation of the thorax may suggest a musculoskeletal component; however, this would not explain the degree of hypoxia
• It should be remembered that all of these are non-specific findings that can also occur in the context of pulmonary embolism

What are the patient's risk factors for thromboembolic disease?

Risk factors for pulmonary embolism are summarised in Table 17.

Table 16 Symptoms and signs of pulmonary embolism

Symptom/sign	Comments
Breathlessness/tachypnoea	Almost invariable in PE; 'true' breathlessness may be difficult to distinguish from shallow breathing due to pain. May come on suddenly or gradually (in the case of multiple PE)
Pleuritic chest pain	Results from pleural irritation due to pulmonary infarction. Usually gradual onset – breathlessness often precedes onset of pain
General malaise/cough/fever	Inflammatory response due to pulmonary infarction may produce constitutional upset which can mimic the symptoms of infection
Haemoptysis	Occurs in the context of pulmonary infarction; usually small volume of blood
Leg swelling	Only around 20% of patients have symptoms/signs of DVT at the time of presentation with PE
Syncope/light-headedness	Drop in blood pressure may accompany significant pulmonary embolism
Tachycardia	Almost invariable following pulmonary embolism
Pleural rub	Not a common finding. Implies pleural inflammation – may also be seen with infective pleural disease

DVT, deep vein thrombosis; PE, pulmonary embolism.

Table 17 Risk factors for thromboembolic disease*

	Risk factor	Comments
Clotting	Thrombophilia (inherited or acquired)	
	Combined oral contraceptive pill	Progesterone-only pill is considered safe
	Nephrotic syndrome	Owing to urinary loss of antithrombin III
	Pregnancy	
	Hormone replacement therapy	
	Cigarette smoking	Probably not an independent risk factor for venous thrombosis
	Malignancy	May result in hypercoagulability as well as reduced mobility or direct compression of pelvic veins
Flow	Immobility	
	Recent surgery/hospital stay	Risk may be reduced by administration of prophylactic doses of heparin or wearing compression stockings
	Long-haul plane flight, coach journey, car trip	Usually journeys of >4-hour duration are considered relevant
	Hyperviscosity states, e.g. polycythaemia, hyperglobulinaemia	
	Abdominal or pelvic mass lesion	Owing to compression of pelvic veins
Vessel	Surgery/trauma to pelvic veins	
	Pelvic radiotherapy	
	Lower limb venous insufficiency	
	Previous DVT/PE	May also imply thrombophilic tendency as well as resulting in damage to lower limb veins

*These are often classified according to 'Verkov's triad': factors relating to blood clotting abnormalities; factors affecting blood flow through the lower limb/pelvic veins; factors affecting the lower limb vessels themselves.

DVT, deep vein thrombosis; PE, pulmonary embolism.

- Mrs Williams takes the oral contraceptive pill
- Mrs Williams has recently undertaken two long-haul plane flights
- The absence of clinical evidence of a DVT should not be seen as reassuring in this case – only around 20% of patients with PE have clinical evidence of DVT at the time of presentation

What is the 'pretest probability' (PTP) score?

As indicated in Table 16, the symptoms and signs of pulmonary embolism are often non-specific. In order to try to improve the objectivity of clinical assessment a number of risk scoring systems have been validated to indicate the likelihood of pulmonary embolism. The most commonly used of these is the Wells score, which is based on the seven factors listed in Table 18.

> The pretest probability score is calculated as 4.5 (1.5 for tachycardia, 3 for 'no alternative diagnosis more likely'), indicating an intermediate probability for pulmonary embolism.

Table 18 Wells pretest probability score

Symptoms and signs of DVT	3.0
Heart rate >100	1.5
Immobilisation ≥3 consecutive days or surgery in past 4 weeks	1.5
Previous DVT/PE	1.5
Haemoptysis	1.0
Alternative diagnosis less likely than PE	3.0
Malignancy (treated in past 6 months or receiving palliative care)	1.0

Interpretation: two or less, 'low probability'; 3–6, 'intermediate probability'; >6, 'high probability' for pulmonary embolism.

DVT, deep vein thrombosis; PE, pulmonary embolism.

Should treatment be prescribed in view of the clinical suspicion of pulmonary embolism?

It is usual practice to prescribe anticoagulant treatment to patients while confirmation is awaited when there is a clinical suspicion of PE.

- Initial treatment usually comprises low molecular weight heparin (LMWH), e.g. enoxaparin 1.5 mg/kg once daily
- Full anticoagulation with warfarin is usually delayed until confirmation of the diagnosis
- Further analgesia may also be required if the effect of the initial dose is wearing off – regular paracetamol and/or ibuprofen may be effective with the addition of codeine or further morphine if required

Mrs Williams is given a single subcutaneous dose of enoxaparin; the pain remains controlled with regular paracetamol and codeine phosphate.

Initial investigation results are now available. The following abnormalities are noted:
- *Neutrophil count 9.8 (normal 3–6)* ↗
- *C-reactive protein (CRP) 93 (normal range <6)* ↗
- *D-dimer 890 (normal range <250)* ↗ ↗
- *ECG: sinus tachycardia, otherwise normal (see Fig. 23).*
- *Chest radiograph: blunting of the costophrenic angle on left side, otherwise normal*

How should the initial investigation results be interpreted?

1 CRP and neutrophil count
- CRP and neutrophil count rise in the context of an inflammatory response
- When elevated these results are often considered indicative of infection
- It should be remembered that pulmonary infarction can also produce an inflammatory response that can result in elevation of CRP and neutrophil levels

2 D-dimer
- D-dimer is a fibrinogen degradation product that is released into the circulation during active fibrin turn-over, as happens during clot formation
- Normal D-dimer levels, particularly in the context of a low clinical suspicion (i.e. low PTP), usually exclude pulmonary embolism, such that further investigation may not be required
- D-dimer is also elevated in the context of infection, other inflammatory processes, malignancy, following surgery and during pregnancy (low 'specificity')
- When D-dimer is elevated in the context of a low clinical suspicion (or low PTP) for PE, it is important to re-evaluate the history, examination and other investigation results to prevent overinvestigation

3 Electrocardiogram

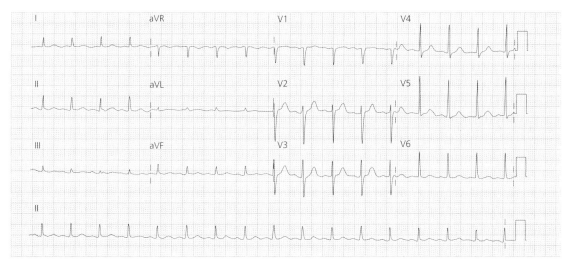

Figure 23 ECG showing sinus tachycardia. P-waves are visible before each QRS complex and the ventricular rate is 100 beats/min (exactly three big squares between each QRS complex – best seen in the rhythm strip at the bottom of the ECG). Sinus tachycardia is the commonest ECG abnormality in patients with pulmonary embolism. The classic S1, Q3, T3 pattern (S-wave in lead I with Q-wave and inverted T-wave in lead III) is rarely seen, and usually indicates a large pulmonary embolism with right ventricular strain.

[handwritten annotation at top: (5) ↑ign INR = high chance of bleeding / (or) Low INR = high chance of having clot.]

The following ECG abnormalities may be noted in patients with pulmonary embolism:

- sinus tachycardia: the commonest abnormality
- other arrhythmias: most commonly atrial fibrillation
- features of right ventricular strain (S-wave in lead I, Q-wave and T-wave inversion in lead III; inverted T-waves in anterior leads; right bundle branch block), usually indicative of large pulmonary embolism

In addition look closely for the following:

- widespread concave ST segment elevation as seen in pericarditis (an alternative explanation for pleuritic chest pain)
- evidence of myocardial ischaemia/infarction – may occasionally mimic the symptoms of pulmonary embolism

4 Chest radiograph

The chest radiograph is rarely diagnostic of pulmonary embolism, but may indicate an alternative explanation for the patient's symptoms. The following points should be considered.

- The chest radiograph may be normal: a normal chest radiograph in association with significant breathlessness and hypoxia is suggestive of pulmonary embolism
- Blunting of the costophrenic angle indicates pleural inflammation, but does not help identify the cause
- Look closely for a pneumothorax: this may explain the patient's symptoms and will save unnecessary investigation
- Peripheral 'wedge-shaped' shadows may be seen where there is segmental pulmonary infarction – on occasions this can be difficult to distinguish from the appearances caused by infection
- Reduced vascular markings on the radiograph may suggest large pulmonary emboli
- Significant abnormalities on the chest radiograph will influence the subsequent choice of investigation

The investigations to date have not found an alternative cause for Mrs Williams' symptoms. The chest radiograph abnormality, sinus tachycardia, elevated D-dimer and inflammatory markers are all compatible with a diagnosis of either pulmonary embolism or infection with pleural irritation. Further investigation is required to confirm or refute the diagnosis of pulmonary embolism.

What confirmatory investigations are required?

The following tests may be used to confirm or exclude pulmonary embolism:

- radionucleotide scintigraphy (Q-scan or V/Q scan)
- CT pulmonary angiography (CTPA)

In addition *lower limb venous duplex scanning* may be helpful in some cases. A detailed summary of the utility of these tests is given in Box 6.

Mrs Williams undergoes a V/Q scan that shows multiple mismatched defects throughout both lung fields indicative of a high probability of pulmonary embolism.

What treatment is indicated following confirmation of pulmonary embolism?

Following confirmation of the diagnosis of pulmonary embolism, the following treatments should be initiated.

- Anticoagulation: daily subcutaneous injections with LMWH (e.g. enoxaparin 1.5 mg/kg once daily) for at least six days. Warfarin: initially 5 mg daily for two days then a variable dose according to daily international normalised ratio (INR) result, aiming for an INR measurement of 2–3 (see below) *[handwritten: Normal 0.8 - 1.2]*
- Continue oxygen until the patient is no longer significantly hypoxaemic *[handwritten: - but aim for higher when on anticoagulant.]*
- Oral analgesia according to requirements: the pleuritic chest pain may continue for several days

Mrs Williams is given daily LMWH injections along with oral warfarin. The pain, breathlessness and tachycardia gradually subside over the next 48 hours, after which Mrs Williams is no longer dependent on analgesia or oxygen with oxygen saturation of 98% while breathing room air. Mrs Williams continues to receive daily LMWH injections until her INR is within the appropriate range (2–3). Follow-up is arranged in the outpatient clinic in six weeks.

Is there a significant underlying cause for the pulmonary embolism?

- If a clear-cut risk factor has been identified, this should be addressed where possible
- In some cases the patient has an underlying 'thrombophilia' (thrombotic tendency) that has resulted in PE. Coagulation abnormalities are usually inherited: recurrent thrombus in a young patient or a family history justifies referral to a haematologist specialising in this area so that further investigation can be undertaken

Box 6 Diagnostic tests for pulmonary embolism

Radionucleotide scintigraphy (Q-scan or V/Q scan)

The test relies on the comparison of images of lung perfusion and ventilation using a radionucleotide scintigraphy technique. Following injection of a radionucleotide, an image of the lungs is obtained ('Q' or 'perfusion scan'). If abnormalities of perfusion are noted the patient inhales a second agent and a 'ventilation' ('V') scan is obtained. In pulmonary embolism defects are noted in lung perfusion, but ventilation of these areas is often maintained – i.e. 'mismatched' defects. Other lung diseases such as pneumonia or chronic obstructive airways disease produce reductions in ventilation and perfusion ('matched' defects) or greater reductions in ventilation than perfusion (reversed mismatch). Unfortunately, matched defects can also occur where there is pulmonary infarction, and interpretation of the images can be difficult in patients with chronic lung disease.

When lung perfusion is normal this excludes pulmonary embolism in around 98% of cases. Where perfusion is abnormal the radiologist will give an indication of the probability of PE (low, intermediate or high probability). This can be compared with the clinical probability to give an overall likelihood of PE (see Table 19).

It should be noted that a 'low probability' V/Q scan result in association with an intermediate or high clinical probability is associated with pulmonary embolism in a significant number of cases. Further investigation is therefore required.

CT pulmonary angiography (CTPA)

This involves a CT scan of the chest, undertaken following the injection of an intravenous contrast agent, allowing visualisation of the pulmonary vessels. Although highly accurate for the diagnosis and exclusion of large PE, this technique has traditionally been limited by difficulties in visualising thrombus in smaller pulmonary vessels ('subsegmental PE'). However, modern spiral CT scanners are increasingly able to produce sensitivity approaching that of V/Q scanning with considerably higher specificity. Furthermore, the scan may identify an alternative explanation for the pain (e.g. pleural tumour, spinal lesion, etc.) that would not have been seen on V/Q.

In many hospitals CTPA has replaced V/Q scanning as the first-line confirmatory investigation for PE. The likelihood of a non-diagnostic V/Q is increased by the presence of chest radiograph abnormalities and prior chronic lung disease; CTPA should always be considered as the first-line investigation in such cases (see Fig. 24).

Lower limb venous investigation

Most PEs originate from thrombus in the lower limbs. However, disappointingly few patients with PE have evidence of lower limb venous thrombosis at the time of presentation. Lower limb venography or lower limb duplex scanning is worth considering for patients with clinical evidence of DVT (see Case 22) or where no clear answer has been obtained following lung scanning.

Presence of a confirmed DVT in the context of recent onset of pleuritic chest pain or breathlessness makes PE a very likely cause for these symptoms.

Table 19 Probability of pulmonary embolism (PE) based on clinical suspicion and V/Q lung scan

| | Clinical suspicion for PE* | | |
V/Q scan result	High (80–100%)	Moderate (20–79%)	Low (0–19%)
High	96 (82–99)	88 (78–94)	56 (21–56)
Intermediate	66 (49–80)	28 (22–34)	16 (8–27)
Low	40 (16–68)	16 (11–22)	4 (1–11)
Normal	0 (0–52)	6 (2–16)	2 (0–9)

*Values represent point estimates with 95% confidence intervals in parentheses. PIOPED Investigators. Value of the ventilation/perfusion scan in acute pulmonary embolism. Results of the prospective investigation of pulmonary embolism diagnosis (PIOPED). *JAMA* 1990; **263:** 2753–9.

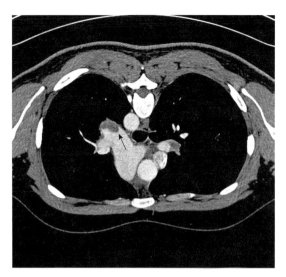

Figure 24 Computed tomography pulmonary angiography showing thrombosis in left pulmonary artery (arrow).

• Up to 10% of patients with DVT or PE have an underlying serious medical condition (particularly malignancy). This is often apparent clinically at the time of presentation, and a careful history with evaluation of suggestive symptoms is required. Breast and prostatic examinations are required, and further investigations including abdominal/pelvic ultrasound and prostate-specific antigen (PSA) are often justified

In this case the oral contraceptive and recent air flights may have contributed. Mrs Williams is advised to stop the oestrogen–progesterone pill and take alternative

contraception (e.g. progesterone-only pill). No clinical features are identified to suggest underlying malignancy.

For how long should the warfarin be continued, and at what dose?

• Warfarin is usually given for a period of six months following pulmonary embolism
• The duration of treatment may need to be longer if the patient is found to have a thrombophilia, recurrent thrombosis, or if the risk factor for PE is not correctable (e.g. patients with chronic illness leading to long-term immobility)
• Maintaining the INR level between 2 and 3 ensures the maximum protective benefit against further thrombosis while minimising the risks of bleeding
• The dose of warfarin required to maintain this level of INR will vary from patient to patient, depending on the efficiency of the liver enzymes and its metabolism
• Patients taking drugs that increase the efficiency of liver enzymes (e.g. carbamazepine) will often require very high doses
• Regular blood testing over the first few weeks will enable the patient's warfarin dose to be stabilised
• Careful communication with the patient's GP is required on discharge to ensure that dose monitoring can continue

Mrs Williams' warfarin dose on discharge is 4 mg daily, with an INR of 2.4; this information is given to the GP, who is asked to repeat the INR measurement after five days and continue monitoring thereafter.

CASE REVIEW

A 35-year-old woman is admitted complaining of severe pleuritic chest pain of gradual onset in association with general malaise, breathlessness and a dry cough. Mrs Williams is significantly hypoxic and tachycardic, but chest examination reveals no focal signs. Mrs Williams' risk factors for pulmonary embolism include recent long-haul plane flights and the combined oral contraceptive pill. Arterial blood gases, taken while she is breathing room air, demonstrate hypoxia and an acute respiratory alkalosis; the hypoxia is corrected by the administration of high-flow oxygen. Initial investigation reveals an elevated D-dimer, CRP and white cell count

with a normal chest radiograph and sinus tachycardia on ECG. The pretest probability score indicates an intermediate clinical probability of pulmonary embolism. Mrs Williams undergoes a V/Q scan, which shows multiple mismatched defects, strongly suggestive of pulmonary embolism. Treatment with LMWH and warfarin is commenced and her symptoms rapidly improve over the next few days. Mrs Williams is advised to stop the combined oral contraceptive pill and use alternative contraception.

This case illustrates the management of a patient presenting with pleuritic chest pain who was found to have pulmonary embolism. In our practice, less than 10% of patients presenting to hospital in this way are found to have PE; for the remainder PE is excluded, either by the combination of a low clinical suspicion with negative D-dimer or by negative V/Q or CT scanning.

Our data indicate a high re-admission rate for patients presenting to hospital with pleuritic chest pain where PE is excluded. 'No PE' does not necessarily mean 'no serious illness'. It is crucial to make a 'positive' diagnosis where possible. The differential diagnoses listed in Table 15 should be carefully considered.

Where no clear cause for the symptoms has been identified, this should be carefully explained to the patient. Simply telling your patient 'I am pleased to tell you that we have ruled out a PE' may do little to reassure them if their symptoms are ongoing. Discussion with the patient's GP and with senior members of the team is essential. The genuine case summarised in Box 7 highlights some of the diagnostic difficulties which can arise in patients presenting with pleuritic chest pain.

Box 7 'It pays to keep an open mind'

A 46-year-old man saw his GP complaining of right-sided pleuritic chest pain associated with mild shortness of breath. The previous day he had been fitting a kitchen and had lifted several heavy boxes. The pain was worsened by rotation of his thorax and there was some chest wall tenderness. The GP made a confident diagnosis of musculoskeletal chest pain and prescribed analgesics.

The following week the patient returned to his GP. He had not felt well since his original visit. He had developed a cough, which produced some pale yellow sputum and mild pyrexia, associated with ongoing breathlessness. He was referred to hospital for assessment. Further questioning revealed a recent long-haul air flight but no other risk factors for PE. Chest examination revealed some right basal crackles and a radiograph revealed significant shadowing at the right base, consistent with right basal pneumonia. D-dimer was elevated at 650. He was mildly hypoxic and tachycardic at 100 beats/min. There were no signs of DVT. An ECG was normal apart from sinus

tachycardia. The symptoms were attributed to pneumonia and he was given oral antibiotics and analgesia.

One week later the GP referred him back to hospital because the symptoms had not improved. He was now breathless with minimal exertion and the pain continued. A repeat chest radiograph showed improvement of the right basal shadowing but with new shadowing at the left base. CTPA was undertaken, which showed multiple large PEs affecting both lungs. He was treated with heparin and warfarin and made a good recovery, with resolution of all his symptoms.

With hindsight this man's symptoms were probably due to PE from the outset, despite the clinical features suggesting musculoskeletal chest pain and infection. It is important to reconsider the diagnosis of PE when a patient fails to respond to treatment of infection or presumed musculoskeletal chest pain: always keep an open mind!

KEY POINTS

- The differential diagnosis for a patient presenting with pleuritic chest pain is wide, although 'exclusion' of PE is often the reason for hospital referral.
- Initial clinical assessment should include an objective measure of clinical risk of PE.
- D-dimer is a sensitive but non-specific test for PE.
- V/Q scanning and/or CTPA are usually required for confirmation of the diagnosis.

- Following confirmation of PE, treatment with heparin and warfarin will usually result in improvement in symptoms; warfarin will usually be continued for six months.
- Following exclusion of PE, always try to make a 'positive' diagnosis as to the cause of the patient's symptoms before discharge from hospital care.

Further reading

European Society of Cardiology. Guidelines on the diagnosis and management of acute pulmonary embolism (2008). http://www.escardio.org/guidelines-surveys/esc-guidelines/Pages/acute-pulmonary-embolism.aspx

Harris T, Meek S. When should we thrombolyse patients with pulmonary embolism? A systematic review of the literature. *Emerg Med J* 2005; **22**: 766–71

PIOPED Investigators. Value of the ventilation/perfusion scan in acute pulmonary embolism. Results of the prospective investigation of pulmonary embolism diagnosis (PIOPED). *J Am Med Assoc* 1990; **263**: 2753

Proudfoot A, Bell D. The diagnostic assessment of suspected pulmonary embolism on the acute medical take: an evidence based guide. *Acute Med* 2007; **6**(1): 20–6

Wells PS, Anderson DR, Rodger M *et al.* Excluding pulmonary embolism at the bedside without diagnostic imaging: management of patients with suspected pulmonary embolism presenting to the emergency department by using a simple clinical model and d-dimer. *Ann Intern Med* 2001; **135**: 98–107

A 50-year-old man presenting with palpitations

A 50-year-old man is referred to hospital by his GP. Mr Frederick Abel awoke in the early hours of this morning with an uncomfortable awareness of a fast heartbeat; the sensation has continued since then. Mr Abel complains that his chest feels 'tight' and he is slightly short of breath. While walking to the GP's surgery Mr Abel felt light-headed, but did not faint. The GP noted a fast, irregular pulse with a rate of around 140 beats/min.

What challenges will this patient present?
• The combination of Mr Abel's description of a rapid heartbeat and the GP's clinical findings suggest some form of tachyarrhythmia
• The differential diagnosis for a patient with 'palpitations' is quite wide (see Table 20); however, if the problem persists, a combination of history, examination and ECG or rhythm strip will usually uncover the underlying cause and enable treatment to be started
• In some cases, a rhythm disturbance may come and go (paroxysmal arrhythmia), in which case the problem may have resolved by the time the patient presents to the doctor; this may present a difficult diagnostic challenge (see Case 15); ambulatory monitoring of the heart rhythm (24-hour tape or Holter monitor) may be diagnostic if the episodes occur frequently

On arrival in hospital Mr Abel is alert and talking, but appears pale and slightly sweaty, with cool peripherae. Initial observations reveal a pulse rate of 140 beats/min, which appears to be irregular. Mr Abel's blood pressure is 130/70. Respiratory rate is increased at 20 breaths/min with oxygen saturation of 94% while breathing room air.

What immediate management is required?
• Check patency of airway and apply high-flow oxygen via a mask

---

Acute Medicine: Clinical Cases Uncovered. By C. Roseveare. Published 2009 by Blackwell Publishing, ISBN: 978-1-4051-6883-0

• Establish intravenous access
• Connect the patient to a cardiac monitor
• Send blood for full blood count, electrolytes, liver function, glucose and thyroid function tests
• Obtain an ECG: if the ECG shows evidence of acute ST elevation myocardial infarction the patient should be managed according to the principles outlined in Case 1
• Request a chest radiograph
Having initiated these measures, it is important to establish the cause of Mr Abel's fast heart rate. A careful history, clinical examination and close inspection of the ECG are required.

The patient's breathing feels more comfortable following application of the oxygen, although the palpitations continue.

Mr Abel describes having a number of similar episodes in the past, usually on waking and settling within about 30 min. Mr Abel has never blacked out during an episode. His chest usually feels 'tight' during the palpitation with slight shortness of breath, but no significant chest pain. The palpitations usually feel irregular and fast, with some beats stronger than others. Mr Abel has never previously had an episode that has persisted and required hospital admission. Mr Abel was investigated one year ago for similar symptoms, at which time an ECG, blood tests and a 24-hour tape were normal.

Mr Abel has recently noticed that he has been getting increasingly breathless on exertion, particularly when walking briskly uphill. He is also slightly breathless when lying flat, which is eased by sleeping with three pillows. Mr Abel's ankles swell during the day but are back to normal by morning.

In the past Mr Abel has suffered from high blood pressure, for which he takes bendroflumethiazide 2.5 mg daily. He also has mild asthma, and uses salbutamol via an inhaler as required. Mr Abel's father had ischaemic heart disease and died from a myocardial infarction at the age of 60. He smokes 20 cigarettes per day and drinks two or

Table 20 Common causes of 'palpitations'

Cause	Symptoms	ECG	Comments
Ectopic beats	Patient describes intermittent, 'missed' beats or erratic 'forceful' beats, usually not fast. Systemically well	Broad or bizarre complexes interspersed within normal sinus rhythm (see p. 16)	Usually benign, but can be uncomfortable if frequent. Often exacerbated by anxiety, caffeine or sympathetic stimulants (e.g. salbutamol)
Atrial fibrillation	Irregular, often fast, heart rhythm. May be associated light-headedness/breathlessness	Irregularly irregular rhythm; no P-waves; QRS complexes all appear similar to each other (see p. 15)	See text
Atrial flutter	Fast, regular palpitation	Rate usually close to 150/min and very regular. May be possible to see jagged 'saw-tooth' flutter waves between QRS complexes (see p. 17)	Atrium 'flutters' at 300 beats/min; ventricular rate determined by degree of 'block' at AV node; commonest is 2 : 1 block resulting in rate of 150 beats/min. 3 : 1 (100/min) or 4 : 1 (75 beats/min) also occur as can variable block leading to symptoms similar to atrial fibrillation
Sinus tachycardia	Fast, regular palpitation – often intermittent. May be symptoms of associated illness (e.g. thyroid disease) or anxiety	Rate usually <150 beats/min. P-waves before QRS complexes; some variability in rate – unlike atrial flutter	Sinus tachycardia is often a feature of other serious illness – e.g. pulmonary embolism, sepsis, hypovolaemia; generally such patients do not present with palpitations as their main symptom. Anxiety is the commonest cause of symptomatic sinus tachycardia
Supraventricular tachycardia	Often very fast ('too fast to count'); very regular; may be associated syncope	Usually narrow QRS complexes (although see Case 4); very regular; rate can be >200 beats/min	Structurally normal heart in the majority of cases; some patients with recurrent episodes may have associated electrical anomalies (e.g. Wolff–Parkinson–White syndrome)
Ventricular tachycardia	Fast, and regular; usually quite unwell – often present with syncope or acute shortness of breath	Always broad QRS complexes (>12 s); regular. If P-waves are visible they do not relate to QRS complexes ('dissociated')	See Case 4 for more detailed discussion of the management of broad complex tachycardia

three glasses of wine most nights. On the night before his admission Mr Abel had consumed about double this quantity. Mr Abel works as a buildings inspector for the council and drives a car to work each day.

On examination he appears overweight, with an irregular pulse of 140–150 beats/min; the strength of the radial pulse appears to vary from beat to beat. Blood pressure remains 130/70. Oxygen saturation is 100% while breathing oxygen. Jugular venous pulsations are not visible.

Heart sounds are normal. Chest examination reveals bibasal inspiratory crepitations and quiet expiratory wheeze throughout both lung fields. There is pitting oedema of both ankles.

Inspection of the cardiac monitor and ECG rhythm strip reveals an irregular tachycardia with a rate between 150 and 170 beats/min. No P-waves are visible and the QRS complexes all appear similar in morphology (see Fig. 25).

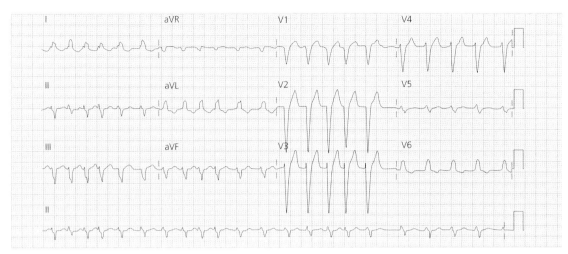

Figure 25 ECG taken on arrival.

What is the likely cause of Mr Abel's symptoms?

Common causes of palpitations, along with their historical and electrocardiographic features, are shown in Table 20.

The symptoms, signs and ECG features point to a diagnosis of *acute-onset, fast atrial fibrillation* as the cause for Mr Abel's palpitations, as indicated by:
- Mr Abel's description of a rapid, irregular heartbeat
- The irregular pulse on examination with variability in pulse volume
- The characteristic ECG findings (see p. 16)

What is the cause of the breathlessness and ankle oedema?

It is likely that Mr Abel has some pre-existing cardiac failure, as suggested by:
- Recent exertional dyspnoea
- Ankle swelling
- Orthopnoea

The onset of fast atrial fibrillation may have exacerbated this problem.
- The lack of coordinated atrial contraction prior to ventricular systole results in reduced cardiac output
- A rapid heart rate reduces the time for ventricular filling during diastole, again reducing cardiac output

What is the relevance of the previous episodes of palpitations?

- Mr Abel's prior symptoms suggest a previous diagnosis of *paroxysmal atrial fibrillation* (see Table 21)

Table 21 Classification of atrial fibrillation (AF)

Terminology	Description
New-onset AF	AF of recent onset
Paroxysmal AF	Episodes of AF, terminating spontaneously within 7 days (and usually within 48 h)
Persistent AF	AF lasting more than 7 days
Permanent AF	AF lasting >1 year, even with attempts to restore sinus rhythm
'Lone' AF	AF occurring in the absence of any structural heart disease or other precipitant

- It is possible that this episode will also resolve spontaneously
- However, given that the symptoms are continuing, with evidence of cardiac failure, Mr Abel will require further inpatient treatment and investigation

Results of further investigations are now available. Blood test results are as follow (for normal ranges see p. 229):
- *haemoglobin 121; white blood cells 11.8; platelets 256*
- *Na 133; K 3.05; urea 6.7; creatinine 75*
- *albumin 38; alanine transaminase 121; alkaline phosphatase 140; bilirubin 13*
- *glucose 4.2*
- *thyroid function normal*

- cardiac troponin I normal (taken 12 h after onset of symptoms)
- chest radiograph: cardiomegaly with evidence of mild pulmonary oedema

What treatment is required?

When considering the treatment of a patient with fast atrial fibrillation, two key questions need to be considered.

- Should an attempt be made to restore sinus rhythm ('rhythm control')?
- Should the heart rate simply be slowed down ('rate control')?
  - the complex issues surrounding rate versus rhythm control are summarised in Box 8
  - in this case there is good evidence that the episode started acutely this morning, which increases the likelihood that sinus rhythm may be restored ('cardioversion')
  - although this may occur spontaneously, this is not guaranteed
  - techniques for cardioversion are summarised below

Box 8 Rate control versus rhythm control

Restoration of sinus rhythm ('rhythm control') is usually considered the 'gold standard' treatment for atrial fibrillation. However, this is not always possible and even where it is achieved, the effect may be only temporary; a large proportion of patients will have reverted back into AF within 1 year. In some cases, therefore, clinicians will choose to adopt an approach which aims simply to control the heart rate ('rate control'), accepting that the patient remains in AF. The patient's symptoms are often well controlled with this approach, and the drugs required to achieve this are often better tolerated than those designed to induce and maintain sinus rhythm.

Although the decision is often complex, the following can be used as a guide.

- Cardioversion is generally recommended for new-onset AF unless the patient is elderly or has structural heart disease
- Rhythm control is preferred in patients with paroxysmal or persistent AF who are highly symptomatic.
- Pharmacological rhythm control of AF does not reduce the risk of stroke
- If drug therapy fails in either rate or rhythm control, referral to a cardiac electrophysiologist for catheter ablation therapy should be considered

---

Are there any 'correctable' precipitating factors?

Potential precipitants for acute atrial fibrillation are summarised in Table 22. Failure to correct a precipitant such as electrolyte imbalance or thyroid dysfunction will reduce the likelihood of the success of other treatment measures, whereas correction may increase the chance of spontaneous resolution.

- In this case Mr Abel is noted to be hypokalaemic (probably as a result of his thiazide diuretic), which may have contributed. Potassium needs to be diluted when infused through a peripheral vein, and care will be required not to give fluid too rapidly in view of his pulmonary oedema
- Mr Abel's heavy alcohol intake the night before his admission may also be implicated as a cause, which may need to be addressed in the future

Does the patient require immediate anticoagulation with heparin?

Atrial fibrillation (AF) results in incomplete emptying of the atrium during systole. Blood may 'stagnate' in the left atrial appendage leading to the formation of thrombus.

Table 22 Causes and precipitants of atrial fibrillation

Cardiac	Ischaemic heart disease
	Valvular heart disease
	Cardiomyopathies
	Hypertensive heart disease
Pulmonary	Pulmonary embolism
	Pneumonia (and other severe systemic infections)
	Bronchial carcinoma
Metabolic	Electrolyte imbalances (e.g. hypokalaemia)
	Acute renal failure
	Thyrotoxicosis
Toxic	Alcohol intoxication
	Caffeine excess
	Drug overdose (e.g. tricyclic antidepressant)
	Recreational drugs (e.g. cocaine)
Iatrogenic	Postoperative (especially following cardiac surgery)
	Sympathetic stimulant drugs (e.g. salbutamol, theophyllines)

If this moves from the heart ('embolisation') it may block an artery resulting in acute ischaemia or infarction of the area that the artery supplies. The commonest and often most devastating manifestation of this is an acute ischaemic stroke.

Embolisation can occur at any time, but is most common following electrical cardioverion, particularly where the AF has persisted for more than 48 h. Formal anticoagulation will reduce the risk of stroke in patients with AF. Recommendations for anticoagulation in AF have been produced by the National Institute for Health and Clinical Excellence (see Table 23). In practice, unless there is evidence of recent or ongoing bleeding, most patients presenting to hospital with acute AF will require treatment with heparin while plans are made for further treatment.

• Mr Abel fulfils these criteria and should be given initial treatment with heparin (e.g. enoxaparin 1 mg/kg twice daily).

Table 23 National Institute for Health and Clinical Excellence recommendations for antithrombotic therapy in acute atrial fibrillation (AF)

1 A patient with acute AF who is receiving no or subtherapeutic anticoagulation therapy
  • In the absence of contraindication, heparin should be started at initial presentation
  • Heparin should be continued until full assessment has been made and appropriate oral antithrombotic has been initiated
2 For a patient with a confirmed diagnosis of acute AF of recent onset (<48 h), oral anticoagulation should be used if:
  • Stable sinus rhythm is not restored within the same 48 h period following onset of acute AF, or
  • There are factors indicating a high risk of AF recurrence or
  • It is recommended by the stroke risk stratification algorithm
3 In a patient with acute AF where there is uncertainty over the precise time of onset, oral anticoagulation should be used as for persistent AF
4 In cases of acute AF where the patient is haemodynamically unstable, any emergency intervention should be performed as soon as possible and the initiation of anticoagulation should not delay any emergency intervention

Mr Abel is given 1 mg/kg of enoxaparin, which is prescribed twice daily. An intravenous infusion of 500 mL of normal saline containing 3 g of potassium chloride is commenced to run in over 4 h.

Following senior review by your consultant, it is decided that an attempt should be made to restore sinus rhythm.

How should sinus rhythm be restored?

• Restoration of sinus rhythm can be achieved by using drugs ('chemical' cardioversion) or by delivering an electric shock to the myocardium ('electrical' cardioversion); the latter usually requires a general anaesthetic
• In the emergency setting, when the patient is severely unwell (hypotensive, persistent tachycardia >160 beats/min, ongoing chest pain, severe pulmonary oedema), immediate electrical cardioversion is recommended
• If the patient is more stable, as in this case, an initial attempt at chemical cardioversion is usually undertaken, followed by electrical cardioversion if unsuccessful. A list of drugs that may be considered for chemical cardioversion is given in Table 24

Mr Abel is treated with an infusion of intravenous amiodarone, 300 mg over 30 min, followed by oral amiodarone 200 mg three times daily. He has been prescribed enoxaparin 1 mg/kg twice daily.

Mr Abel's heart rate is noted to slow to 110 beats/min over the next 2 h, but he remains in atrial fibrillation.

Repeat measurement of electrolytes after 12 h reveals correction of the potassium concentration (now 4.1 mmol/L).

Mr Abel is observed on a cardiac monitor in the medical admissions unit. He is noted to be less breathless while breathing oxygen, which is reduced to 28% via a Venturi mask, maintaining his saturation at 99%. Examination of Mr Abel's chest reveals clearing of the bibasal crackles.

A transthoracic echocardiogram is undertaken, which reveals dilatation of the left ventricle and left atrium with moderate left ventricular systolic dysfunction. There is no evidence of valvular heart disease.

What further treatment options are available?

Initial attempts at chemical cardioversion have apparently failed, although Mr Abel's heart rate has reduced, which may have accounted for the improvement in the symptoms of cardiac failure.

A number of further treatment options can now be considered.

Table 24 Drugs used for 'chemical' cardioversion

Drug	Dosage/administration	Comments
Amiodarone	300 mg intravenously or oral loading with 200 mg tds for 1/52, bd for 1/52 then 200 mg daily	Will require administration via a central venous cannula if prolonged intravenous use required; long half-life – slow onset of action following oral administration
Flecainide	300 mg orally or 2 mg/kg by intravenous infusion over 30 min	Avoid in ischaemic or other structural heart disease
Sotalol	80–240 mg bd orally	Avoid in asthma and uncontrolled heart failure
Propafenone	150 mg tds orally	Avoid in structural heart disease
Esmolol	5–200 µg/kg/min i.v.	Avoid in asthma and uncontrolled heart failure

Inpatient electrical cardioversion prior to discharge

This has the advantage of potentially restoring sinus rhythm before discharge from hospital. In this case there is good reason to believe that the onset of AF occurred shortly before admission. If cardioversion can be performed within 48 h of the onset of AF (or if anticoagulation was initiated shortly after the onset of AF) the risk of embolisation is minimal. If the duration of AF is more prolonged, or is uncertain, it is usually recommended to anticoagulate the patient for at least three weeks before electrical cardioversion. If more urgent cardioversion is required, a transoesophageal echocardiogram can be used to confirm the absence of clot from the atrium before cardioversion.

Continuation of amiodarone and oral anticoagulation with warfarin, followed by outpatient electrical cardioversion if sinus rhythm is not restored (additional rate control as required)

This approach has the advantage of giving the patient the opportunity of spontaneous cardioversion (assisted by amiodarone), thereby avoiding the potential risk of the anaesthesia. However, the patient may remain symptomatic while in AF, particularly if rate control is difficult.

Long-term rate control and anticoagulation with warfarin

Adequate symptom control can often be achieved simply by controlling the heart rate. Furthermore, a large proportion of patients whose sinus rhythm is restored by cardioversion will revert to AF within one year. Although the patient will usually have to take anti-arrhythmic drugs lifelong as well as warfarin, some patients may prefer this to cardioversion.

This approach is generally preferred in older patients who are relatively asymptomatic, those with a longer duration of AF and those with structural or valvular heart disease.

Where possible it is important to involve the patient in this decision in relation to the risks and benefits of drugs, long-term anticoagulation and general anaesthesia.

Following discussion with Mr Abel it is decided to undertake inpatient electrical cardioversion. This is conducted under general anaesthesia the following day. Following 3 DC shocks at 200 J, sinus rhythm is restored; however, shortly after returning to the ward Mr Abel is noted to be back in AF with a heart rate of 110 beats/min. This is confirmed by 12-lead ECG, which shows no new acute ischaemic changes.

Mr Abel is no longer breathless at rest, and is not aware of any palpitations. He mobilises uneventfully on the ward with mild dyspnoea on exertion.

It is decided that further management should concentrate on providing rate control.

How can the heart rate be controlled for patients who remain in atrial fibrillation?

• Rate control in AF is achieved by reducing the transmission of electrical impulses from the atrium to the ventricle at the atrioventricular (AV) node
• A variety of drugs that can block transmission at the AV node are available and are listed in Table 25
• The choice will be dependent on factors related to the individual patient

Table 25 Drugs used for rate control in atrial fibrillation

Drug name	Dosage/administration	Comments
Digoxin	1.5 mg orally in three divided doses over 24 h followed by 125–250 µg daily Or 500 µg i.v. infusion over 30 min	Slow onset of action – intravenous administration rarely justified. Lower doses in elderly patients or those with renal impairment
Beta-blockers	Bisoprolol 2.5–5 mg daily orally; atenolol 25–50 mg daily orally	Avoid in asthma and uncontrolled heart failure
Calcium antagonists	Verapamil 40 mg orally tds or diltiazem 90–180 mg bd	Avoid in severe heart failure
Amiodarone	200 mg orally tds for 1/52 reducing to bd for 1/52 then 200 mg daily	Generally avoided for rate control due to long-term side effects

Severe asthma is an absolute contraindication to treatment with beta-blockers. Mr Abel's 'asthma' is described as mild, and may in fact represent smoking-induced chronic obstructive pulmonary disease (COPD) rather than 'true' asthma. The wheeze noted on admission may have been related to pulmonary oedema rather than bronchospasm. This should be considered a 'relative' contraindication and a small dose of a cardioselective beta-blocker (e.g. bisoprolol 2.5 mg daily) may be tolerated. The patient must be advised to stop immediately if they become wheezy.

> Mr Abel's amiodarone is stopped. He starts taking digoxin, with three oral doses of 500 µg, followed by 125 µg daily. Mr Abel also starts taking ramipril 2.5 mg daily, in view of his left ventricular failure, and his bendroflumethiazide is stopped. Mr Abel is given warfarin, orally. It is decided not to commence beta blockade unless the above measures fail to control the heart rate.
>
> Over the next two days Mr Abel's heart rate settles to 80/min, although he remains in atrial fibrillation. Mr Abel is mobile around the ward without breathlessness and is weaned off his oxygen.

What further management/follow-up is required following discharge from hospital?

A number of issues need to be considered on discharge.

• **Anticoagulation monitoring**: warfarin requires regular blood testing to measure the international normalised ratio (INR). Stabilisation of the dose usually requires at least five days of treatment with daily monitoring. If the patient has already been on the drug for more than five days the stable dose may already have been established. Further testing after discharge is normally undertaken by the patient's GP. It is often helpful to speak directly to him/her to discuss the timing of the next blood test

• **Monitoring of electrolytes**: Mr Abel was hypokalaemic on admission; although the bendroflumethiazide has been stopped, he has started taking ramipril, which can also cause electrolyte imbalances. Digoxin toxicity may be precipitated by hypokalaemia, which may also increase the risk of further arrhythmias

• **Digoxin level**: although not essential if the patient's heart rate is controlled, measurement of digoxin level after one week of treatment may give an indication whether the dose is appropriate. This is more important for elderly patients and those with renal impairment, in whom accumulation of the drug may result in toxicity

• **Heart rate control**: confirmation that the heart rate is controlled following discharge may be achieved by asking the GP to review the patient after one week. A 24-hour tape will also help to identify episodes of poor rate control, which may necessitate the introduction of a beta-blocker or increase in the digoxin dose (if the level is subtherapeutic)

• **Alcohol**: heavy alcohol intake may precipitate arrhythmias, and chronic use may result in a cardiomyopathy; the patient should be advised to cut down alcohol consumption to <21 units per week (14 units for women)

• **Cigarette smoking**: discontinuation of smoking should reduce thrombotic risk and may also be important if there is underlying ischaemic heart disease. The patient may require help to do this, such as with the use of nicotine replacement

• **Caffeine**: excessive caffeine consumption should be avoided; ideally the patient should be advised to consume decaffeinated coffee, although complete abstinence from caffeine consumption is not an absolute requirement

• **Driving:** if the patient has experienced any syncopal episodes they should cease driving for a period of three months. In the absence of syncope (as in this case) the patient may drive providing the symptoms from the arrhythmia are not likely to impair their driving ability in the view of the doctor treating them

• **Consideration of underlying myocardial ischaemia:** this is an important cause of atrial fibrillation and Mr Abel has risk factors for ischaemic heart disease: cigarette smoking, hypertension and a family history of myocardial infarction. Exercise testing, myocardial perfusion scanning or coronary angiography should be considered following discharge

Mr Abel returns to the outpatient clinic six weeks after discharge. He has felt much better for the past two weeks with no further feelings of 'palpitation'. Mr Abel's exercise tolerance has improved and he no longer experiences orthopnoea. Mr Abel has reduced his alcohol intake dramatically since discharge and has stopped smoking. Clinical examination reveals that his pulse now feels regular and ECG demonstrates that he has reverted to sinus rhythm. Chest examination is normal with a blood pressure of 135/70. Mr Abel has not needed to use the salbutamol since discharge. His digoxin is stopped and he starts taking bisoprolol 2.5 mg daily, as a means of reducing the risk of further episodes. Mr Abel is advised to stop this immediately if he becomes wheezy. It is determined to continue his warfarin in view of his previous history, which was suggestive of 'paroxysmal' atrial fibrillation. Mr Abel is booked for an outpatient treadmill ECG and further follow-up to establish whether there is evidence of myocardial ischaemia.

CASE REVIEW

This case describes a 50-year-old man who presented to his GP with a prolonged episode of palpitations. ECG revealed fast AF, and symptoms suggested that there was co-existent cardiac failure. Possible precipitants for the arrhythmia included heavy alcohol consumption on the previous night, hypokalaemia (probably diuretic induced) and underlying myocardial ischaemia.

After initial stabilisation with oxygen and correction of the hypokalaemia Mr Abel was given intravenous amiodarone in an attempt to restore sinus rhythm. Mr Abel was also prescribed subcutaneous LMWH to reduce the risk of thrombus formation during the arrhythmia and subsequent embolisation. Although the heart rate slowed following the amiodarone he remained in atrial fibrillation. An echocardiogram confirmed a degree of left ventricular

impairment with dilatation of the left atrium and ventricle. Electrical cardioversion was attempted, but only restored sinus rhythm for a short period; he was therefore commenced on digoxin to control his heart rate and discharged from hospital on this combined with warfarin and ramipril for the heart failure. He was advised to reduce his alcohol intake and stop smoking at the time of discharge from hospital.

At follow-up he had 'spontaneously' reverted to sinus rhythm, enabling the digoxin to be stopped. He was started on a small dose of the beta-blocker bisoprolol as prophylaxis against further episodes. An outpatient treadmill ECG was arranged to investigate the possibility of underlying myocardial ischaemia.

KEY POINTS

• Palpitations usually imply a cardiac tachyarrhythmia.
• Careful history, clinical examination and ECG during the episode will usually enable identification of the causative rhythm disturbance.
• AF is a common arrhythmia that can compromise cardiac output, particularly when the rate is very fast.
• Treatment of AF can involve either rate control or attempts to restore sinus rhythm.

• Anticoagulation should be considered for all patients presenting to hospital with AF to reduce the risk of systemic embolisation.
• Precipitating factors, such as electrolyte imbalances, should always be sought and, where possible, corrected.
• Underlying valvular, ischaemic or other structural heart disease should be sought by careful investigation including echocardiography and exercise testing.

Further reading

AHA/ACC/EHC 2006 guidelines for the management of patients with atrial fibrillation. *Eur Heart J* 2006; **27**: 1979–2030

Atrial Fibrillation Follow up Investigation of Rhythm Management (AFFIRM) Investigators. A comparison of rate control and rhythm control in patients with atrial fibrillation. *N Engl J Med* 2002; **347**: 1825–33

National Institute for Health and Clinical Excellence (NICE). Guidelines for the management of atrial fibrillation (2006). http://www.nice.org.uk/guidance/index.jsp

PART 2: CASES

A 60-year-old man with a broad complex tachycardia

The doctor working in the accident and emergency department phones to refer a 60-year-old man who has been brought into hospital having collapsed at home. Mr Garth Dale became unwell while gardening, when he suddenly felt breathless with light-headedness and a feeling of chest tightness. On arrival of the ambulance Mr Dale was noted to be pale, sweaty and tachycardic with a pulse of 160 beats/min and blood pressure 100/50. The cardiac monitor has shown a broad complex tachycardia (BCT).

What is a broad complex tachycardia?

• BCT is defined as a pulse rate >100 beats/min, and where the QRS complexes are more than 120 ms in duration (>3 mm on standard ECG settings)
• BCT results from either ventricular tachycardia (VT) or supraventricular tachycardia (SVT) combined with a bundle branch block (BBB) (see Box 9)
• BCT is a potentially life-threatening medical emergency, particularly when caused by VT. Loss of cardiac output ('pulseless VT') or degeneration into ventricular fibrillation can result in cardiopulmonary arrest
• Although generally less serious than VT, tachycardia caused by SVT can also result in reduced cardiac output because of reduced cardiac filling time during diastole

On your arrival in the emergency department Mr Dale remains unwell. Mr Dale is conscious and breathing spontaneously with a respiratory rate of 20/min. He is complaining of central chest tightness and a feeling of breathlessness. Oxygen saturation is 99% while breathing oxygen via a re-breath mask. Mr Dale's pulse feels weak and thready, but regular with a rate >160 beats/min, which is confirmed on the cardiac monitor. Blood pressure is now 90/40.

Acute Medicine: Clinical Cases Uncovered. By C. Roseveare. Published 2009 by Blackwell Publishing, ISBN: 978-1-4051-6883-0

What immediate management is required?

• **Administer oxygen** (15 L via a re-breath mask)
• **Establish intravenous access:** if a cannula has already been inserted, confirm that it is patent
• **Administer opiate analgesia if required** (e.g. morphine sulphate 1–5 mg i.v. until pain is controlled) combined with an antiemetic (e.g. cyclizine 50 mg i.v.)
• **Ensure continuous cardiac monitoring, pulse oximetry, regular measurement of blood pressure and assessment of conscious level**
• **Perform a 12-lead ECG**
• **Request a chest radiograph**
• **Send venous blood to the laboratory** for full blood count (FBC), urea and electrolytes (U&E), liver function tests (LFT), serum magnesium level, thyroid function and cardiac enzymes (e.g. troponin – may need to be repeated later if patient is presenting less than 12 h after the onset of symptoms)
• **Try to obtain any previous hospital records,** including any old ECG readings
Provided the patient's condition is not deteriorating it is important to obtain further history and conduct a clinical examination, including careful inspection of the ECG. This must be done quickly.

Mr Dale describes feeling well before the episode of collapse 2 h ago. He has been experiencing episodes of light-headedness, associated with a feeling of 'palpitations' every few days for the past month, although these usually last a few seconds only and have never resulted in collapse or loss of consciousness. Between the attacks Mr Dale has felt well. Mr Dale had a myocardial infarct one year ago, for which he was treated with thrombolytic drugs and subsequently underwent coronary angiography and stent insertion. Mr Dale has not experienced any chest pain or breathlessness since that time. He has no other significant past medical history. Mr Dale takes aspirin, clopidogrel, bisoprolol, ramipril and simvastatin. He is an ex-smoker and only occasionally drinks alcohol.

Box 9 Mechanisms of broad complex tachycardia

The QRS complex represents the wave of depolarisation travelling across the ventricular wall, resulting in contraction of the ventricle (ventricular systole). The width of the QRS complex is determined by the speed at which the wave travels through the ventricle.

Specialised conducting fibres in the interventricular septum (the left and right bundles of His) carry the wave at the maximum speed; when the impulse travels by this route the calibre of the complex is usually <120 ms. When the cardiac impulse arises 'above' the atrioventricular node (AVN), it is able to enter the bundle of His resulting in a narrow-calibre QRS complex.

- **For this reason narrow-calibre QRS complexes (and therefore narrow complex tachycardias) are almost always supraventricular in origin.**

On occasion, conduction of the impulse through the bundle of His is slower than normal. The usual cause for this is an abnormality of one of the bundles, termed a left or right bundle branch block. The result is that the QRS complex becomes wider than normal, resulting in a 'broad' complex (see p. 24).

- **If a supraventricular tachycardia is combined with a left or right bundle branch block the result is a BCT.**

Broad complexes may also occur when the origin of the impulse is in the ventricular wall, outside the normal conducting system. All cardiac myocytes are capable of producing spontaneous electrical activity, although this is normally 'overridden' by the beats arising within the pacemaker cells. When a QRS complex arises from within the ventricular wall, the resulting wave of depolarisation travels relatively slowly across the myocardium, resulting in a broad complex. A tachycardia arising in the ventricular wall will therefore almost always comprise broad complexes.

- **Ventricular tachycardia is almost always a broad complex tachycardia.**

PART 2: CASES

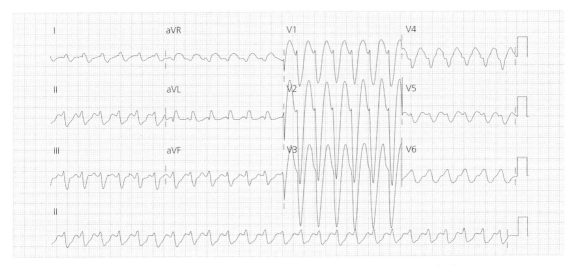

Figure 26 ECG taken on arrival; note the broad complexes and concordance of electrical polarity in leads v1–v6.

Examination reveals the persistent tachycardia with hypotension as described above. There are bibasal crepitations and mild pitting ankle oedema.

Mr Dale's serum potassium level is slightly low at 3.15 mmol/L; other blood results are normal, including serum magnesium.

The ECG is shown in Fig. 26.

Is the tachycardia caused by VT or SVT with bundle branch block?

Clinical clues to the cause of the tachycardia are described in Table 26.

- In this case the prior history of ischaemic heart disease combined with the significant haemodynamic compromise are both suggestive of VT as the cause for the BCT

Table 26 Clinical clues to distinguish ventricular tachycardia (VT) from supraventricular tachycardia (SVT) with bundle branch block

	VT	SVT	Comments
History	Previous VT Recent MI, previous IHD or any other structural heart disease makes VT much more likely than SVT; BCT in patients with previous IHD or any other structural heart disease is VT in >95% of cases Often older age group (e.g. age >40)	Previous documented SVT or cardioversion of arrhythmia with AVN blocking agents (e.g. adenosine) Often younger age group (e.g. age <40)	Patients with VT tend to be more unwell than those with SVT, although this cannot be relied upon: patients with SVT can be severely compromised if the rate is very rapid, while some patients can tolerate VT for many hours without significant haemodynamic effects
Examination	Often severe haemodynamic compromise with hypotension, raised JVP and pulmonary oedema 'Cannon' waves sometimes seen in JVP due to contraction of right atrium against closed tricuspid valve Pulse rate rarely >200/min	Usually better tolerated than VT, unless rate very rapid	Any patient who is haemodynamically compromised should be treated as having VT until proven otherwise Patients with a well-tolerated tachycardia can usually undergo diagnostic tests provided resuscitation equipment is rapidly available if required

AVN, atrioventricular node; IHD, ischaemic heart disease; JVP, jugular venous pressure.

Further clues can be obtained from close inspection of the patient's ECG. Helpful distinguishing features of the ECG in VT and SVT with BBB are given in Table 27.

This patient's ECG would support the diagnosis of VT on the basis of:
• QRS complex width >150 ms
• concordance across chest leads
Administration of intravenous adenosine is worth considering if there is any ongoing doubt about the diagnosis (see Box 10), provided there are no contraindications.

> Adenosine is not considered appropriate in this case, given the high likelihood of VT combined with the history of asthma.

What are the treatment options if the likely diagnosis is VT?

Restoration of sinus rhythm ('cardioversion') should be achieved as soon as possible if VT is considered likely, as in this case. Options to achieve this include:
• Pharmacological cardioversion, using drugs such as amiodarone
• Electrical cardioversion, by administration of a DC shock to the chest wall
Electrical cardioversion is the most rapid and effective method, and is therefore the required treatment when the

Table 27 ECG clues to distinguish ventricular tachycardia from supraventricular tachycardia with bundle branch block

Features which make ventricular tachycardia more likely

'Concordance' of polarity across the chest leads (all QRS complexes across chest leads point in the same direction – see Fig. 26)

Broader QRS complexes (especially if >150 ms)

P-waves visible but dissociated from QRS complexes

Capture beats

Fusion beats

Features which make supraventricular tachycardia more likely

QRS duration 120–150 ms

Rate >200 beats/min

Classic left or right bundle branch block morphology

P-wave visible (or inverted) and associated with QRS complex

Resolution following administration of adenosine

patient is pulseless, severely compromised or rapidly deteriorating. If patients are conscious they will usually require general anaesthesia, which will have some risk attached in this clinical setting. For this reason, if

Box 10 Administration of intravenous adenosine

Intravenous administration of adenosine results in rapid and total blockage of the atrioventricular node. Because of the short half-life of the drug this only lasts for a few seconds. However, if a tachycardia is supraventricular in origin the rate will usually be temporarily slowed. In cases where the tachycardia has arisen within the atrioventricular node (e.g. nodal re-entrant tachycardia), adenosine may result in cardioversion to sinus rhythm.

Procedure for administration

- confirm no contraindications (see below)
- site a cannula in a large peripheral vein (e.g. antecubital fossa)
- warn the patient that they may experience a feeling of extreme light-headedness or chest pain following administration (although this should be extremely short-lived)
- ensure the patient is connected to a cardiac monitor with the ability to print the trace for later review if required: press the 'print' button immediately before administration of the drug
- administer 6 mg by rapid intravenous bolus, followed by 20 mL of normal saline flush
- if there is no change in the rate or rhythm after 2 min, administer a further 12 mg of the drug.

If no response is seen after administration of 12 mg it is likely that the tachycardia is ventricular in origin; if there is still a strong clinical suspicion of supraventricular origin it may be worth administering an 18 mg bolus if there is no response after 12 mg.

Contraindications to adenosine

- severe haemodynamic compromise
- asthma: may cause acute bronchospasm
- Wolf–Parkinson–White (WPW) syndrome: may result in paradoxical increase in heart rate – discuss with local cardiology team before use of adenosine in patients with known or suspected WPW
- Denervated heart following cardiac transplantation.

a patient is more stable, as in this case, an attempt at pharmacological cardioversion is usually made in the first instance.

Intravenous amiodarone is the usual drug of choice for **pharmacological cardioversion**, and has the added advantage of increasing the sensitivity of the myocardium to, and therefore the effectiveness of, subsequent electrical cardioversion, if required.

In addition to these measures it is important to correct any potentially contributing factors (e.g. electrolyte abnormalities).

Mr Dale is given an intravenous infusion of 300 mg of amiodarone over 30 min via a cannula in the antecubital fossa. A second cannula is sited and an infusion of 500 ml of normal saline containing 3 g of potassium chloride is commenced, infusing over 3 h.

The heart rhythm is unchanged 10 min after completion of the amiodarone infusion. Furthermore, Mr Dale now appears more breathless. His oxygen saturation has fallen to 94% despite high-flow oxygen, and his blood pressure has fallen to 85/40.

The on-call anaesthetist is contacted and attends urgently. After informed consent, Mr Dale is anaesthetised and undergoes synchronised DC cardioversion. After two shocks at 200 J the sinus rhythm is restored.

What further investigation is required after restoration of sinus rhythm?

It is crucial to establish whether there is a treatable underlying cause for the arrhythmia. This will help to guide further treatment. If no clear reversible cause is identified, it is likely that the patient will require long-term anti-arrhythmic therapy or insertion of an implanted cardiac defibrillator (ICD).

- Repeat the ECG
- Recheck electrolytes
- Check cardiac enzymes (e.g. troponin I, 12 h after onset of the original collapse)
- Review other blood test results (e.g. thyroid function) when available

The repeat ECG shows sinus rhythm with left BBB at a rate of 70 beats/min. Mr Dale's blood pressure is now 130/70 and he looks and feels much better. The repeat serum potassium level is 4.1 mmol/L after completion of the saline/potassium infusion. Cardiac troponin is slightly elevated at 0.75 ng/mL (normal <0.15 ng/mL), 12 h after admission.

How should the elevated troponin be interpreted in this situation?

Elevated troponin indicates some degree of myocardial damage; this may have resulted from:

- Myocardial ischaemia or infarction prior to Mr Dale's admission

• Rate-related ischaemia: reduced coronary artery filling during the shortened diastole resulting from the tachyarrhythmia

• Minor myocardial damage during electrical cardioversion

It is likely that Mr Dale will require coronary angiography and electrophysiological studies, which may be required prior to discharge from hospital. This will help to determine his requirement for an ICD. Mr Dale should be referred for review by a cardiologist in the hospital or regional centre.

What further monitoring/treatment is required while awaiting cardiology review?

• Maintain the patient on continuous cardiac monitoring

• Restart the patient's regular medication (especially the antiplatelet therapy – aspirin and clopidogrel)

• Commence regular low molecular weight heparin (e.g. enoxaparin 1 mg/kg twice daily)

• Commence regular oral amiodarone (initially 200 mg tds for one week; this will then be reduced to 200 mg twice daily and then once daily after a further week)

Mr Dale is reviewed by the cardiologist, who agrees to transfer him to a bed on the cardiac unit as soon as possible. Mr Dale is prescribed oral amiodarone and enoxaparin as well as his regular medication. He remains in sinus rhythm on his cardiac monitor. Mr Dale undergoes cardiac catheterisation 24 h after admission, which reveals a significant stenosis in his left anterior descending artery; a stent is inserted with good effect. At the same time, an ICD is sited enabling Mr Dale to discontinue treatment with amiodarone. Mr Dale is discharged from hospital after five days of inpatient observation having had no further arrhythmias.

CASE REVIEW

A 60-year-old man with a past history of ischaemic heart disease is brought to the accident and emergency department after collapsing in his garden. The admission ECG reveals a broad complex tachycardia. Mr Garth Dale is hypotensive and sweaty with cool peripherae. Examination reveals signs consistent with mild pulmonary oedema. Examination of the ECG reveals broad complexes in a left BBB pattern and a heart rate of 160 beats/min. There is also concordance of polarity across the chest leads. Combined with the past history of ischaemic heart disease and haemodynamic compromise, it is felt that the BCT is likely to reflect ventricular tachycardia.

Mr Dale is noted to have low potassium and he is given infusions of amiodarone and saline with potassium via a separate cannula. Mr Dale's rhythm is unchanged and his condition appears to be deteriorating, with falling blood pressure and increasing respiratory rate. He therefore undergoes emergency synchronised DC cardioversion, which restores sinus rhythm on the second shock at 200 J.

Following restoration of sinus rhythm, Mr Dale is noted to have a left bundle branch block and slightly elevated troponin 12 h after admission to hospital. He starts regular low molecular weight heparin and oral amiodarone, pending transfer to the cardiac ward. Mr Dale undergoes cardiac catheterisation 24 h after admission, revealing a significant stenotic lesion in his left anterior descending artery, which is stented by the cardiologists. An implantable cardiac defibrillator is also inserted.

This case highlights some of the diagnostic dilemmas encountered when managing a patient with a BCT. In some cases the distinction between VT and SVT with BBB is much less clear-cut. When the ECG is more suggestive of SVT or if the patient's condition is stable, it is often advisable to administer a short-acting atrioventricular node (AVN) blocking agent, such as adenosine. This is given by rapid intravenous bolus injection and produces temporary blockage of the AVN. Incremental doses of 6, 12 and, sometimes, 18 mg are given; if the patient has a supraventricular tachycardia, the rate will be slowed or reverted to sinus rhythm. There will be no response in VT, where the rhythm is generated from below the AVN. This drug therefore acts as both a diagnostic and therapeutic agent for patients with SVT.

KEY POINTS

- Broad complex tachycardia is a potentially life-threatening medical emergency.
- Broad complex tachycardia implies either ventricular tachycardia or supraventricular tachycardia with BBB.
- VT is more serious than SVT, mainly because of the risk of degeneration into pulseless VT or ventricular fibrillation.
- Distinction of VT from SVT with BBB requires careful consideration of the history, examination findings and ECG appearances.
- Where doubt remains, administration of adenosine may be helpful as a diagnostic agent: reversion to sinus rhythm or slowing of the rate implies a supraventricular source.

- When the patient is acutely unwell or deteriorating, DC cardioversion is the most rapid and effective means of re-establishing sinus rhythm.
- Underlying causes such as myocardial ischaemia, myocardial infarction and electrolyte imbalances should be sought and corrected where possible.
- Referral to the cardiology team for consideration of coronary angiography and insertion of an ICD is recommended for all patients when VT is the likely diagnosis.

Further reading

ACC/AHA/ESC. Guidelines for the management of patients with ventricular arrhythmias and the prevention of sudden cardiac death (2006). http://www.escardio.org/guidelines-surveys/esc-guidelines/Pages/ventricular-arrhythmias-and-prevention-sudden-cardiac-death.aspx

O'Neill MD, Davies DW. Cardiac arrhythmias part II: Broad complex tachycardia. *Acute Med* 2005; **4**(1): 3–9

Resuscitation Council UK. Resuscitation guidelines (2005). http://www.resus.org.uk/pages/guide.htm

PART 2: CASES

A GP calls to refer a 25-year-old woman whom he has just seen in his surgery. Jennifer Gardner has suffered with asthma since childhood and was well controlled until the past year, during which she has had two admissions to hospital. According to the GP records Jennifer Gardner normally takes regular beclomethasone and salmeterol inhalers along with salbutamol as required, although Ms Gardner has apparently not picked up a repeat prescription for the beclomethasone or salmeterol for over six months.

This morning Ms Gardner woke with an extremely tight chest and unable to catch her breath. This was not eased by taking her usual inhalers. Ms Gardner's partner brought her to the surgery, where she was unable to give any history because of severe shortness of breath. The GP administered a salbutamol nebuliser and called an ambulance, which is bringing her to hospital.

What challenges will this patient present?

• Acute asthma remains a life-threatening medical emergency, despite major advances in therapy over the past few decades

• Failure to recognise the severity of the attack has been identified as the commonest reason for death in patients with asthma

• Factors that predict a higher likelihood of fatal or near-fatal asthma exacerbation are listed in Table 28; these will need to be considered when obtaining the initial history

• Immediate therapy will be required when Ms Gardner arrives in hospital to ensure she survives

On arrival in the medical admissions unit Ms Gardner is alert and breathing spontaneously with a respiratory rate of 40/min. An audible expiratory wheeze is apparent from the end of the bed, and Ms Gardner is clearly in respiratory distress.

Acute Medicine: Clinical Cases Uncovered. By C. Roseveare.
Published 2009 by Blackwell Publishing, ISBN: 978-1-4051-6883-0

Oxygen saturation is recorded as 90% while breathing room air. Ms Gardner's pulse is 120 beats/min with blood pressure 110/70. She is not currently able to speak to you because of the severity of her respiratory distress.

What immediate management is required?

• Ensure patency of Ms Gardner's airway (in this case she is alert and therefore the airway is unlikely to be in danger; if the patient is drowsy, immediate anaesthetic support should be sought in case intubation is required)

• Apply oxygen: if the patient is truly 'asthmatic' (as in this case) this should be delivered at the highest rate possible (e.g. 15 L/min via a non-rebreath mask). Be aware that some patients labelled with asthma may in fact have chronic obstructive pulmonary disease (COPD) (see p. 71): patients with COPD may require a more controlled flow (e.g. 28% via a Venturi mask – see p. 72)

• Administer nebulised salbutamol (5 mg) and ipratropium bromide (500 µg) using oxygen as the driving gas

• Ensure continuous pulse oximetry, cardiac monitoring and regular measurement of the blood pressure

• Insert an intravenous cannula

• Take venous blood for full blood count (FBC), urea and electrolytes (U&E)

• Give steroids: if the patient is able to swallow, administer 40–60 mg of oral prednisolone; if the patient is unable to swallow, give 200 mg hydrocortisone intravenously

• Take an arterial blood gas sample

• Obtain an ECG

Ms Gardner's oxygen saturation has improved to 98% while receiving nebulised salbutamol/ipratropium via high-flow oxygen. She remains tachycardic (pulse 125 beats/min) and tachypnoeic (respiratory rate 35 breaths/min). Ms Gardner is still unable to speak. Examination of her chest reveals air entry throughout with widespread expiratory wheeze. On completion of the nebuliser she manages a peak flow

Table 28 Factors that predict the higher likelihood of fatal or near-fatal asthma

Severe asthma recognised by one or more of:

- previous near-fatal asthma (e.g. previous ventilation or respiratory acidosis)
- previous admission for asthma especially in the last year
- requiring three or more classes of asthma medication
- heavy use of beta-2 agonist
- repeated attendances at accident and emergency for asthma care in the past year
- 'brittle' asthma

AND

adverse behavioural or psychosocial factors, recognised by one or more of:
- non-compliance with treatment or monitoring
- failure to attend appointments
- self-discharge from hospital
- psychosis, depression, other psychiatric illness or deliberate self-harm
- current or recent major tranquilliser use
- denial
- alcohol or drug abuse
- obesity
- learning difficulties
- employment problems
- income problems
- social isolation
- childhood abuse
- severe domestic, marital or legal stress

---

recording of 160 L/min (predicted peak flow 450 L/min). She has been given 40 mg of prednisolone orally.

Arterial blood gases (while breathing 15 litres O_2) are as follows: pH 7.49; pCO_2 3.15; pO_2 14.9; HCO_3 22; base excess −0.4; saturation 96%; ECG shows sinus tachycardia.

How severe is the exacerbation?

- Acute asthma is usually graded according to the scale shown in Table 29
- Grading the severity of asthma will give a guide as to the treatment and prognosis, as well as the need for involvement of the critical care team
- Ms Gardner has indicators of *acute severe asthma* following the initial treatment
- In addition, Ms Gardner's peak flow is still only 35% of predicted even after completion of nebulised bronchodilators, which is borderline for classification as *life threatening*

- The low pCO_2 and raised pH indicate that Ms Gardner is adequately ventilating her lungs at present; however, this needs to be repeated if Ms Gardner's condition fails to improve rapidly. A normal or rising pCO_2 in the context of acute asthma may imply that the patient is tiring and in danger of respiratory arrest
- The presence of wheeze on auscultation implies that Ms Gardner is moving reasonable volumes of air with each breath; *absence of wheeze*, or 'silent chest', in the context of acute asthma suggests inadequate ventilation and is a poor prognostic sign
- Anxiety and the effect of salbutamol (stimulation of the sympathetic nervous system) may have contributed to the increasing sinus tachycardia; however, increasing tachycardia may also be a sign of clinical deterioration

Thirty minutes after completion of the nebuliser Ms Gardner's condition has not changed.

What further treatment/investigation is required?

- **Administer further nebulised salbutamol**: repeated nebulised salbutamol can be given ('back-to-back nebulisers') at a dose of 5 mg every 15–30 min. There is no benefit to repeating administration of ipratropium bromide more frequently than 6 hourly
- **Consider an intravenous salbutamol infusion**, if the patient's chest is so tight as to make inhalation of nebulised salbutamol unreliable: use 5 mg of salbutamol in 500 mL of saline at an initial infusion rate of 30 mL/h
- **Administer 2 g of magnesium sulphate** by intravenous infusion over 20 min: this has been shown to be effective in patients with acute severe and life-threatening asthma
- **Arrange an urgent portable chest radiograph** (see Box 11)
- **Check for evidence of urticarial rash**: if present this may suggest that the condition is caused by anaphylaxis rather than acute asthma
- **Try to obtain a more detailed history** and perform a general physical examination as soon as the patient's condition allows

Following administration of a second salbutamol nebuliser and 2 g of magnesium sulphate intravenously Ms Gardner says she is feeling better. Her pulse rate has fallen to 110 beats/min and her respiratory rate is now 25 breaths/min. Ms Gardner appears much less distressed and is able to talk in complete sentences.

Table 29 Levels of severity of acute asthma exacerbations

Near-fatal asthma	Raised $PaCO_2$ and/or requiring mechanical ventilation with raised inflation pressures
Life-threatening asthma	Any one of the following in a patient with severe asthma:
	PEF <33% best or predicted
	SpO_2 <92%
	PaO_2 <8 kPa
	Normal $PaCO_2$ (4.6–6.0)
	Silent chest
	Cyanosis
	Feeble respiratory effort
	Bradycardia
	Dysrhythmia
	Hypotension
	Exhaustion
	Confusion
	coma
Acute severe asthma	Any one of:
	PEF 33–50% best or predicted
	Respiratory rate ≥25 breaths/min
	Heart rate ≥110 beats/min
	Inability to complete sentences
Moderate asthma exacerbation	Any of:
	Increasing symptoms
	PEF 50–75% of best or predicted
	No features of acute severe asthma
Brittle asthma	Type 1: wide variability of PEF (>40% diurnal variation for >50% of the time over a period of >150 days) despite intense therapy
	Type 2: sudden severe attacks on a background of apparently well-controlled asthma

PEF, peak expiratory flow.

Box 11 Chest radiograph and acute asthma

The chest radiograph rarely provides diagnostic information in the initial management of acute asthma. Most cases of exacerbation are caused by viral infection, where the chest radiograph is almost invariably normal. The chest radiograph may show evidence of hyperinflation of the lung fields but this will not alter the clinical management. Occasionally there may be evidence of pulmonary consolidation, indicating likely bacterial infection, or an unexpected finding such as a lung tumour (more common in older patients).

For young patients with regular hospital admissions for exacerbations of their asthma repeated radiographs should be avoided because of the cumulative effect of radiation exposure.

The main purpose of undertaking a chest radiograph in this situation is the exclusion of pneumothorax, which is more common in patients with asthma. This will require specific treatment, which is very different from the treatment of an acutely wheezy asthmatic. When pneumothorax complicates asthma the patient usually presents with abrupt onset of shortness of breath accompanied by pleuritic chest pain; examination will reveal reduced breath sounds over the affected side of the chest, although this may be difficult to assess in the patient with acute severe asthma, where the breath sounds are generally reduced.

If the patient has features of acute severe or life-threatening asthma a radiograph should be undertaken on the ward ('portable' chest radiograph) rather than moving the patient to the radiology department, where observation may be difficult. Although the quality of a portable radiograph may be lower than if undertaken in the radiology department, it should be adequate for the exclusion of pneumothorax.

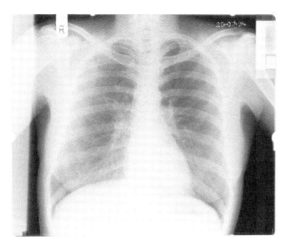

Figure 27 Chest radiograph showing hyperinflation of the lungs, but no pneumothorax and no focal consolidation.

A portable chest radiograph reveals hyperinflation of both lungs with no focal consolidation and no pneumothorax (see Fig. 27).

Further history reveals that Ms Gardner was diagnosed with asthma at the age of 12, at which time she started regular inhaled steroid therapy along with a salbutamol inhaler if required. Ms Gardner regularly attended the asthma clinic at her GP's surgery in the past, but since leaving home she has stopped going despite regular requests from her new GP. In the past year Ms Gardner has had two similar admissions to hospital, but did not require mechanical ventilation or admission to the intensive care unit. Following the second admission, a follow-up appointment was made in the asthma clinic, but she failed to attend. Ms Gardner was prescribed a regular long-acting beta-agonist inhaler (salmeterol) following this admission along with her regular steroid inhaler (beclomethasone). Ms Gardner admits that she often forgets to use these. She uses salbutamol when required and her use of this has increased over recent months.

Ms Gardner has never smoked cigarettes and works in an office. She has been under some financial stress recently since her partner became unemployed.

Over the past three days she had developed coryzal symptoms, with sore throat and mild fever. She has been expectorating a small quantity of sputum that is pale yellow in colour. She noticed herself becoming more wheezy, particularly in the mornings, and initially found some relief from her salbutamol inhaler. Ms Gardner slept poorly last night and this morning became suddenly much more wheezy, with no relief from her inhaler.

Examination reveals widespread expiratory wheeze with a resonant percussion note throughout. Cardiovascular examination is unremarkable apart from the tachycardia, and the abdominal examination is also normal.

What is the likely cause of the 'exacerbation of Ms Gardner's asthma'?

Common causes of asthma exacerbation are listed in Table 30.

• In this case viral upper respiratory tract infection is the most likely cause

• Bacterial infection is an uncommon precipitant of acute asthma (unlike COPD – see Case 6); for this reason, antibiotics are not usually administered unless the patient is expectorating thick purulent sputum or there are clinical or radiological signs to suggest pulmonary consolidation

• The poor compliance with medication and follow-up may have contributed to the likelihood/severity of this attack and will need to be addressed on discharge

• Remember to consider and exclude other causes of acute shortness of breath (particularly pulmonary embolism, pneumothorax and pneumonia – see Table 36, p. 82 for a more comprehensive list of causes of breathlessness)

What ongoing treatment and monitoring is required once Ms Gardner's condition has been stabilised?

• Prescribe regular bronchodilators: salbutamol 2.5–5 mg 4 hourly and in between if required; ipratropium 500 µg 6 hourly (all nebulisers delivered with oxygen as the driving gas)

• Continuous oxygen as required to maintain saturation >95% (use of a humidified mask may make this easier to tolerate for the patient)

• Ensure prescription of daily prednisolone (40–60 mg orally in the morning)

• Ensure continuous pulse oximetry and cardiac monitoring

• Hourly recording of respiratory rate, conscious level and blood pressure: any fall or rise in respiratory rate or drop in conscious level should be acted upon immediately

You are called back to Ms Gardner 2 h after her arrival in hospital. The nursing staff are concerned about the change in her condition over the last 15 min. Ms Gardner's

Table 30 Common causes of acute exacerbation of asthma

Cause	Symptoms/signs	Comments
Viral infection	Fever, sore throat or other coryzal symptoms Expectoration of mucoid or clear sputum	The commonest cause of an asthma exacerbation
Bacterial respiratory tract infection	Expectoration of thick, green/brown or purulent sputum Signs of pulmonary consolidation (coarse crackles or bronchial breathing)	Uncommon cause of exacerbation
Acute allergy (e.g. pollen, house dust mite, pets)	History of previous allergy precipitating asthma or seasonal changes with worsening in summer (pollen) Recent exposure to new potential allergen (e.g. new pet, etc.) Damp or dusty home may lead to exposure to house dust mite	Distinguish from the acute wheeze associated with anaphylaxis (usually associated with urticarial rash and circulatory collapse) – while this may also require bronchodilator treatment, anaphylaxis will also require antihistamine and adrenaline administration if severe
Smoke inhalation	Usually clear history of worsening after entering smoky environment	Asthmatics who smoke cigarettes are at much higher risk of deterioration and should be actively supported in giving up. Smokers who share a house with the patient should also be encouraged to quit

respiratory rate has slowed to 12 breaths/min. She appears more drowsy and oxygen saturation has dropped to 92% despite continuing to receive 60% humidified oxygen. Ms Gardner remains tachycardic at 120 beats/min, and her blood pressure has fallen to 90/50.

When you arrive you note that Ms Gardner's airway is patent and her breathing appears 'laboured'. Ms Gardner's eyes are open to command and she obeys commands; however, she is unable to speak due to respiratory compromise. Ms Gardner is currently receiving a further 5 mg of salbutamol by nebuliser. Breath sounds are more quiet than before with a soft wheeze throughout; however, there are no clinical signs of pneumothorax.

Repeat arterial blood gases show the following: pH 7.28; pCO_2 5.4; pO_2 8.9; HCO_3 21; base excess −4.4; saturation 92%; lactate 5.5

Why has Ms Gardner's condition deteriorated and what immediate actions are required?

Causes of deterioration following admission are listed in Table 30.

- In this case the patient is showing signs of fatigue and continued bronchospasm
- The raised lactate and low base excess are suggestive of poor tissue oxygenation
- Reduced breath sounds on examination and the rising pCO_2 (despite being within the 'normal range') suggest deteriorating alveolar ventilation – the patient may be in imminent danger of respiratory arrest if the problem cannot be corrected immediately
- Falling blood pressure may be due to hypovolaemia, sepsis or raised intrathoracic pressure

Immediate actions should include:

- Contact the critical care team and ask for them to attend immediately to review the patient
- Continue with back-to-back salbutamol nebulisers, delivered via oxygen
- Commence an intravenous infusion of aminophylline (see Box 12)
- Commence intravenous fluid therapy (e.g. normal saline 500 mL over 30 min)

Box 12 Intravenous bronchodilators and acute asthma

The use of intravenous bronchodilators in acute asthma is the subject of considerable controversy; at present there is no clear consensus on which, if any, drug is more appropriate in this clinical setting. Two drugs are available.

1 Intravenous salbutamol

Although salbutamol is usually administered via a nebuliser, an intravenous preparation is also available for use in acute severe asthma.

This form of administration is particularly useful where the bronchospasm is so severe that the patient is unable to inhale the nebulised solution.

There is limited additional benefit from intravenous use in addition to nebulised salbutamol, and this may result in severe tachycardia, tremor and anxiety.

2 Intravenous aminophylline

Intravenous aminophylline can be used in addition to nebulised salbutamol to provide additional bronchodilatation where the patient has failed to respond to initial therapy.

All patients receiving aminophylline should be connected to a cardiac monitor because of the risk of cardiac arrhythmias during administration.

Caution should be exercised in patients who are already taking oral theophylline drugs (aminophylline, Nuelin, Phyllocontin, etc.) in whom toxicity and therefore arrhythmia are more likely. Administration of a loading dose should be avoided in these patients.

The dosing regimen is as follows.

Loading dose: 250 mg in 100 mL of 5% dextrose over 30 min (avoid in patients already taking oral theophylline)

Maintenance dose: 0.5 mg/kg/h (i.e. 500 mg of aminophylline in 500 mL of 5% dextrose running at 30 mL/h for 60 kg patient)

Because of the combined effect of these drugs on the heart rate, combinations of intravenous aminophylline and salbutamol should be avoided.

Despite these measures Ms Gardner's condition fails to improve; on arrival of the critical care team the respiratory rate is noted to drop further and Ms Gardner's conscious level and oxygen saturation are falling. The anaesthetist decides to intubate Ms Gardner and commence bag-and-mask ventilation; he comments that the intrathoracic pressure is very high. Ms Gardner is connected to a mechanical ventilator and transferred to the intensive care

unit. Within 48 h her condition has improved enough to enable extubation and return to the ward.

Shortly after Ms Gardner's return to the ward the nurses ask you to review her as she is asking if she can go home.

What should be considered before the patient goes home from hospital?

Has the exacerbation settled adequately?

• Serial measurement of peak expiratory flow rate (PEFR) will give a guide to recovery. Ideally the patient's PEFR should be consistently measured at 75% of predicted/best prior to consideration of discharge

Has Ms Gardner been 'weaned off' her nebulised salbutamol and ipratropium?

• It is important that Ms Gardner is observed to be taking the medication which she would normally be taking at home, prior to discharge; ideally the patient should be converted to inhaled therapies for 24 h prior to discharge

• The most likely time for deterioration is early morning – if the patient is discharged too early, re-admission may be required if there is a sudden increase in bronchospasm on the morning after they arrive home

Has the cause of the 'exacerbation' been addressed?

• In this case the cause was felt to be a viral infection, which would normally resolve spontaneously within 48–72 h. Bacterial infection may require more prolonged treatment

• If the exacerbation resulted from allergy, it may be possible to remove the potential allergen from the home environment prior to discharge (e.g. new pets, etc.)

Have other 'contributory factors' been considered?

• As outlined in Table 28, a number of behavioural or psychosocial factors may contribute to the risk of re-admission because of severe or life-threatening asthma

• In this case Ms Gardner's poor compliance with medication, failure to attend hospital or GP appointments and recent financial and domestic stresses may need to be addressed

• Most hospitals and many general practitioners have access to asthma specialist nurses, who represent a valuable resource for patient education and support following discharge. Poor compliance with medication may reflect poor understanding of the nature and severity of the condition and the beneficial effects of taking regular inhaled corticosteroids to prevent deterioration. Discussion with the GP prior to discharge may be useful to ensure that non-medical issues are properly addressed after discharge

Has the patient's inhaler technique been assessed and optimised?

• Inhaled steroid and bronchodilator treatment will be less effective if the drug fails to reach the small and medium airways. The commonest form of inhaler (the metered dose inhaler, or MDI: see Plate 2) requires a long, consistent inhalation of breath to coincide with administration. However, even with perfect technique only a relatively small proportion of the drug (around 11%) will reach the smaller airways. A sharp inhalation may also induce coughing, particularly in the context of a recent viral infection. Delivery can be improved by the use of a large volume 'spacer' device, attached to the mouthpiece of the device (e.g. aerochamber or volumatic: see Fig. 28). Other devices are also available to make administration easier, and may be of use for older patients and those with rheumatic diseases for whom manual dexterity may be problematic

• The patient should be observed using their inhaler by a member of the team with expertise to provide advice where necessary. An asthma specialist nurse is often best placed to provide this

How long should the patient continue taking oral corticosteroids?

• Corticosteroid drugs have unpleasant side effects when taken in the long term, and the course should therefore be kept as short as possible. A total of two weeks' treatment with prednisolone at a dose of 30 or 40 mg daily is usually adequate. At the end of this course the patient can be advised to discontinue the drug

• Occasionally the patient may require a more prolonged course, in which case the patient should be weaned off the drug slowly, reducing the dose by 5 or 10 mg each week. Prolonged courses of steroids cause depression of the patient's adrenal gland preventing production of their own natural steroid; weaning the prednisolone dose slowly allows re-establishment of the patient's own steroid production

What follow-up is required?

• Follow-up of the patient within a few weeks of discharge is essential. This will enable reinforcement of the importance of compliance with medication, re-checking of inhaler technique and monitoring of disease severity

• Where this follow-up takes place is dependent on local resources and should also be discussed with Ms Gardner; she may have difficulty attending the hospital due to transport problems or other social factors, and may prefer to be seen in the GP's asthma clinic

• Given Ms Gardner's previous record of poor attendance, the importance of this should be clearly emphasised

Does Ms Gardner have an 'asthma management plan'?

• Patients should be able to recognise the symptoms of poor control and know what to do if their asthma is deteriorating. A formal, written asthma management plan with actions based on symptoms and peak flow recordings should be given to the patient on discharge

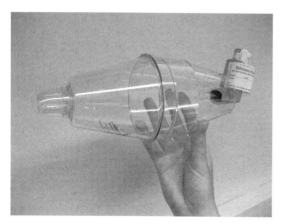

Figure 28 Volumatic device, used to improve delivery of metered dose inhaler.

Measurement of the peak flow is demonstrated to be >75% of Ms Gardner's predicted level. Ms Gardner is converted to a regular salbutamol inhaler (two puffs of salbutamol 6 hourly via a volumatic), along with regular salmeterol and beclomethasone (two puffs twice daily via a volumatic). Ms Gardner is given the option of a nebuliser if required. Her peak flow is monitored for 24 h during which she experiences no significant early morning dip in recordings and does not require any nebulised salbutamol. Ms Gardner is visited on the ward by the asthma specialist nurse who checks her technique. She is also given a peak flow meter, recording chart and asthma management plan. She feels she would rather be followed up by her GP, as she has no means of transport to get to hospital. You telephone the GP to discuss this prior to discharge and he agrees to an appointment the following week, which Ms Gardner promises to attend. Ms Gardner is allowed home later that day.

CASE REVIEW

A 25-year-old woman with known asthma is referred to hospital with the third exacerbation of her condition in the past year. On arrival in hospital Ms Jennifer Gardner has features consistent with acute severe asthma. The history suggests that this has been precipitated by a viral upper respiratory tract infection; in addition Ms Gardner's compliance with regular inhaled medication and outpatient follow-up has been poor over recent months.

Ms Gardner is given salbutamol and ipratropium bromide via nebuliser, delivered using high-flow oxygen, along with oral prednisolone and intravenous magnesium sulphate. Initial arterial blood gases reveal a respiratory alkalosis with adequate oxygenation. After a second salbutamol nebuliser Ms Gardner's condition appears to be improving; however, while being observed on the ward Ms Gardner deteriorates with apparent respiratory muscle fatigue and ongoing bronchospasm resulting in inadequate alveolar ventilation. Ms Gardner is reviewed urgently by the critical care team, who arrange for immediate transfer to the intensive care unit, where she is ventilated for 24 h.

Ms Gardner returns to the ward having been extubated 24 h earlier and is weaned on to inhalers after 24 h. Prior to discharge from hospital she undergoes counselling on inhaler technique by the asthma specialist nurse, who also reinforces the importance of compliance with prophylactic medication in the longer term. Ms Gardner is advised to use her inhalers via a volumatic device and is given a total of two weeks' prednisolone. Ms Gardner is given a peak flow meter and a home management plan prior to discharge. A follow-up appointment with the GP's asthma clinic is arranged.

KEY POINTS

- Acute asthma is a life-threatening condition that requires prompt recognition and treatment when presenting to hospital.
- Immediate treatment should include high-flow oxygen, nebulised bronchodilator drugs, oral or intravenous corticosteroids and intravenous magnesium sulphate.
- Characterisation of severity will enable the identification of patients who are at risk of deterioration in hospital and require transfer to a high-dependency unit.
- Close observation is essential – deterioration or failure to respond to initial therapy should prompt immediate review by the critical care team for consideration of mechanical ventilation.
- Factors which may have contributed to the admission should be addressed prior to discharge, with the use of a home asthma management plan where appropriate.
- Follow-up by the GP or hospital-based asthma clinic is essential following discharge from hospital.

Further reading

BTS/SIGN. British guideline on the management of asthma (2008). http://www.brit-thoracic.org.uk/Portals/0/Clinical%20Information/Asthma/Guidelines/asthma_final2008.pdf

Holgate ST, Polosa R. The mechanisms, diagnosis and management of severe asthma in adults. *Lancet* 2006; **368**; 80–93

Ramsay C. Acute exacerbation of asthma in adults. *Acute Med* 2003; **2**(2): 41–7

A 60-year-old woman with an 'exacerbation' of chronic obstructive pulmonary disease

The emergency department contacts you to say that a 60-year-old woman has been brought in by ambulance from home. Mrs Geetha Sinha is a lifelong smoker and has a long history of chronic obstructive pulmonary disease (COPD), with many previous admissions to hospital. Mrs Sinha had been more breathless than normal over the past few days with a cough, producing green sputum. In the early hours of the morning, Mrs Sinha became acutely short of breath. She tried using her nebuliser at home, but did not improve and dialled 999. The paramedic crew gave Mrs Sinha a further salbutamol and ipratropium bromide nebuliser, and 15 L of oxygen via a non-rebreath mask. The referring doctor believes that this illness represents an exacerbation of COPD.

What is an 'exacerbation of chronic obstructive pulmonary disease'?

• COPD or chronic obstructive airways disease (COAD) is a common condition, usually induced by smoking

• The condition usually follows a slowly progressive course over many years, characterised by exertional breathlessness, cough, wheeze and regular sputum production. This can usually be managed by the patient's GP, sometimes with the support of a specialist respiratory team and community nurses

• The course of the illness is frequently punctuated by 'exacerbations', which may require hospital admission. In most (but not all) cases the exacerbation is caused by infection, which may be viral or bacterial

• Because of the relapsing/remitting nature of the condition, the underlying diagnosis of COPD is often well defined. As in this case the patient may have had many previous similar hospital admissions and have been extensively investigated in the past

However, the diagnosis of 'exacerbation of COPD' is not always clear-cut, so always consider the following points:

Acute Medicine: Clinical Cases Uncovered. By C. Roseveare.
Published 2009 by Blackwell Publishing, ISBN: 978-1-4051-6883-0

• The patient may have been misdiagnosed in the past

• The patient may have asthma rather than COPD (see Box 13 and Table 31)

• There may be an alternative explanation for the increase in breathlessness (see Table 36, p. 82)

On your arrival Mrs Sinha is drowsy and disorientated but responding to voices and obeying commands. Mrs Sinha's respiratory rate is 8 breaths/min, with a prolonged expiratory phase and 'pursed lip' breathing. Saturations read 97% on 15 L of oxygen via a non-rebreath mask. Mrs Sinha's heart rate is 130 beats/min, with a blood pressure of 130/70 and she is apyrexial. Auscultation of the lung fields reveals generally poor air entry throughout with a few scattered wheezes but no other added sounds.

What immediate management is required?

• Assess the patency of Mrs Sinha's airway, oxygen saturation and circulatory status

• Attach a cardiac monitor and pulse oximeter

• Perform urgent arterial blood gas analysis

• Administer salbutamol (5 mg) and ipratropium bromide (500 μg) via a nebuliser

• Establish intravenous access and give fluid as required to correct hypovolaemia

• Obtain an ECG

Why is the patient drowsy/confused?

Drowsiness and confusion are common features in patients presenting with exacerbation of COPD. Possible causes include:

• Hypoxia
• Carbon dioxide (CO_2) narcosis
• Sepsis
• Drugs
• Co-existent cerebral pathology (e.g. cerebrovascular disease, dementia, etc.)

Of these causes, the first two represent the greatest immediate priority.

Hypoxia and CO_2 narcosis

Hypoxia (hypoxaemia) is a life-threatening medical emergency requiring rapid correction. Failure to correct hypoxia in the acute setting can result in permanent brain damage and can be rapidly fatal. When an ambulance crew finds a breathless patient to be hypoxic, they will usually apply high-flow oxygen in an attempt to reverse this.

Patients with COPD are often *chronically* hypoxic, in many cases maintaining and tolerating capillary oxygen saturation of <90% while allowing CO_2 levels to rise above the normal range. In healthy individuals, a rise in CO_2 would trigger an increased respiratory rate; however, patients with COPD and chronic hypoxaemia lose this trigger, relying instead on the low oxygen level to trigger respiration (*hypoxic drive*). Aggressive correction of hypoxia in this situation leads to a loss of this drive, resulting in slowing of the respiratory rate and a further rise in the CO_2 level. As the CO_2 level rises the patient may become confused and drowsy (*CO_2 narcosis*). Failure to correct this can also result in brain damage and death. The clinical features of CO_2 narcosis are summarised in Table 32.

Rising CO_2 levels can also result from respiratory muscle fatigue (the usual cause in patients with asthma rather than COPD – see Case 5) and from problems with gas exchange, such as bronchospasm, infection and sputum plugging.

A difficult balance has to be found between, on the one hand, correcting hypoxia adequately while not allowing CO_2 levels to rise and cause narcosis. Management will require careful evaluation of the patient's clinical condition in combination with their arterial blood gas results.

In managing this challenge consider the following.
- **Look at the patient**: if she is very drowsy/unresponsive (e.g. Glasgow Coma Score <8) she may require intubation and further management on the intensive care unit. Contact the critical care team immediately
- **Look at the oxygen saturation/pO_2** on arterial blood gases: if the patient is significantly hypoxic (pO_2 <8 kPa;

> ### Box 13 Is it asthma or chronic obstructive pulmonary disease?
>
> Asthma and COPD share many similarities: both are characterised by wheezing and periodic exacerbations and may respond to bronchodilators and anti-inflammatory drugs. However, there are also key differences in the initial and ongoing management, which requires that an early attempt is made to distinguish the predominant pathology. Confusion regarding the diagnosis can arise for a number of reasons.
> - Some patients with COPD may have been told that they have 'asthma'.
> - Some patients with asthma may develop COPD as they get older.
> - The two conditions can co-exist.
> - The management of acute asthma is dealt with in Case 5.
>
> Some of the features which may help in this distinction are highlighted in Table 31.

Table 31 Some features that distinguish between asthma and chronic obstructive pulmonary disease (COPD)

	Asthma	COPD
Onset	Childhood/adolescence	Over 40
Smoking history	Often minimal/non-smoker	Usually a smoker or significant smoking history
Airway obstruction	Largely reversible	Largely irreversible
Allergy	Association with atopy/eczema	No associated allergy
Lung parenchymal involvement	No	Often
Inflammatory cells/markers	Eosinophils/CD4	Neutrophils/CD8
Symptoms	Wheezing predominates and can be worse at night with symptoms intermittent	Cough and sputum predominate, progressively worsening

Table 32 Features of CO_2 narcosis

Examination	Findings
General appearance	Sweating
	Facial 'flushing'
Fundoscopy	Papilloedema
Neurology	Myoclonus
	Asterixis
	Seizures
Level of consciousness	Drowsiness
	Confusion
	Coma

Table 33 Guide to Venturi valves

Venturi valve (colour)	Oxygen flow rate needed (L/min)	Oxygen delivered (%)
Blue	2	24
White	4	28
Yellow	6	35
Red	8	40
Green	12	60

saturation <85%) she almost certainly will require more oxygen. This may require mechanical ventilatory support (see below)

• **Look at the pH**: if this is low (<7.35), in combination with an elevated CO_2 level, it suggests that the raised CO_2 is (at least in part) 'acute'. In the chronic setting, the pH would be corrected by retention of bicarbonate in the kidneys ('metabolic compensation'); however, this usually takes at least 48–72 h to take effect

• **Look at the bicarbonate** (HCO_3, standard bicarbonate, SBC) level: if this is raised it suggests an element of chronic CO_2 retention (and therefore chronic hypoxia). Even if the pH is normal the patient will be at risk of further CO_2 retention and therefore will require close observation and monitoring of arterial blood gases

> The arterial blood gas (ABG) results, taken on arrival with Mrs Sinha breathing high-flow oxygen via a non-rebreath mask, are as follows (normal ranges shown in brackets):
> pH 7.29 (7.35–7.45); pO_2 12.3 (12–16); pCO_2 9.1(4.7–6.3); HCO_3 34.5 (22–24); base excess +9.5 (–2 to +2); saturation 99%.
> Mrs Sinha is well oxygenated but the CO_2 level is elevated with a low pH, suggesting that acute CO_2 narcosis is the cause of her confusion. The elevated bicarbonate indicates that Mrs Sinha is a 'chronic' CO_2 retainer and would probably tolerate lower oxygen saturation.

How can CO_2 narcosis be corrected?

• **If the patient is well oxygenated:** reduce inhaled oxygen concentration (FiO_2) – initially to 28%. A Venturi mask is the most reliable means of controlling FiO_2. The

oxygen flow rate required to deliver the desired FiO_2 is summarised in Table 33

• **Improve gas exchange where possible:** reverse bronchospasm with bronchodilators/steroids; reduce sputum plugging with physiotherapy, if the patient is awake enough to tolerate this

• **Repeat arterial blood gas measurement after 30 min to assess the response to treatment:** a rise in pH and fall in pCO_2 without a significant fall in pO_2 implies a good response to treatment. Close monitoring is still required. If the pH/pCO_2 has not corrected or has worsened further the patient is likely to require mechanical ventilatory support (see below)

In addition, remember the following

• **If the patient is significantly hypoxic (pO_2 <8; saturation <85%), do not reduce their oxygen delivery**. The patient will die from hypoxia faster than hypercapnia.

• **A rising pCO_2 in a patient with *asthma* is managed very differently**: this usually requires immediate mechanical ventilation; reduction of the oxygen delivery would be completely *inappropriate* in this situation

> Ms Sinha is changed to 28% oxygen via a Venturi mask and given salbutamol and ipratropium bromide via a nebuliser. Oxygen saturation falls to 92%, but Mrs Sinha appears to become more alert and the respiratory rate increases to 12 breaths/min. The repeat ABG after 30 min while breathing 28% oxygen is as follows: pH 7.33, pCO_2 6.7, PO_2 8.4, HCO_3 33.7.
> The CO_2 has fallen with a corresponding rise in pH; although the pO_2 has fallen, it is likely that Mrs Sinha will tolerate this. She needs to be monitored closely. Attention can now be switched to determining the underlying cause of the exacerbation.

What further information/investigation is required?

Following initial stabilisation, a more detailed history, examination and investigation should focus on the following.

- What is the cause of this exacerbation?
- How severe is the exacerbation?
- How severe is Mrs Sinha's underlying COPD?

Prior to this admission Mrs Sinha had been unwell for approximately one week. She had seen her GP initially complaining of a productive cough with green sputum along with fever and increased shortness of breath. The GP had prescribed oral amoxicillin and prednisolone 30 mg daily, which had produced some improvement in Mrs Sinha's symptoms for a couple of days with a lightening in the colour of the sputum; however, in the past three days the breathlessness had worsened, with continued coughing, although the fever had settled. Mrs Sinha's usual inhalers and nebulisers had been having very little effect during this period. Although this has been the third similar admission to hospital in the past year Mrs Sinha says this is the worst she has ever felt.

Mrs Sinha has been diagnosed with COPD for approximately five years. During this period she had been becoming gradually more breathless and immobile. She smoked 20 cigarettes per day for the last 40 years, although she had cut down to five per day in the last year. Following Mrs Sinha's last admission to hospital she was given a nebuliser to use at home and was told that she would be considered for home oxygen if she were able to give up smoking. Mrs Sinha has been housebound for the past two months because of ongoing shortness of breath.

Examination reveals Mrs Sinha to be sitting on the edge of her bed using her accessory muscles of respiration and exhibiting pursed-lip breathing. The respiratory rate is 14 breaths/min. There is widespread expiratory wheeze on auscultation with generally poor air entry throughout both lung fields. Percussion note is resonant throughout. Mrs Sinha's jugular venous pressure (JVP) is elevated at 5 cm and her ankles are swollen with pitting oedema to level of the knee.

What is the cause of this 'exacerbation'?

Causes of increased breathlessness in patients with COPD are summarised in Table 34.

In this case the combination of general malaise, gradual worsening of wheeze and breathlessness with discolouration of the sputum is suggestive of bacterial infective exacerbation.

Common bacterial pathogens include:
- *Streptococcus pneumoniae*
- *Haemophilus influenzae*

and less commonly
- *Staphylococcus aureus*
- *Moxarella catarrhalis*

How severe is the exacerbation?

Features indicating that this is a severe exacerbation include:
- Mrs Sinha's description of this being the 'worst ever' exacerbation
- Pursed-lip breathing and using the 'accessory' muscles of respiration (sternomastoid and abdominal) at rest

If Mrs Sinha's condition fails to improve with treatment, she will need to be reviewed by the critical care team, and should be considered for transfer to a high-dependency unit (HDU) setting.

How severe is the patient's underlying chronic obstructive pulmonary disease?

The severity of Mrs Sinha's underlying COPD is indicated by:
- Repeated hospital admissions in the past year
- Poor exercise tolerance and requirement to be 'house-bound' in recent months
- Lack of response to bronchodilator and corticosteroid treatment prior to admission
- Ankle oedema and elevation of JVP, suggestive of right heart failure because of cor pulmonale

As Mrs Sinha has previously been admitted to hospital on several occasions it is very likely that the severity of her airways disease may have been quantified objectively with pulmonary function testing in the past. Serial measurements of FEV_1 (forced expiratory volume in 1 second) and FVC (forced vital capacity) may give a guide to the speed of deterioration. Considering the severity of the underlying disease may be important if Mrs Sinha's condition deteriorates further, as it may help to inform the decision on the appropriateness of mechanical ventilation.

What further investigation is required?

- Full blood count
- Urea and electrolytes
- C-reactive protein
- Chest radiograph
- ECG
- Sputum culture (if the cough is productive)

Table 34 Causes of increased breathlessness in patients with chronic obstructive pulmonary disease

Cause	Characteristic symptoms	Signs
Bacterial infective exacerbation	Fever/malaise Gradual increased breathlessness and wheeze Increased sputum production Increased sputum purulence or change in colour of sputum	Pyrexia (may be absent if patient on corticosteroids) Widespread wheeze Reduced breath sounds
Viral/non-infective exacerbation	As above without increased sputum production/purulence	As above
Pneumothorax	Sudden onset of breathlessness Pleuritic chest pain	Absent breath sounds Hyperresonant percussion Asymmetrical chest expansion
Pneumonia	Fever/rigors Malaise/lethargy Anorexia	Pyrexia Bronchial breathing Dull percussion note Increased vocal resonance
Pulmonary embolus	Sudden onset of breathlessness Pleuritic chest pain Haemoptysis Syncope	Tachycardia Hypotension Raised JVP Evidence of DVT in some cases
Pleural effusion	Progressive dyspnoea Other symptoms can depend on cause	Decreased breath sounds Dull percussion note Decreased vocal resonance

A full blood count reveals an elevated haemoglobin (179 mg/L) and high white cell count (14.5, neutrophils 11.3). Potassium is slightly low at 3.15 mmol/dL but renal function is otherwise normal. C-reactive protein (CRP) is elevated at 65 mg/L.

A chest radiograph reveals hyperinflated lung fields with no focal consolidation and no evidence of pneumothorax (see Fig. 29).

The ECG shows a sinus tachycardia with prominent P-waves and atrial ectopic beats (see Fig. 30).

Sputum culture reveals a heavy growth of Haemophilus influenzae, sensitive to amoxicillin.

• The raised haemoglobin is likely to be a result of chronic hypoxia
• The elevation of the white cell count probably reflects infection (also supported by the elevation of CRP) but can also occur simply because of steroid treatment
• The low potassium level is commonly due to increased urinary potassium loss as a result of steroid and salbutamol
• The chest radiograph is frequently normal or shows simply hyperexpanded lung fields; careful inspection for

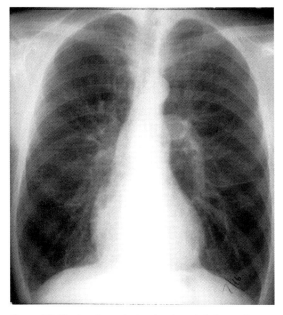

Figure 29 Chest radiograph showing hyperinflation and prominent pulmonary arteries, typical of chronic obstructive pulmonary disease, but no focal inflammation, and no evidence of pneumothorax.

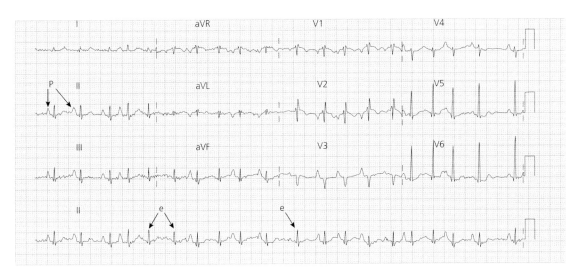

Figure 30 ECG showing sinus tachycardia with prominent P-waves (P). In addition there are atrial ectopic beats (e), resulting in slight irregularity.

signs of pneumothorax is necessary as this would require specific management and can easily be missed
• The ECG features are suggestive of right atrial enlargement and increased pulmonary venous pressure, consistent with chronic lung disease
• Sputum culture may help to guide antibiotic treatment, but is often negative and may take several days to be available; antibiotic treatment is therefore usually commenced on the basis of the most likely pathogens. Most hospitals have local antibiotic guidelines based on evidence of current pathogens and sensitivities

What further treatment is required?
In this case, Mrs Sinha is deemed likely to have a bacterial exacerbation of COPD. The following treatment should be commenced (see Table 35).
• Regular inhaled bronchodilators
• Corticosteriods
• Antibiotics
• Chest physiotherapy may be indicated if the patient is experiencing difficulty expectorating sputum, or if there is concern that the patient's airways are obstructed by a sputum plug. Humidification of oxygen and a regular nebuliser may also help with expectoration

Mrs Sinha starts taking regular nebulised salbutamol, 5 mg 4 hourly, and ipratropium bromide 500 μg 6 hourly. She is prescribed 40 mg of oral prednisolone daily and amoxicillin 500 mg tds intravenously. Mrs Sinha continues to receive humidified 28% oxygen via a Venturi mask.

How and where should the patient be monitored?
All patients should be observed closely in a monitored bed in an acute medical unit or specialist respiratory unit.

Careful monitoring is required, as transfer to a HDU may be indicated if Mrs Sinha's condition deteriorates.

Monitoring should include:
• Continuous pulse oximetry
• Continuous ECG monitoring
• Hourly recording of pulse, blood pressure, respiratory rate and conscious level

How frequently should arterial blood gases be repeated?
Repeated arterial puncture is painful for the patient, so needs to be considered carefully. Following initial assessment it may be necessary to repeat the ABG measurement several times to ensure that the patient is adequately oxygenated with stable CO_2 and pH. Insertion of an arterial cannula can facilitate regular sampling, but usually requires that the patient be managed in an HDU setting. For most patients this is not necessary.

Once the patient has been stabilised on oxygen, repeated ABG analysis is usually not required. However, ABG measurement is always required in the following situations.
• Following a change in inhaled oxygen concentration
• Following a fall in oxygen saturation

Table 35 Drug treatment

Drug	Rationale	Dose	Delivery	Cautions
Salbutamol	Bronchodilatation	2.5–5 mg as needed	Inhaled (usually via nebuliser, initially)	Tachycardia Tremor
Ipratopium bromide	Bronchodilatation	500 µg, 6 hourly	Inhaled (usually via nebuliser, initially)	
Prednisolone	Reduce airway inflammation	30–60 mg once daily	Oral	Oedema Insomnia (if given late in evening)
Hydrocortisone	Reduce airway inflammation (if unable to take oral prednisolone)	100–200 mg 8 hourly	Intravenous	
Antibiotics*	Treat bacterial infection	Variable	Oral or intravenous	Allergic reactions Previous culture showing resistance

*Refer to local microbiology or British Thoracic Society guidelines.

• Following a deterioration in the patient's conscious level
• Following a change in respiratory rate

You are called back to the ward to review Mrs Sinha 2 h later. The nurses are concerned that her condition has deteriorated. Mrs Sinha has become less responsive (Glasgow Coma Score 11/15) and her breathing is more laboured. The oxygen saturation has fallen to 80% on 28% oxygen. The pulse is 110 beats/min with blood pressure 130/70. Auscultation of the lungs reveals poor air entry throughout with a few scattered wheezes.

Repeat blood gases reveal the following: pH 7.15; pCO_2 10.2; pO_2 6.57; HCO_3 35.9.

Why has Mrs Sinha deteriorated and what action should be taken?

Mrs Sinha has developed a respiratory acidosis, this time in association with a fall in her pO_2. Possible causes include:
• Fatigue: Mrs Sinha may be tiring, resulting in respiratory muscle fatigue
• A further problem with gas exchange in the lung, such as acute bronchospasm, pneumothorax or sputum plugging
The following measures should be instigated.
• Increase FiO_2: although Mrs Sinha developed CO_2 nar-

cosis when given high-flow oxygen previously, the current hypoxia needs to be corrected
• Administer a further salbutamol nebuliser; if there is a marked wheeze consider intravenous aminophylline as an additional bronchodilator (see p. 67)
• Contact the critical care or high-dependency unit team – Mrs Sinha is likely to require mechanical ventilatory support if she does not respond immediately to these measures
• Arrange a repeat portable chest radiograph (Mrs Sinha is not well enough for transfer to the radiography department) to exclude pneumothorax

Mrs Sinha's condition has not improved following these measures. Repeat arterial blood gas after 20 min on 60% O_2 is as follows: pH 7.12; pCO_2 11.3; pO_2 7.8; HCO_3 34.8.

Although the pO_2 has risen slightly Mrs Sinha remains acidotic with rising CO_2. She will therefore require mechanical support for ventilation.
Two options may be considered:
• Invasive ventilation on the intensive care unit
• Non-invasive ventilation in a HDU or specialist respiratory ward
Invasive ventilation requires that the patient is anaesthetised and undergoes insertion of an endotracheal tube. This is the usual practice for patients with acute asthma

who deteriorate in this way (see Case 5). For patients with COPD, non-invasive ventilation is usually employed initially when type II respiratory failure fails to respond to the above measures. Biphasic positive airway pressure (BiPAP) is the most commonly used form of non-invasive ventilation, and is often effective at improving oxygenation and reversing respiratory acidosis. Patients receiving BiPAP will require close monitoring, regular arterial blood gas measurement and careful observation by a skilled nursing team, familiar with its use.

A detailed description of BiPAP is beyond the scope of this chapter. For further reading on this subject see the British Thoracic Society guidelines (BTS 2002) and Cooper *et al.* (2006).

Mrs Sinha commences BiPAP and is moved to respiratory HDU. She slowly improves over the following week, and is weaned off the non-invasive ventilator. Fourteen days later Mrs Sinha is discharged home, where she unfortunately starts smoking again. Two weeks later she is re-admitted with similar symptoms.

CASE REVIEW

A 60-year-old woman with a documented history of COPD has been brought to the emergency department by ambulance. Mrs Geetha Sinha has had a number of previous admissions with exacerbations of COPD, but has become more unwell over the past few days, with increased breathlessness, wheezing and sputum purulence. Mrs Sinha has not responded to treatment with antibiotics, nebulised salbutamol and corticosteroids prescribed by her GP. Having been found to be hypoxic by the ambulance crew, she is given high-flow oxygen, but on arrival she is drowsy with evidence of acute respiratory acidosis. Reduction of the inhaled oxygen concentration to 28% with further nebulised salbutamol and ipratropium results in an improvement in Mrs Sinha's conscious level and reduction of the pCO_2.

Mrs Sinha's condition initially stabilises, with symptoms, signs and investigations consistent with an infective exacerbation of COPD. No alternative cause for Mrs Sinha's symptoms is identified and the sputum culture confirms that the infection is likely to be sensitive to the amoxicillin which has been prescribed. However, during Mrs Sinha's observation on the ward her condition deteriorates and she develops hypoxia and hypercapnia. This probably relates to a combination of poor gas exchange from ongoing bronchospasm and infection, along with respiratory muscle fatigue. Mrs Sinha is transferred to the HDU where she is managed with non-invasive ventilation and makes a good recovery, allowing discharge from hospital after two weeks.

KEY POINTS

- Exacerbation of COPD is a common cause for hospital admission, particularly during winter months.
- Most exacerbations of COPD are caused by respiratory tract infections.
- Alternative explanations for increased breathlessness should always be sought and treated where appropriate.
- Controlled oxygen delivery via a Venturi mask is usually recommended in the initial stages of assessment to reduce the risk of CO_2 narcosis.

- Bronchodilatation with nebulised salbutamol, reduction of airway inflammation with corticosteroids and antibiotic therapy are the usual treatments required.
- A rising CO_2 level or deteriorating level of conscious are indications for transferring the patient to a HDU for consideration of mechanical ventilatory support.

Further reading

British Thoracic Society (BTS). Chronic obstructive pulmonary disease: national clinical guideline on management of chronic obstructive pulmonary disease in adults in primary and secondary care. (March 2004) http://thorax.bmj.com/content/vol59/suppl_1

British Thoracic Society (BTS). Non-invasive ventilation in acute respiratory failure, *Thorax* 2002; **57**: 192–211

Cooper N, Forrest K, Cramp P. *Essential guide to acute care*, Chapter 4, 2nd edition. Blackwell Publishing, Oxford, 2006.

Gomersall CD, Joynt GM, Freebairn RC *et al*. Oxygen therapy for hypercapnic patients with chronic obstructive pulmonary disease and acute respiratory failure, a randomised controlled pilot study. *Crit Care Med* 2002; **30**: 113–16

Ram FSF, Picot J, Lightowler J, Wedzicha JA. Non-invasive positive pressure ventilation for treatment of respiratory failure due to exacerbations of chronic obstructive pulmonary disease. Cochrane systematic review and metanalysis. *BMJ* 2003; **326**: 185

An 86-year-old woman with acute shortness of breath

A GP telephones to ask you to admit an 86-year-old woman whom he has been called to see at home. Mrs Margaret McDonald has been getting increasingly breathless over the past few months and woke in the early hours of the morning with an acute onset of severe breathlessness. Mrs McDonald's husband called for an ambulance, but on its arrival she refused to go into hospital and the breathlessness appeared to be settling. However, this morning Mrs McDonald has become more breathless again and she is becoming confused. Mrs McDonald now seems agreeable to hospital admission and the GP feels that this is the only option in order to establish the cause of Mrs McDonald's breathlessness and provide some treatment.

What challenges will this patient present?

Breathlessness resulting in hospital admission in an older person often presents a series of interesting challenges.

• There is often a broad differential diagnosis
• Some patients have combinations of several pathologies, all of which may be contributing to the breathlessness
• Symptoms are often atypical or non-specific
• A history may be difficult to establish, particularly if there is an element of chronic cognitive impairment, or an acute confusional state
• Clinical examination and investigation may be difficult if the patient is confused and uncooperative

Mrs McDonald is brought into the admissions ward by the ambulance crew, accompanied by her husband and daughter. Mrs McDonald looks very short of breath at rest and appears agitated and confused. She is reluctant to use the oxygen, which the ambulance crew have been trying to administer during transit to hospital. Mrs McDonald's initial

observations reveal an oxygen saturation of 88% while breathing room air, with a respiratory rate of 25 breaths/min and a pulse rate of 120/min. Mrs McDonald blood pressure is 120/70. She is apyrexial.

What immediate management is required?

• **Confirm patency of the airway**: in this case Mrs McDonald is alert and talking so the airway is not likely to be in danger. Listen carefully for evidence of stridor (harsh, inspiratory noise) indicating laryngeal or tracheal obstruction
• **Administer oxygen**: Mrs McDonald is breathless and hypoxic and therefore needs oxygen. How much oxygen to give in this situation is a subject of some controversy. This is discussed in more detail in Case 6. In practice if the patient is deemed likely to have chronic obstructive pulmonary disease (COPD) it is advisable to give 28% oxygen via a Venturi mask in the first instance. If there is no history of prior COPD, the hypoxaemia should be rapidly corrected by administering high-flow oxygen (e.g. 15 L/min via a reservoir mask). If the patient will not comply with use of an oxygen mask, administration of oxygen via nasal cannulae ('nasal specs') should be considered. Although this will not deliver as much oxygen as a mask, an agitated patient may tolerate this better, and correction of hypoxaemia may reduce their level of confusion
• **Insert an intravenous cannula and check circulatory status**: although the blood pressure appears reasonable, if the patient is normally hypertensive this may still represent 'shock' (see Case 8). Check capillary refill time, skin temperature and peripheral pulses
• **Connect the patient to a cardiac monitor** and confirm that the pulse is regular: a regular tachycardia at this rate is likely to represent sinus tachycardia, but a fast irregular pulse may reflect rapid atrial fibrillation (see Case 3) which may have contributed to the breathlessness

Acute Medicine: Clinical Cases Uncovered. By C. Roseveare.
Published 2009 by Blackwell Publishing, ISBN: 978-1-4051-6883-0

- **Formally assess conscious level** using the Glasgow Coma Scale (see p. 127)
- **Obtain an ECG**: sometimes this may show diagnostic features, such as evidence of ST elevation myocardial infarction (STEMI) (Case 1) or an arrhythmia (Case 3&4)
- **Obtain blood for arterial blood gas analysis**: this is particularly important for patients with suspected COPD in whom there is a danger of CO_2 narcosis (see p. 71). However, it will also provide useful information about the degree of correction of hypoxaemia, as well as electrolyte levels (sodium and potassium). Most blood gas analysers will also measure the lactate level, which gives an indication of tissue perfusion. The haemoglobin level is also often provided

Mrs McDonald remains tachypnoeic and agitated but there is no stridor. She will not tolerate an oxygen mask, despite encouragement from her family, but with administration of 3 L/min via nasal specs Mrs McDonald's oxygen saturation improves to 94%. Mrs McDonald is cool and clammy peripherally, with increased capillary refill time of 4 s. The cardiac monitor demonstrates a regular heart rate of 110 beats/min, which the ECG confirms to be sinus tachycardia; there is evidence of an old inferior myocardial infarction (MI), but no ST segment elevation (see Fig. 31).

Arterial blood gases (while breathing 3 L of oxygen via nasal specs) are as follows: pH 7.34, pCO$_2$ 3.8, pO$_2$ 9.87, HCO$_3$ 21.5, base excess −3.2, lactate 2.4, haemoglobin 98 mg/L.

Mrs McDonald is too confused to give a reliable history, but with the help of her husband and daughter and a letter provided by her GP you obtain the following information.

Over the past few years Mrs McDonald's family have noticed that she has been getting gradually more breathless on exertion, which Mrs McDonald has been told was caused by obesity and smoking-related lung disease. Two months ago Mrs McDonald was able to walk to local shops and climb a flight of stairs slowly, but this has become more difficult, and she has not been out of the house for the past month. Over the past two weeks even minor exertion around the house has resulted in breathlessness and Mrs McDonald has been sleeping downstairs in her armchair as she found lying flat made the breathlessness worse. Mrs McDonald's GP has visited her several times during this period and initially prescribed her a salbutamol inhaler and a course of antibiotics, which had little effect. Two weeks ago he commenced a diuretic drug (furosemide 40 mg daily), which seemed to improve the symptoms initially. However, Mrs McDonald stopped using this drug in the past week as she found that she was having difficulty getting to the toilet in time. Mrs McDonald has been coughing up thin, white sputum, which has turned yellow in the past few days, since when she has been noticeably more breathless.

Mrs McDonald's past medical history includes a myocardial infarction at the age of 70. Mrs McDonald has experienced occasional angina since this time. She has diet-controlled diabetes and is treated for hypertension. Mrs McDonald smoked 30 cigarettes per day until the age of 70, after

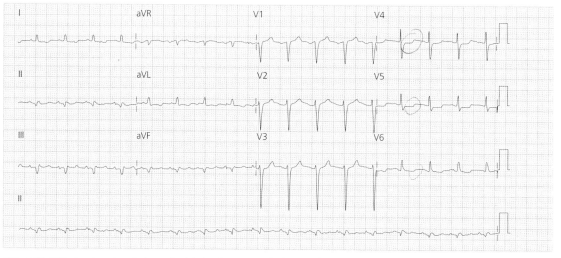

Figure 31 ECG showing sinus tachycardia, inferior Q-waves and minor ST depression in leads V4–V6. There is also evidence of T-wave inversion in the lateral leads (I, AVL, V5, V6).

which she cut down to around five per day. She has not smoked for the past month.

Mrs McDonald's current medication is as follows: aspirin 70 mg daily; ramipril 2.5 mg daily; atenolol 25 mg daily; simvastatin 40 mg daily; furosemide 40 mg daily (prescribed two weeks ago but not taken for the past week); glyceryl trinitrate (GTN) spray and salbutamol inhaler as required. Mrs McDonald has no known allergies.

On examination Mrs McDonald appears overweight (approx 100 kg). Examination of her lungs reveals coarse bibasal crackles and widespread expiratory wheeze. Mrs McDonald's jugular venous pulsation is not visible because of her obesity, and there is bilateral pitting ankle oedema. There are no heart murmurs. Abdominal and central nervous system examination is unremarkable.

What is/are the likely cause(s) of Mrs McDonald's breathlessness?

Table 36 lists some of the common causes of breathlessness and their presenting symptoms/signs. A patient in this age group may have more than one cause for breathlessness, so it is essential to keep an open mind.

In this case the differential would be as follows.

Pulmonary oedema/acute left ventricular failure
- The past history of ischaemic heart disease may suggest some underlying congestive cardiac failure, which would be supported by the history of increasing breathlessness on exertion with orthopnoea and improvement with furosemide
- The history of sudden worsening in the early hours of the morning is also typical of acute left ventricular failure. It is important to consider an acute cardiac event (e.g. myocardial infarction or arrhythmia) as the cause for the sudden worsening in symptoms
- The examination finding of bibasal crackles and ankle oedema supports this diagnosis, although these are non-specific findings in this age group
- Expiratory wheeze is also sometimes a sign of pulmonary oedema (often termed cardiac asthma)

Exacerbation of chronic obstructive airways disease
- As a lifelong smoker Mrs McDonald will be at risk of COPD, although there has been no formal diagnosis of this in the past. This can also manifest with worsening shortness of breath, and patients with COPD also often complain that lying flat exacerbates their breathlessness. Wheeze and expectoration also support this diagnosis
- The recent change in colour of Mrs McDonald's sputum may suggest infection as a cause for the exacerbation. The sudden increase in symptoms overnight may

have resulted from acute bronchospasm, sputum plugging or pneumothorax
- The ankle oedema may reflect right heart failure resulting from raised intrapulmonary pressure (cor pulmonale), which often complicates COPD

Community-acquired pneumonia
- Although the gradual worsening of symptoms is suggestive of a more chronic problem, there has been a clear-cut worsening in the past few days that coincides with a change in colour of Mrs McDonald's sputum
- Infection may also explain the combination of tachycardia and relative hypotension, and does not always produce pyrexia, particularly in patients of this age group
- Pneumonia could also have caused decompensation of cardiac failure resulting in acute pulmonary oedema

Pulmonary embolism
- Multiple pulmonary emboli (PE) occurring over a long period may result in gradually worsening shortness of breath. This is not uncommon in older patients, particularly if they are relatively immobile and overweight as in this case
- Multiple PE could also account for the elevated jugular venous pressure (JVP) and ankle oedema, due to right heart strain
- Bibasal coarse crackles may reflect pleural 'rub' resulting from pulmonary infarction and subsequent inflammation of the pleura, although this is normally associated with pleuritic type chest pain (see Case 2)
- Alternatively, a PE could have complicated one of the above conditions as a result of immobility resulting from her recent breathlessness

Anaemia
- Although not likely to be the sole cause for this patient's symptoms, Mrs McDonald's low haemoglobin (98 mg/L on arterial sample) may be contributing to her breathlessness
- Anaemia may also precipitate cardiac failure. The finding of anaemia should also raise suspicions about other potentially serious underlying pathology (e.g. renal impairment or blood loss from undiagnosed gastrointestinal malignancy)

What further investigations may be helpful?

- Blood tests: suggested blood tests, along with their justification and interpretation, are listed in Table 37
- Repeat arterial blood gases (after Mrs McDonald has been on oxygen for around 30 min to ensure that there is no rise in her CO_2 level, given the possibility of previous COPD)

Table 36 Common causes of acute shortness of breath presenting on the acute medical take

Cause	Symptoms	Signs	Comments
Acute pulmonary oedema	Typically starts in early morning/when lying flat May be prior history of ischaemic heart disease/MI May describe orthopnoea/PND in build-up to onset Cough productive of thin' frothy' sputum Examination findings	Coarse bibasal crackles: often both inspiratory and expiratory May be expiratory wheeze Elevated JVP/ankle oedema	May coexist with other pathologies
Acute asthma	May be prior history of asthma or previous admissions	Prolonged expiratory phase with expiratory wheeze (may disappear as symptoms become more severe)	See Case 5
Exacerbation of COPD	Usually prior history of smoking or similar hospital admissions Productive cough (sputum not necessarily purulent)	Globally reduced breath sounds; hyperinflated lungs; expiratory wheeze May be evidence of right heart failure (raised JVP/ankle swelling)	See Case 6
Community-acquired pneumonia	General malaise and fever; productive cough; sometime pleuritic chest pain	Pyrexia Signs of pulmonary consolidation	
Pulmonary embolism	May be co-existent pleuritic chest pain and haemoptysis Risk factors for thromboembolic disease	Tachycardia May be pleural rub; more commonly chest sounds clear Signs of DVT (in approximately 20%)	See Case 2
Spontaneous pneumothorax	Abrupt onset; usually with associated pleuritic chest pain Usually tall, thin stature	Reduced breath sounds and hyper-resonance on affected side	May complicate asthma or COPD/emphysema
Metabolic acidosis	Deep, sighing respiration (Kussmaul breathing) Symptoms of underlying pathology (e.g. sepsis, diabetic coma, renal failure)	Normal oxygen saturation (unless co-existent pulmonary disease)	See Case 18
Hyperventilation	Episodic breathlessness, often occurring at rest and not associated with exertion Dry mouth, light-headedness, paraesthesia in hands, feet and around mouth May be history of anxiety or other neurosis	Oxygen saturation normal and lung fields clear Sinus tachycardia and other features of anxiety (sweating, etc.)	

COPD, chronic obstructive pulmonary disease; DVT, deep vein thrombosis; JVP, jugular venous pressure; MI, myocardial infarction; PND, paroxysmal nocturnal dyspnoea.

Table 37 Suggested blood tests for an older patient presenting with breathlessness

Test	Justification	Comments
Full blood count	Anaemia may cause/exacerbate breathlessness Raised white cell count suggestive of infection Neutropenia may be associated with more severe infection	Neutrophilia may be seen in any acute physiological response – not specific to infection
Urea and electrolytes	Renal impairment may cause fluid overload or may complicate treatment Hyponatraemia/hypokalaemia common in elderly patients, particularly if taking diuretic drugs	Chronic renal impairment is common in older patients; comparison with previous blood test results is important
Liver function tests	Hypoalbuminaemia associated with sepsis; abnormalities of liver enzymes or raised bilirubin may suggest co-morbidity	
C-reactive protein	Usually raised in bacterial infection	Should not be interpreted in isolation as non-specific: elevation is also associated with pulmonary infarction and other inflammatory disorders
Troponin I or T	Myocardial infarction may precipitate pulmonary oedema	Peak not seen until 10–12 h after a cardiac event; may be necessary to delay blood sampling for troponin or repeat later Modest elevations may be seen in association with pulmonary embolism, following arrhythmia and in other serious illness
Thyroid function	Hyper- or hypothyroidism may precipitate heart failure	Thyroid disease may be difficult to diagnose clinically in elderly patients; symptoms may be non-specific (breathlessness, confusion, weight loss, etc.)

- Chest radiograph

  A high-quality chest radiograph may provide diagnostic information in this scenario. Specifically the chest radiograph should enable:
  - exclusion/diagnosis of pneumothorax
  - diagnosis of lobar consolidation or collapse
  - measurement of the cardiac size: enlarged in the context of congestive cardiac failure (but see below)
  - identification of evidence of pulmonary oedema: upper lobe venous diversion, interstitial shadowing, fluid in the horizontal fissure and septal lines ('Kerly B-lines')

    However, there are a number of caveats.
  - the patient may be too unstable to move to the radiology department. A portable chest radiograph on the ward will be of lower quality and therefore of more limited use
  - if the patient is still very breathless and confused the patient may not be able to take and hold an adequate inspiration, again reducing the quality of the film
  - most patients undergoing chest radiography in the acute setting will have the film taken from in front (anteroposterior, AP, projection) rather than the preferable posteroanterior (PA) projection. This will tend to magnify the size of the heart and result in the scapulae overlying the lung fields
  - Mrs McDonald is quite overweight; soft tissue shadowing may mimic the appearances of pulmonary oedema and complicate the interpretation of the appearances
  - chest radiograph may be normal in patients with exacerbations of COPD and pulmonary embolism

Venous blood has been sent to the laboratory as above, and a chest radiograph has been requested; however, there is likely to be an approximately 1 h delay before the radiograph is carried out because of a backlog in the radiography department. Although Mrs McDonald's condition has not deteriorated and she is maintaining her oxygen saturation at 94% with 3 L oxygen via nasal specs, she remains noticeably breathless and distressed.

The repeat arterial blood gases are as follows: pH 7.29, pCO_2 5.1, pO_2 9.9, HCO_3 19, base excess –4.2, lactate 2.9.

Mrs McDonald's daughter asks if anything can be done to make her more comfortable while awaiting the radiograph.

Should treatment be started before a radiograph is available?

Although it is always preferable to obtain diagnostic information before starting treatment, delays are not uncommon in the clinical setting. The rise in Mrs McDonald's pCO_2 is probably a reflection of her tiring and this, combined with the rise in her lactate, probably accounts for the fall in Mrs McDonald's pH (uncompensated metabolic acidosis). Treatment should therefore not be delayed in this case. Commencing treatment may also make the patient more stable for transfer and improve the quality of the radiograph obtained.

In this case pulmonary oedema seems the most likely cause of the patient's symptoms; in addition, the patient is wheezy and may have some underlying COPD with bronchospasm.

It would be reasonable to administer the following:
- intravenous diuretic, e.g. furosemide 40 mg
- nebulised bronchodilator, e.g. salbutamol 2.5 mg combined with ipratropium bromide 500 µg (assuming Mrs McDonald will now tolerate a mask)

Following administration of the treatments Mrs McDonald's condition appears to stabilise. Her respiratory rate slows to 16/min although her pulse remains >100/min. Oxygen saturation now reads 96%. Mrs McDonald passes 200 mL of urine into a catheter bag over the next hour but her blood pressure remains stable at 120/60. Examination of Mrs McDonald's chest reveals that the wheeze has gone although there are still bibasal crackles.

The chest radiograph shows appearances consistent with pulmonary oedema, although interpretation is complicated by the presence of overlying soft tissue shadowing. The cardiac size also appears to be enlarged (see Fig. 32).

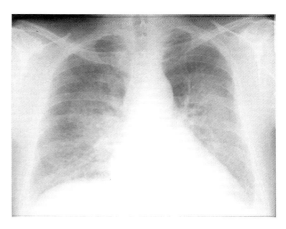

Figure 32 Chest radiograph.

Blood results are now available and are as follows:
- *haemoglobin 96, white blood cells 14.5 (neutrophils 12.1), platelets 195, mean corpuscular volume 88*
- *Na 134, K 3.9, urea 12.7, creatinine 140*
- *C-reactive protein (CRP) 37*
- *troponin I <0.15 (taken 6 h after acute deterioration during the night)*
- *thyroid function normal*
- *liver function tests normal*

How should the results be interpreted?

- The chest radiograph appearance supports the clinical diagnosis of pulmonary oedema as the predominant pathology. This does not exclude co-existent COPD or infection. Pulmonary embolism appears less likely given the improvement in Mrs McDonald's condition following diuretic and bronchodilator treatment
- Mrs McDonald has a normocytic anaemia and renal impairment; both of these may be chronic. The renal impairment may have been exacerbated by the recent diuretic treatment prior to admission and will need to be monitored closely during Mrs McDonald's hospital stay, particularly if she is going to be treated with further diuretic. It is important to try to obtain previous blood test results for comparison (from either the hospital database or the GP)
- The neutrophil count is elevated: although this is often seen in association with infection, any acute physiological stress may result in elevation of the neutrophil count. The C-reactive protein is slightly elevated, which may reflect infection or some other acute inflammatory process
- The troponin level is normal but may continue to rise for about 12 h following a myocardial infarction. It

would be worth repeating this test later in the day to assess whether it has risen further. A repeat ECG should also be undertaken

What further treatment and monitoring are required?

• **Commence an infusion of glyceryl trinitrate (GTN):** this acts as a vasodilator, which reduces the 'preload' on the heart, reducing pulmonary oedema

A total of 50 mg of GTN is mixed with 48 mL of normal saline and administered via a syringe driver. An initial infusion rate of 1 mL/h (i.e. 1 mg) is usual. The GTN will tend to lower the systemic blood pressure, which should be measured every 10–15 min, aiming to maintain the systolic pressure at >90 mmHg. The dose should be increased to a maximum of 10 mg/h if tolerated. Cranial vasodilatation often results in a headache that may require analgesia (avoid non-steroidal anti-inflammatory drugs (NSAIDs) as these may cause fluid retention, exacerbating pulmonary oedema)

• **Prescribe a further daily dose of furosemide** (e.g. 40 mg once daily, oral or i.v.). The renal function will need to be monitored daily, and if deteriorating on this treatment, the furosemide may need to be withheld

• **Prescribe an appropriate antibiotic**: it remains possible that respiratory infection was the precipitant for Mrs McDonald's deterioration and this is supported by the raised neutrophil count and CRP. Remember that this age group is at particularly high risk of *Clostridium difficile* infection after broad-spectrum antibiotic use (especially with cephalosporins) – use a narrow-spectrum antibiotic such as amoxicillin 500 mg tds orally (or doxycycline 200 mg daily if the patient is allergic to penicillin)

• **Prescribe a salbutamol nebuliser** to be given if required. Although the wheeze may have been related to pulmonary oedema there may be co-existent broncho-spasm. Remember that salbutamol may exacerbate tachy-cardia, which may reduce cardiac output; therefore, keep the dose low (2.5 mg rather than 5 mg) and infrequent (maximum 4 hourly)

• **Prescribe thromboprophylaxis**. Although PE is considered an unlikely cause of Mrs McDonald's acute presentation she will be at high risk of deep vein thrombosis (DVT) and subsequent PE during admission in view of her immobility, obesity and cardiac failure. Subcutaneous heparin (e.g. enoxaparin 40 mg daily) and thromboembolic disease (TED) stockings should be prescribed in the absence of contraindications

• **Withhold atenolo**l: although beta-blockers may be beneficial in chronic heart failure they may exacerbate acute pulmonary oedema and also worsen broncho-spasm. Remember other drugs that may exacerbate pulmonary oedema, including NSAIDs and thioglitazones (used in treatment of diabetes)

• **Keep the patient on a cardiac monitor** and maintain continuous pulse oximetry

Mrs McDonald commences a GTN infusion and manages to tolerate an infusion rate of 3 mg/h. Mrs McDonald is also prescribed oral amoxicillin and salbutamol nebulisers as required, along with a prophylactic dose of enoxaparin and TED stockings. A repeat troponin level later that day remains normal and Mrs McDonald's ECG is unchanged. Mrs McDonald is monitored in an observation bed in the medical admissions unit.

Two hours later you are called back to the ward to review Mrs McDonald, because her condition has suddenly deteriorated. Her oxygen saturation has dropped to 86% and her respiratory rate has increased to 30/min. Mrs McDonald's blood pressure is 90/50. The nurses report that her breathing sounds 'bubbly'. She has just completed a 2.5 mg salbutamol nebuliser with no effect. Mrs McDonald is awake, but more drowsy than before and remains confused. She is expectorating thin frothy sputum and clinical examination now reveals coarse crackles throughout both lung fields with minimal wheeze. A repeat ECG shows sinus tachycardia but no other new changes.

You ask the nurses to administer a further intravenous dose of furosemide – this time 80 mg.

Mrs McDonald's family have been called into the ward and are currently sitting in the relatives' room.

What is the cause of Mrs McDonald's deterioration and what further treatment is required?

• The symptoms and signs are again consistent with acute pulmonary oedema, which has recurred despite the fairly intensive therapy Mrs McDonald is receiving

• Positive pressure ventilation, e.g. continuous positive airway pressure (CPAP), may be beneficial in reducing pulmonary oedema; however, this requires a tightly fitting mask and Mrs McDonald may struggle to tolerate this given her earlier intolerance of an oxygen mask and ongoing confusion

• It is worth considering whether there may be a reversible cause for the cardiac failure (e.g. cardiac tamponade from pericardial effusion, or acute valvular rupture); an urgent echocardiogram should be requested

• A small dose of morphine (or diamorphine) may be worthwhile: this acts in part as a vasodilator (adding to the effects of the GTN) and also reduces the distress that the symptoms of acute pulmonary oedema often produce

• Discussion with her family about the appropriateness of further escalation of treatment should be considered at this point

The further dose of furosemide produces little improvement in Mrs McDonald's condition but she appears more settled following the administration of 2.5 mg of morphine sulphate intravenously. Mrs McDonald's respiratory rate is now 25/ min and saturation 90% on high-flow oxygen via a mask. The on-call cardiology registrar attends and performs an echocardiogram on the ward, which reveals poor left ventricular function with no regional wall abnormalities, no valvular abnormality and no significant pericardial effusion.

You talk to Mrs McDonald's husband and daughter and explain the current situation, describing the sudden build-up of fluid on Mrs McDonald's lungs resulting from chronic weakness of the heart, perhaps exacerbated by a recent chest infection. You explain that the long-term outlook is

poor and so far Mrs McDonald is not responding to treatment. Although Mrs McDonald has not signed a formal living will her daughter says that she has previously expressed a wish not to be resuscitated in the event of a cardiac arrest, and feels that Mrs McDonald would not want to be ventilated in intensive care.

You agree with the family that you will conduct a trial of non-invasive CPAP on the ward, but that Mrs McDonald's treatment will not be escalated beyond this.

Mrs McDonald commences CPAP, which she tolerates surprisingly well. After one hour her chest sounds much clearer. The CPAP and GTN are continued for 24 h. Mrs McDonald remains in hospital for a total of 10 days, during which she starts taking regular oral furosemide, and the dose of her ramipril is increased to 5 mg daily. A small dose of bisoprolol (2.5 mg daily) is introduced and does not cause any significant bronchospasm. Mrs McDonald's renal function remains unchanged and iron studies reveal no evidence of iron deficiency to account for the anaemia, which is attributed to her chronic renal impairment. Mrs McDonald continues to take aspirin and simvastatin at the same doses as on admission.

At the time of discharge Mrs McDonald is able to walk unaided on the flat but as she cannot manage stairs some modifications are required at home to enable her to sleep downstairs.

CASE REVIEW

An 86-year-old woman with a past history of myocardial infarction and possible smoking-induced chronic lung disease is referred to hospital after a sudden worsening of her breathlessness the previous night. Mrs Margaret McDonald has been getting increasingly breathless for the past few months and has noticed that this is worsened by lying flat. Recently she has also started to expectorate yellow sputum. On arrival in hospital Mrs McDonald is noted to be hypoxic, agitated and confused. Initially she does not tolerate oxygen by mask, which is therefore administered by nasal specs. Chest examination reveals a combination of bibasal crackles and widespread expiratory wheeze.

A provisional diagnosis of pulmonary oedema complicating pre-existing congestive cardiac failure and COPD is made. Mrs McDonald is given a combination of furosemide 40 mg i.v. and nebulised salbutamol, which produces some initial improvement. A chest radiograph

supports the diagnosis of pulmonary oedema, and inflammatory markers and white cell count are slightly elevated suggesting co-existent respiratory infection. ECG and troponin reveal no evidence of acute myocardial infarction as a cause for Mrs McDonald's admission.

Treatment with an intravenous GTN infusion is commenced, along with oral amoxicillin and regular daily furosemide. However, 2 h later Mrs McDonald's condition deteriorates dramatically with recurrence of acute pulmonary oedema. Following discussion with Mrs McDonald's family it is agreed to try CPAP but not to escalate her treatment further. Mrs McDonald makes a dramatic response to this treatment, and she is weaned off CPAP and GTN over the next 24 h. Mrs McDonald stays in hospital for a total of 10 days before being discharged on a combination of ramipril, bisoprolol, furosemide, aspirin and simvastatin.

KEY POINTS

- Older people with breathlessness present difficult diagnostic challenges to the admitting team.
- Combinations of several causes of breathlessness should be considered, although there is usually a predominant problem that has precipitated admission.
- A variety of treatment options are available for the treatment of pulmonary oedema.

- If initial therapy with a diuretic fails to resolve the symptoms, an infusion of GTN is often effective for symptom control by reducing the cardiac preload.
- CPAP is often highly effective in treatment of pulmonary oedema in the acute setting.

Further reading

Cooper N, Forrest K, Mulley G. *ABC of geriatric medicine*. Blackwell Publishing, Oxford, 2008

ESC guidelines for the diagnosis and treatment of acute heart failure (2008). http://www.escardio.org/guidelines-surveys

Gehlbach BK, Geppert E. The pulmonary manifestations of left heart failure. *Chest* 2004; **125**: 669–82

PART 2: CASES

You are called by a GP who has just seen a patient at home. Mr Geoffrey Field is a 68-year-old man with a past history of ischaemic heart disease and hypertension. Mr Field has been unwell for about 48 h with a productive cough and has become gradually short of breath. This morning Mr Field was dizzy and fell. The GP is concerned that Mr Field looks unwell and has a high respiratory rate with a blood pressure of 85/50. He is concerned that Mr Field may be 'shocked'.

What is meant by a 'shocked' patient?

• The term *shock* can cause confusion because of frequent use by the lay press to indicate a psychological state induced by a traumatic event
• In medical terminology, shock implies a state of inadequate perfusion of the vital organs with blood
• It is important to realise that a low blood pressure alone does not necessarily indicate a shocked state: for some patients a systolic blood pressure of 85 mmHg may be entirely normal and result in adequate perfusion of all organs
• Conversely, a person who is normally hypertensive may be shocked with a relatively 'good' blood pressure
• From a practical perspective, we can assess the perfusion of three main organs
    ○ perfusion of the brain can be assessed by monitoring conscious level
    ○ perfusion of the renal system can be assessed by monitoring the urine output
    ○ perfusion of the skin can be assessed by measuring capillary refill time (normally less than 2 s)
The physiological principles behind shock are summarised in Box 14.

Mr Field arrives in the medical assessment unit. The admitting nurse calls you over because she is very concerned about Mr Field. Mr Field is able to tell you that he feels very unwell. He has a respiratory rate of 35 and is pale and

---

Acute Medicine: Clinical Cases Uncovered. By C. Roseveare.
Published 2009 by Blackwell Publishing, ISBN: 978-1-4051-6883-0

clammy. His tympanic temperature is 38.8°C. Mr Field's blood pressure is 85/50 and his pulse rate is 120, with a capillary refill time of 4 s. Mr Field's oxygen saturation on air is 85%

What immediate management is required?

Shocked patients can be extremely unwell and unstable. Systematic assessment of the airway, breathing and circulation provides a useful starting point.
• **Check patency of the airway**: if Mr Field is talking it is unlikely to be compromised but it may be at risk if his conscious level deteriorates. Certain infections such as epiglottitis and tracheitis may compromise the airway directly; listen carefully for evidence of stridor (a harsh inspiratory noise)
• **Check respiratory rate**: a rising respiratory rate is a sign of more severe illness, whereas a falling rate may indicate fatigue
• **Measure oxygen saturation**, although this may be unreliable if the tissue perfusion is poor: apply appropriate levels of oxygen to correct hypoxia
• **Repeat measurement of blood pressure and pulse rate**
• **Examine the jugular venous pulsation** to determine fluid status
• **Assess conscious level** using the Glasgow Coma Score (GCS) (p. 127)
• **Ensure that adequate intravenous access is maintained**: insert the largest bore cannula that the peripheral circulation will permit and commence intravenous fluid resuscitation using crystalloid (e.g. normal saline) or colloid (e.g. gelofusine)
• **Send blood to the laboratory** for full blood count (FBC), urea and electrolytes (U&E), blood cultures, liver function test (LFT), clotting profile
• **Obtain an arterial blood gas sample**: this provides an accurate measure of oxygenation and also may enable measurement of lactate and acid–base status, which are useful predictors of prognosis

> ### Box 14 Physiology of blood pressure
>
> To appreciate the different causes of shock, it is necessary to understand what determines blood pressure (BP).
>
> In its simplest form the blood pressure is determined by the following equation:
>
> BP = CO (cardiac output) × SVR (systemic vascular resistance)
>
> Cardiac output can be further defined as:
>
> CO = SV (stroke volume) × HR (heart rate)
>
> In some cases shock results from reduction of cardiac output, through failure of the heart muscle to pump fluid (cardiogenic shock) or reduced fluid volume (hypovolaemic shock); for other causes the problem may be reduction of SVR (septic shock, anaphylactic shock). Understanding the physiology may help to understand the physical signs associated with the different causes of shock, summarised in Table 38.

• **Insert a urinary catheter** with the ability to measure the urine output hourly
• **Send a urine sample for culture**
• **Obtain an ECG and request a chest radiograph**

Mr Field's airway is not compromised and there is no stridor but he remains hypotensive and tachycardic. He is now receiving 15 L/min oxygen via a rebreath mask and his oxygen saturation is reading 94%. Mr Field appears less breathless, although his respiratory rate remains high at 30 breaths/min. A jugular venous pulse is not visible. The GCS is 14/15 (eyes open to command). Mr Field has a 16 guage (grey) cannula in situ and 500 mL of normal saline is infused over 30 min after which his blood pressure has risen to 95/40.

Arterial blood gas analysis reveals pH 7.33, pCO₂ 5.5, pO₂ 8.3, base excess −4.5, lactate 3.7 (normal <1.5).

A urinary catheter is inserted and 50 mL of residual concentrated urine is drained. A sample is sent for culture.

The ECG reveals sinus tachycardia (see Fig. 33).

The patient is exhibiting features of shock with evidence of poor organ perfusion as indicated by:
• Reduced conscious level
• Poor skin perfusion
• Low urine output
• Raised lactate and base deficit

What further management is necessary?
• Initial resuscitative measures are now under way and Mr Field is starting to show signs of improvement with a reduction in the respiratory rate, improved oxygenation and a rise in blood pressure
• It is now important to obtain further information from history, examination and investigations, in order to try to determine the cause. This will help to guide further treatment

Mr Field tells you that he has felt unwell for the last few days and has been feverish intermittently. He has felt quite nauseated and has not been drinking too well. Mr Field has been coughing up green sputum and has become very short of breath. For the last few hours he has been feeling dizzy and light-headed. Mr Field tells you that he has had two heart attacks in the past, and his exercise tolerance is normally limited to around half a mile. On examination there are coarse crepitations and bronchial breathing in the middle and upper zones of the right hemithorax.

Blood tests reveal raised white cell count (19.5/mm, neutrophils 12.7); C-reactive protein (CRP) is elevated at 299 (normal <6); renal function is deranged: urea 12.5, creatinine 135; albumin is low (29); international normalised ratio (INR) is slightly elevated at 1.4, with activated partial thromboplastin ratio (APTR) 1.3; platelets are slightly reduced at 110.

A chest radiograph reveals consolidation of the right upper lobe (see Fig. 34).

What is the cause of the shock?
Common causes of shock are listed in Table 38.

In this case the most likely cause is septic shock precipitated by a right upper lobe pneumonia, as evidenced by:
• Pyrexia, tachycardia and low jugular venous pressure
• Symptoms of productive cough preceding onset of shock
• Clinical signs in left lung, confirmed by radiograph findings
• Raised white cell count and CRP

What is the significance of the other abnormal blood test results?
• Low serum albumin level is common in patients with sepsis
• Mr Field's renal function is impaired: this may simply relate to poor renal perfusion or pre-existing disease

Table 38 Common causes of shock

Classification	Specific cause	Physiology	Symptoms/signs
Hypovolaemic shock	Dehydration Acute blood loss Burns	Reduced cardiac output due to reduced circulating volume	May be symptoms of fluid loss (e.g. diarrhoea, vomiting, haematemesis, melaena) Cold peripherae; weak, thready pulse Low JVP Skin pallor (especially with blood loss); dry mucous membranes
Cardiogenic shock	Myocardial infarction Cardiac arrhythmia	Reduced cardiac output due to reduced stroke volume or reduced filling time in diastole	Chest pain, palpitations, history of ischaemic heart disease or previous arrhythmia Cold, sweaty peripherae; weak pulse; JVP raised. Tachycardia >150 beats/min suggests arrhythmia (see Cases 3&4); pulmonary oedema
Septic shock	Any severe infection, e.g. pneumonia, meningococcus, Gram-negative septicaemia	Reduced SVR causing reduced blood pressure	Symptoms of underlying infection preceding collapse. Exposure to severe infection (e.g. meningococcus) Warm peripherae, bounding pulse with low diastolic pressure; low JVP. Pyrexia (or hypothermia) Signs of underlying infection
Anaphylactic shock	Severe allergy to drug or other allergen: bite, sting or food, especially nuts	Reduced SVR causing reduced blood pressure	Previous anaphylaxis or exposure to potential allergen (e.g. new drug, insect bite, etc.); itching, rash and SOB preceding onset of collapse Urticarial rash, wheeze; low JVP; low diastolic blood pressure

JVP, jugular venous pulse; SOB, shortness of breath; SVR, systemic vascular resistance.

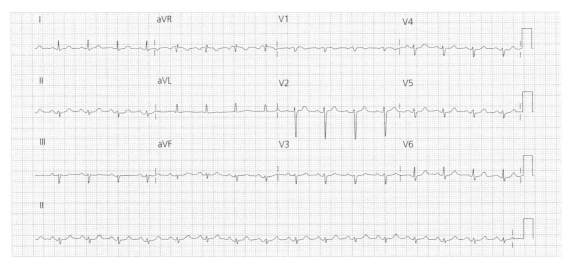

Figure 33 ECG showing sinus tachycardia. The R waves are small in the anterior leads (v2–v4) which may indicate previous myocardial infarction. There are no other acute changes.

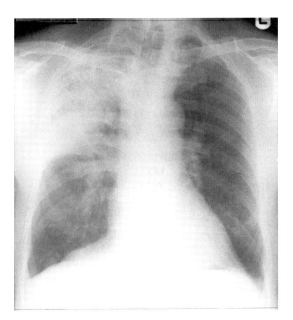

Figure 34 Chest radiograph showing right upper lobe consolidation.

• The blood clotting abnormality may suggest the development of early disseminated intravascular coagulation (DIC), where clotting factors and platelets are consumed by clot formation in the peripheral circulation. This is a poor prognostic sign in patients with septic shock

How will you manage Mr Field?

Initial management of septic shock is vital. If the basics are done well, then deterioration of the patient may be prevented.

Fluid management

• Optimising preload to the heart is the first priority
• This will be achieved by giving boluses of fluid and assessing their impact on blood pressure and signs of poor perfusion
• Large amounts of fluid may be needed
• In younger patients with no cardiovascular disease administration of large volumes of fluid will not normally cause complications
• In older patients with cardiovascular or renal disease, fluid management can be more difficult
• Insertion of a central venous cannula may be helpful in assessing the fluid status of the patient by measuring the central venous pressure (CVP)

• If a patient is adequately filled with fluid, then their CVP should rise and stay elevated following a fluid challenge
• If the CVP either doesn't rise or rises transiently and then falls, this indicates the patient is 'under-filled' and the fluid challenge should be repeated
• The aim of the fluid management is to achieve a blood pressure which is adequate to perfuse the internal organs such as the brain and the kidneys. Hourly measurement of urine output will give a good guide to renal perfusion
• If fluid status has been optimised but the blood pressure or end organ perfusion remains compromised, this is an indication for inotropic/vasopressor support (see below)

Antibiotics

• Early administration of intravenous antibiotics should be the aim, alongside fluid resuscitation
• Blood cultures should be taken *before* the antibiotics are given, as this will maximise the potential of a positive result
• Antibiotic therapy should be targeted at the most likely source of infection
• Antibiotic guidelines vary from hospital to hospital, and you should be familiar with the local policy

The 'surviving sepsis' campaign has produced guidelines (termed sepsis resuscitation bundles) designed to improve outcomes in patients with septic shock. These are summarised in Box 15.

Mr Field is being treated in an observation bed on the acute admissions ward. A central venous cannula has been inserted and Mr Field has received 3 L of intravenous fluid since his arrival on the ward two hours ago. Mr Field was given 1.5 g of cefuroxime and 500 mg of clarithromycin intravenously in accordance with the hospital's antibiotic prescribing policy for severe community-acquired pneumonia. Despite this treatment Mr Field's blood pressure remains low at 80/50. He remains tachycardic (pulse 100) and tachypnoeic (respiratory rate 30 breaths/min) with oxygen saturation of 96% on 15 L of oxygen via a rebreath mask. Mr Field's conscious level has not changed. His CVP is now 12, and rises to 20 following a further 500 mL of fluid challenge. Mr Field has passed 15 mL of concentrated urine in the past two hours.

Repeat arterial blood gas reveals pH 7.28, pCO_2 5.9, pO_2 9.9, base excess −7.5, lactate 5.9 mmol/L.

PART 2: CASES

Box 15 The 'Surviving Sepsis' Resuscitation Care Bundle

Surviving Sepsis Campaign

This is an international campaign to try and improve outcomes in sepsis

It has an excellent website which discusses the management of sepsis in depth (www.survivingsepsis.org)

A helpful guide to the initial management of sepsis is the 'Sepsis Resuscitation Bundle'

This consists of five elements

Element 1

Serum lactate to be measured: most acute units have access to a near patient analyser, which enables measurement of lactate on a venous or arterial sample

Serum lactate of >4 mmol/L indicates poor tissue perfusion

Element 2

Obtain blood cultures prior to antibiotic administration

Element 3

Administer broad-spectrum antibiotics within three hours of admission to hospital

Element 4

If lactate >4 mmol/L, or patient is hypotensive then deliver an initial 20 mL/kg of crystalloid or equivalent

Apply vasopressors for hypotension not responding to initial fluid resuscitation to maintain a mean arterial pressure of >65 mmHg

Element 5

In the event of persistent hypotension despite fluid resuscitation (septic shock) and/or lactate of >4 then achieve a CVP of >8 mmHg

Achieve a central venous oxygen saturation of >70%, or a mixed venous oxygen saturation of >65%

How and where should Mr Field now be managed?

- Mr Field's condition has deteriorated, despite aggressive fluid resuscitation and administration of appropriate antibiotics
- Mr Field now appears to be adequately filled with fluid (as evidenced by a sustained rise in CVP following fluid challenge), but blood pressure and urine output remain low, indicating continued poor organ perfusion
- Mr Field is likely to require drug therapy with drugs designed to produce peripheral vasoconstriction (vasopressor drugs). This will increase his blood pressure by increasing systemic vascular resistance (see Box 14); however, Mr Field will require very close monitoring
- Mr Field's rising lactate, falling pH and base excess and failure to respond to initial fluid resuscitation place him in a poor prognostic group: mortality rate in this situation is >50%
- Urgent involvement of the critical care team should be requested: this patient is likely to require transfer to the intensive care or high dependency unit for further care

The intensive care team arrives on the medical assessment unit. They agree with your assessment and feel that Mr Field would be best managed on the HDU with vasopressor support. Mr Field is transferred. Over the next few days his condition slowly improves. Mr Field's blood cultures grow Streptococcus pneumoniae sensitive to penicillin. Mr Field's antibiotic therapy is changed to benzylpenicillin 1.2 g four times daily. His vasopressor support is weaned off and he is returned to a general medical ward. Ten days after Mr Field's admission he is discharged home having made a full recovery. Follow up chest x-ray six weeks later is entirely normal.

CASE REVIEW

A 68-year-old man is admitted with a two-day history of worsening breathlessness, a productive cough and fever. On the morning prior to Mr Geoffrey Field's admission he had deteriorated significantly, and become dizzy on standing and unsteady on his feet. On presentation Mr Field displays signs of septic shock. He is tachypnoeic, tachycardic and hypotensive. Mr Field has a fever and is coughing up green sputum. Examination reveals signs of right upper lobe consolidation, which is confirmed on a chest radiograph.

Mr Field responds to initial fluid resuscitation, with an improvement in his clinical state. Cultures of blood and sputum are taken and Mr Field starts broad-spectrum intravenous antibiotics. Following an initial improvement, Mr Field deteriorates further. Arterial blood gases reveal him to have a significant metabolic acidosis with a lactate level of 5 mmol/L. Despite optimal fluid management with the aid of a central venous cannula, Mr Field remains hypotensive with evidence of inadequate end organ perfusion. He is transferred to the HDU for vasopressor therapy, where his condition stabilises and then gradually improves. The causative organism is cultured from sputum and blood, and Mr Field's antibiotic regime is altered accordingly. He makes a full recovery and is discharged home.

This case illustrates that the patient presenting with septic shock requires rapid assessment and treatment. The prompt use of broad-spectrum intravenous antibiotics in addition to appropriate fluid resuscitation is the key to stabilising the patient. Even if this is all done quickly and appropriately a proportion of patients will deteriorate and require high dependency or intensive care. Mortality rates remain high. Early senior review and involvement of the critical care team in the patient's management are essential to optimise the outcome.

KEY POINTS

- Rapid initial assessment of a shocked patient should use the ABC approach.
- Adequate fluid resuscitation is essential; central venous cannulation will enable accurate titration of fluid requirements.
- Careful clinical evaluation should enable distinction of the major causes of shock.

- Rapid administration of intravenous antibiotics is essential;. Use of the Surviving Sepsis Campaign Resuscitation Care Bundles may help to guide early management
- Early involvement of the critical care team and consideration of transfer to the HDU are essential if the patient's condition fails to improve following fluid resuscitation.

PART 2: CASES

Further reading

BTS Pneumonia Guidelines Committee. BTS guidelines for the management of community acquired pneumonia in adults – 2004 update. http://www.brit-thoracic.org.uk/Portals/0/Clinical%20Information/Pneumonia/Guidelines/MACAPrevisedApr04.pdf

Dellinger RP, Levy MM, Carlet JM *et al.* Surviving sepsis campaign: international guidelines for the management of severe sepsis and septic shock. *Crit Care Med* 2008; **36**: 296–327 (also surviving sepsis website http://www.survivingsepsis.org/node/156)

Case 9) A 55-year-old man with suspected upper gastrointestinal bleeding

You receive a call from a GP regarding a 55-year-old male patient. Mr Nick Gross has been experiencing upper abdominal pains after meals for some time, which have previously settled with antacids. Today Mr Gross attended the GP's emergency surgery and described two days of black, tarry stools. Mr Gross also vomited a small quantity of bright red blood this morning. According to the GP Mr Gross appears pale and is slightly tachycardic, although his blood pressure is normal at 135/70. There is mild epigastric tenderness. The GP has arranged for an ambulance to bring him directly to the acute medical unit.

What challenges will this patient present?

• Mr Gross has attended his GP's surgery giving a fairly classic history for upper gastrointestinal (GI) bleeding

• The stool, described as black and 'tarry', is the hallmark of melaena, resulting from the bacterial digestion of blood in the small bowel

• The presence of melaena usually suggests that a significant bleed has occurred. Co-existent haematemesis is further evidence that the origin of Mr Gross's bleeding is in the upper intestine

• Upper GI bleeding carries a significant mortality, up to 15% in some studies, although there is some evidence to suggest that appropriate management in a specialist unit can have a significant impact on this figure

• Upper GI bleeding has many causes, although peptic ulcer is the commonest cause of significant bleeding requiring hospital admission (see Table 39)

While en route to hospital Mr Gross's condition deteriorates. He has a further large haematemesis and the ambulance crew report that he became pale, sweaty and lost consciousness for a few seconds. The paramedic has

inserted an intravenous cannula and infused 500 mL of saline. On arrival on the ward Mr Gross remains pale and sweaty with a thready pulse at a rate of 120 beats/min. The blood pressure is measured at 80/40 mmHg. Mr Gross is conscious, alert and orientated, and is maintaining his airway with a respiratory rate of 14 breaths/min.

• Mr Gross is now exhibiting features consistent with hypovolaemic shock

• It is likely that he has sustained a further significant bleed

• Mr Gross requires **urgent fluid resuscitation**

• Acquisition of a detailed history and full examination should be deferred until Mr Gross's condition has been stabilised

What immediate management is required?

• **Ensure patency of the airway**: given that Mr Gross is awake and alert this should be safe for now; however, this should be kept under review – if Mr Gross continues to vomit and his conscious level falls, he will be at risk of aspiration, which is associated with a high mortality. Early senior or critical care review and intubation should always be considered

• **Apply high-flow oxygen** by mask

• **Check the patency of the cannula** inserted by the ambulance crew and insert another (12 or 14 gauge). Use the cannula to take blood for full blood count (FBC), urea and electrolytes (U&E), liver function tests (LFT), clotting and cross-match (4 units initially is adequate for most cases)

• **Commence intravenous resuscitation** with a further 500–1000 mL of 0.9% saline or Hartmann's solution by rapid infusion. Replace this with cross-matched blood as soon as this is available. For severely shocked patients it may be more appropriate to use group O-negative blood, which should be immediately available from the emer-

Acute Medicine: Clinical Cases Uncovered. By C. Roseveare.
Published 2009 by Blackwell Publishing, ISBN: 978-1-4051-6883-0

gency blood fridge. Alternatively, the laboratory should be able to provide group-specific blood without full cross-match within about 15 min

Further resuscitation will depend on the response to this treatment, but should include:

Table 39 Causes of acute upper gastrointestinal haemorrhage

Diagnosis	Approximate percentage
Peptic ulcer	35–50
Gastroduodenal erosions	8–15
Oesophagitis	5–15
Oesophageal varices	5–10
Mallory–Weiss tear	15
Upper gastrointestinal malignancy	1
Vascular malformations	5
Other	5

• **Regular review of blood pressure/pulse and fluid balance**: the volume of fluid required will vary from patient to patient. Ideally a blood pressure of >100 systolic and a pulse <100 beats/min should be achieved
• **A urinary catheter** will enable monitoring of urine output, which will help to guide fluid management
• **Consideration of central venous cannulation**. This will enable more accurate assessment of the volume of fluid required, which is particularly important for older patients, and for those with co-existent renal or cardiac failure (see Table 40)
• **ECG and chest radiograph** to exclude co-existent pulmonary or cardiac pathology. An abdominal radiograph is rarely required

Mr Gross's condition has improved after administration of 1 L of 0.9% saline over 30 min. His systolic blood pressure is now 110 with a pulse of 95 beats/min. A further 1000 mL of normal saline is prescribed to run over the next hour. Mr Gross has not vomited since his arrival in hospital.

The patient confirms the GP and ambulance history of tarry, offensive smelling black stools, followed by several

Table 40 Indications for insertion of a central venous pressure (CVP) line

Indication	Specific problems	Comments
To ensure adequate fluid resuscitation	Large volume bleed/ongoing bleeding Persistent hypotension/tachycardia	These patients have a significant mortality; central monitoring will give a more accurate guide to fluid requirements than measurement of blood pressure/pulse
Risk of fluid overload	Cardiac failure Renal failure Elderly patients	Overresuscitation is common in these patients and carries significant morbidity
Difficulties with fluid balance management	Suspected variceal bleeding Patients on beta-blockers	Overtransfusion of patients with bleeding varices can result in continued bleeding by refilling the bleeding vessel Beta-blockers and some other drugs can prevent tachycardia which hampers interpretation of the pulse rate
To ensure adequate venous access	For patients with poor peripheral venous access	Peripheral venous access is usually achievable and preferable for the infusion of large volumes of fluid. Occasionally CVP insertion may be required
As 'early warning' for rebleeding	Following endoscopy, where high risk of the patient having further bleeding has been identified	Drop in the CVP will usually precede the appearance of blood in vomit or stool and often implies further bleeding, which will require treatment

episodes of vomit containing bright red blood. Mr Gross estimates that he vomited around 500 mL in total.

Mr Gross has had no similar episodes in the past, but describes a long history of acid reflux relieved by antacids. Recently he has sustained a shoulder injury for which he has been taking ibuprofen 400 mg three times daily for three weeks. Over the past three days Mr Gross has developed upper abdominal pain. He is otherwise well and takes no other regular medication. Mr Gross drinks approximately 20 pints of beer per week and is a non-smoker. Examination reveals no stigmata of chronic liver disease and no evidence of portal hypertension. There is mild epigastric tenderness but no peritonism. A rectal examination reveals black, tarry stool with the characteristic pungent aroma of melaena.

While obtaining the history and conducting clinical examination, it is important to consider the questions below.

Is the suspicion of upper gastrointestinal bleeding correct?

Characteristic clinical features of upper GI bleeding are listed in Table 41.
• The combination of haematemesis and characteristic melaena stool is strongly supportive of an upper GI source for bleeding
• Some caveats are summarised in Box 16

How severe is the bleeding?

• The presence of melaena usually suggests a minimum of 250 mL of blood has entered the intestine
• The patient has estimated approximately 500 mL of blood in the vomit
• The presence of hypovolaemic shock is further evidence of a large volume bleed

What is the likely cause of the patient's bleeding?

• This patient has recently developed upper abdominal pain, suggesting the development of an ulcer
• Alcohol excess and the recent use of ibuprofen may have precipitated the development of a peptic ulcer

Could the patient be bleeding from oesophageal varices? (see Box 17)

• Although Mr Gross consumes large quantities of alcohol, there is no evidence of chronic liver disease or portal hypertension. The likelihood of oesophageal varices is therefore low

---

Box 16 Diagnostic dilemmas for the unwary

The coffee-ground vomit
Whereas fresh haematemesis has a distinctive bright or dark red colour, blood that has been 'altered' in the stomach is frequently described as 'coffee-ground' vomit. This terminology can be confusing. Gastric contents are frequently dark brown ('coffee coloured'), particularly in the context of delayed emptying or stasis, which occurs with a variety of serious illnesses (e.g. septic shock, myocardial infarction, pulmonary embolism, etc.).
If this dark colour is misinterpreted as implying altered blood, there is a danger that a collapsed patient with another serious condition is mislabelled as having had an upper GI bleed. 'True' altered blood has a thick, black, grainy appearance – for a coffee analogy look at the contents of your cafetière after pouring all the liquid out. Always be wary of the shocked patient described as having 'coffee-ground' vomit; consider alternative explanations for the shock before jumping to what may be the wrong conclusion.

The fresh rectal bleed
Fresh, red rectal bleeding usually implies a lower gastrointestinal (GI) source, for which the management is often very different. On occasions, however, brisk upper GI blood loss can result in rapid intestinal transit such that the rectal loss is red, rather than black. Such patients will usually be shocked and unwell, which is relatively uncommon in lower gastrointestinal haemorrhage. Conversely, if the patient is haemodynamically stable with fresh rectal bleeding, the source is almost invariably the distal colon, unless the patient has a shortened bowel following previous surgery. If in doubt, the urea–creatinine ratio may be helpful. Blood in the small bowel acts as a high-protein meal, resulting in a rise in urea; a urea : creatinine ratio of >1 : 15 may suggest proximal intestinal bleeding.

'Black stool without a pungent odour'
Patients frequently do not volunteer information about the odour of their stool; however, in the context of upper GI bleeding this is as characteristic as its colour. In the absence of this odour remember:
• Iron tablets produce a 'charcoal grey' colour to the stool; this is usually solid (rather than 'tarry') in consistency. A careful drug history should reveal the cause
• Bleeding from the proximal colon can also produce black stool. Bleeding will often have been chronic so the patient is often anaemic with evidence of iron deficiency (e.g. low mean corpuscular volume); urea–creatinine ratio should be normal.

Table 41 Important considerations in the history for a patient with suspected upper gastrointestinal (GI) bleeding

Reason	Historical features	Comments
Confirmation of suspicion of upper gastrointestinal bleed	Colour, consistency and odour of stool	Patient often will not volunteer information about odour
	Colour and consistency of vomit	Ask the patient to describe what they saw: be wary of the statement: 'the GP said it looked like coffee grounds' (see Box 16)
Assessment of severity	Volume of blood loss in vomit/stool	Terms such as 'cupful' , 'bowlful', 'a few streaks' may give an idea of volume of blood loss
	History of syncope/collapse/light-headedness	Implies haemodynamic compromise: suggests larger bleed
Assessment of cause	History of 'indigestion', abdominal pain, heartburn	May imply peptic ulcer disease/reflux
	Previous peptic ulcer disease/endoscopic abnormalities	Peptic ulcer disease is often recurrent
	Drugs: aspirin, non-steroidals, steroids	May precipitate peptic ulceration; remember that aspirin and non-steroidal anti-inflammatory drugs can be bought over the counter
	Previous varices or portal hypertension	Higher risk of varices as cause
	Weight loss, poor appetite, dysphagia, early satiety	May imply malignancy
	Previous episodes with normal endoscopies	Suspicious of vascular malformation
	Normal vomit immediately prior to vomit containing blood	May suggest Mallory–Weiss tear
Complicating factors	History of alcohol excess	Increases risk of many of the above causes: gastritis, ulceration, varices; may experience withdrawal symptoms in hospital
	Anticoagulant drug use	Make bleeding more likely; ensure international normalised ratio is measured and clarify reason for taking these drugs
	Recreational drug use	Risk factor for hepatitis/chronic liver disease
	Beta-blocker/diltiazem	May mask tachycardia
	Co-existent cardiac/renal/liver disease	Increase morbidity/mortality; fluid balance consideration of central venous cannula
	Previous cardiac valve replacement	May require antibiotic prophylaxis prior to endoscopy; often on anticoagulants

Mr Gross's blood pressure and pulse have remained under control (pulse 80–90 beats/min, blood pressure 120–130 systolic) in the two hours since admission. Mr Gross was catheterised on arrival and is passing 50–100 mL/h urine. He is now completing his first unit of blood. Mr Gross has had one further episode of melaena, but no further haematemesis.

Laboratory investigations are now available and reveal haemoglobin (Hb) 105, platelets 235, urea 13.5, creatinine 86, normal liver function and clotting.

Box 17 Oesophageal varices

Oesophageal varices occur when blood is diverted away from the portal circulation as a result of portal hypertension, usually due to chronic liver disease.

If bleeding occurs, this is associated with a significant mortality of up to 50%.

Management differs from that of bleeding peptic ulceration, because of the need for earlier endoscopic intervention and difficulties with fluid balance.

Oesophageal varices should be considered if the patient has any of the following:

- clinical evidence of chronic liver disease: jaundice, spider naevi, palmar erythema, etc.
- evidence of portal hypertension: ascites, caput medusa
- history of previous oesophageal varices
- history of previous portal vein thrombosis

If oesophageal varices are considered a likely cause of bleeding:

- reconsider insertion of a central venous cannula – accurate fluid balance is crucial, and may be difficult in the context of chronic liver disease
- move the patient to a high-dependency area
- contact the on-call endoscopist as early as possible – early endoscopic intervention may be required in order to stop the bleeding
- Prescribe a drug to lower portal pressure once fluid resuscitation is under way, e.g. terlipressin 2 g 6 hourly – this acts as a splanchnic vasoconstrictor, reducing variceal blood flow.

Box 18 When to endoscope a patient with suspected upper gastrointestinal bleeding

Many hospitals provide an on-call endoscopy service, although in most cases the procedure can be undertaken within 12 h of admission. However, it is important not to miss the 'window of opportunity' that resuscitation has provided, since further bleeding remains possible, and would be associated with a significant mortality.

Advantages of immediate endoscopy include:

- early diagnosis: can start appropriate treatment
- early endoscopic treatment: may prevent further/ ongoing bleeding
- reduces any delay if the patient rebleeds as the cause has already been identified

Disadvantages of 'immediate' endoscopy may include:

- lack of trained endoscopy nursing staff – often not available out of hours
- higher risk to procedure if patient inadequately resuscitated
- views may be impaired by blood/stomach contents

In general, immediate endoscopy should be undertaken in the following situations:

- evidence of ongoing bleeding: persistent hypotension/ tachycardia despite fluid resuscitation; continuing haematemesis
- suspected variceal bleeding
- suspected 'rebleed': drop in blood pressure/central venous pressure/rise in pulse or further haematemesis following initial stabilisation

---

How should the blood results be interpreted?

- The Hb level is often difficult to interpret in the context of an acute bleed
- In this case the Hb is only slightly reduced. This is not uncommon in the acute setting, and should not detract from the diagnosis of significant GI bleeding
- Raised urea with a normal creatinine level can occur as a result of absorption of protein from digested blood; this supports the clinical diagnosis of upper GI bleeding

What further investigation is required?

- Mr Gross now requires the diagnosis to be confirmed by urgent upper GI endoscopy (oesophagogastroduodenoscopy or OGD)
- The timing of endoscopy will partly depend on the available facilities, which may vary in different hospitals
- Other factors that will help to determine the urgency of endoscopy are summarised in Box 18

What can be done while awaiting endoscopy?

- Keep the patient 'nil by mouth'
- Monitor closely with hourly pulse, blood pressure and (where a urinary catheter or central venous pressure (CVP) line has been inserted) urine output measurement and central venous pressure recording
- Correct abnormalities of clotting/platelets by infusion of platelets or fresh frozen plasma. This may require discussion with the on-call haematology team
- If variceal bleeding is suspected consider use of drugs designed to lower portal pressure (e.g. glypressin, somatostatin); however, for suspected peptic ulcer haemorrhage no specific drug therapy has been shown to affect mortality at this stage

Mr Gross has undergone upper GI endoscopy, which has shown a large duodenal ulcer. The endoscopist has reported stigmata of recent haemorrhage. The ulcer was injected with adrenaline and a vessel was cauterised using thermal coagulation. There was a small amount of fresh blood in the stomach, but no active bleeding at the time of the procedure. The endoscopist has documented a Rockall score of 5.

What are 'stigmata of recent haemorrhage'?

These provide evidence of recent bleeding from a lesion in the stomach and include:
• A 'visible vessel' protruding from the base of an ulcer
• Active bleeding from an ulcer base – either a venous 'ooze' or an arterial 'spurt'
• Fresh blood clot overlying an ulcer – usually implies a recent bleed from a vessel: sometimes deliberately dislodged by the endoscopist to enable treatment of the vessel beneath

The presence of stigmata of haemorrhage influences the likelihood of ongoing bleeding/rebleeding and is usually an indication for endoscopic therapy (see Plate 3).

What is endoscopic therapy?

Endoscopic therapy in the context of a recent upper GI bleed is designed to stop bleeding or to reduce the risk of rebleeding. Endoscopic therapy may take the form of:
• Injection of the submucosa with dilute adrenaline (epinephrine). This results in vasoconstriction of vessels supplying this area. The submucosal 'bleb' may also provide a direct tamponade effect, compressing the relevant vessel (see Plate 3)
• Application of a 'band' to the bleeding vessel. This is the treatment of choice for bleeding oesophageal varices (see Plate 4)
• Cauterisation of bleeding vessel with diathermy ('heater probe') or argon plasma coagulation
• Sometimes a combination of the above techniques may be used

What is the Rockall score?

This widely used scoring system enables assessment of risk of further bleeding and mortality following endoscopy. The score is derived from six criteria, and the risk of rebleed and death can be calculated from a graph (see Box 19 and Fig. 35). Although the fully validated total score requires the results of endoscopy, it may be possible to get an idea of the score from the pre-endoscopic criteria (age, haemodynamics and co-morbidities).

Patients with a total score of 5 or more are at high risk and should be observed in a high dependency unit or specialist GI bleeding unit.

Conversely, patients with a score of 0 or 1 are at very low risk and may be suitable for early discharge.

In Mr Gross's case a score of 5 predicts a rebleed rate of 25% and mortality 10%. He clearly requires close observation and is transferred to the high dependency unit for further management.

What further treatment/observation is now required?
Prevention of rebleeding
• **Acid suppression** with an intravenous proton pump inhibitor (e.g. omeprazole 80 mg over 30 min followed by an infusion of 8 mg/h over 72 h) has been shown to reduce rebleeding when there is endoscopic evidence of peptic ulceration with stigmata of haemorrhage (as in this case)
• **Tranexamic acid** has been shown to reduce rebleeding in a meta-analysis in 1999; however, the prothrombotic tendency may increase the risk of deep vein thrombosis (DVT) and this treatment is not widely used. Consider this for patients at high risk of rebleed where surgery would be particularly dangerous
• **Pressor agents (e.g. terlipressin 2 mg 6 hourly):** useful for patients with variceal bleeding, but of no benefit in peptic ulcer bleeding

Identification of rebleeding
• Regular measurement of blood pressure/urine output
• Continuous cardiac monitoring
• Reconsider CVP line insertion, given the high risk of rebleed (see Table 40)

Inform the on-call surgical team
Surgical intervention may be required if the patient rebleeds. Many hospitals therefore provide a joint medical/surgical management approach to such patients. Early discussion gives the on-call surgical team the opportunity to assess the patient and may speed up management later if rebleeding should occur.

You are called back to see Mr Gross on the high-dependency unit (HDU). Mr Gross's blood pressure has dropped to 80/50 with a pulse rate of 120 beats/min. The nurses report that Mr Gross used the commode 10 min ago and passed 300 mL of dark red blood. He has not vomited.

Box 19 The Rockall score

Variable	Score 0	Score 1	Score 2	Score 3
Age	<60 years	60–79 years	80+ years	
Shock	No shock Heart rate <100	Tachycardia Heart rate >100	Hypotension Heart rate >100	
	Systolic >100 mmHg	Systolic BP >100 mmHg	Systolic BP <100 mmHg	
Co-morbidity	None		Congestive cardiac failure Ischaemic heart disease Major morbidity	Renal failure Liver failure Metastatic malignancy
Endoscopic stigmata of recent haemorrhage	None Red spot on lesion		Blood in upper gastrointestinal tract Adherent clot Active spurting vessel Visible vessel within ulcer	
Diagnosis	Mallory–Weiss tear No lesion	All other non-malignant diagnoses	Malignancy of upper gastrointestinal tract	

Add the scores for each line to produce the 'total' score.

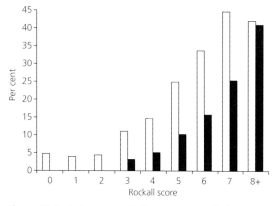

Figure 35 Rockall score graph. Percentage mortality/ rebleeding rate. □, Rebleed; ■, mortality. Reproduced from Rockall *et al.* (1995) with permission from BMJ Publishing Group Ltd.

What is the cause of the deterioration and what treatment is required?

Mr Gross has probably re-bled from his ulcer.

Further managments should be as follows:

• Initiate resuscitative measures (as above)

• Contact the blood bank and ensure a further 4 units of blood are available: cross-match further blood if required

• Recheck blood clotting and correct as required

• Contact the on-call surgical team and on-call endoscopist

• Insert central venous cannula

The options now include repeat endoscopy and surgery – the decision of which to undertake is complex and will require careful discussion at a senior level. The key is to ensure that the patient is adequately resuscitated for whichever approach is taken.

Following appropriate resuscitation the decision was taken to repeat the endoscopy. The vessel was injected again and cauterised with diathermy. Mr Gross returned to the high dependency unit and was treated for 72 h with intravenous omeprazole. Mr Gross had no further rebleeds during this time. An immediate urease test taken at the time of the second endoscopy was positive, indicating the presence of Helicobacter pylori. After four days on the HDU Mr Gross has now been transferred to the general ward and discharge is being planned for tomorrow.

What final considerations are there on discharge?

• **Treatment of *Helicobacter pylori* (Hp):** this is a possible cause of Mr Gross's ulcer. Eradication of this bacterium will reduce the risk of recurrence. A variety of antibiotic combinations are effective – refer to your hospital's local policy/formulary to identify the regimen used locally. Confirmation of eradication by the urea breath test 6–8 weeks after initial eradication should always be considered

• **Acid suppression with an oral proton pump inhibitor (PPI)** should follow Hp eradication, or be used in isolation if the patient was Hp negative (e.g. omeprazole, 20–40 mg daily)

• **Stop non-steroidal anti-inflammatory drugs (NSAIDs) (and aspirin if relevant)** and prescribe alternative analgesia where appropriate. Mr Gross was taking ibuprofen for a shoulder injury. A paracetamol/codeine mixture should be safe from a gastrointestinal perspective

Should a repeat endoscopy be arranged following discharge?

• A repeat endoscopy is not normally required to confirm healing of a duodenal ulcer, unless there is a need to restart NSAID treatment or anticoagulants

• Patients with gastric ulcers should usually undergo repeat endoscopy following 6–8 weeks' treatment with PPI since around 10% are malignant. A repeat endoscopy with biopsy if unhealed may enable these to be identified

• Patients with varices will require a repeat endoscopy and further banding to ensure eradication of the varices as well as follow-up to investigate the cause of their portal hypertension

CASE REVIEW

This case describes a 55-year-old man who is referred urgently by his GP after describing two episodes of melaena and a small fresh haematemesis. During transit to hospital Mr Nick Gross's condition deteriorates with further fresh haematemesis, resulting in features suggestive of hypovolaemic shock. Mr Gross is resuscitated initially with normal saline and subsequently cross-matched blood, which restores his blood pressure. The history is suggestive of a peptic ulcer, based on a background of recent ibuprofen use and heavy alcohol consumption. An endoscopy confirms this diagnosis, with evidence of recent haemorrhage requiring endoscopic therapy. Mr Gross is transferred to the high dependency unit and starts an intravenous infusion of omeprazole. Despite this he experiences a further drop in his blood pressure, associated with the passage of dark red stools. Following discussion with the gastroenterology and surgical teams, Mr Gross undergoes repeat endoscopy with further ulcer injection, which successfully controls the bleeding. Mr Gross is noted to be *H. Pylori* positive and starts eradication therapy prior to discharge five days after admission. Mr Gross makes an uneventful recovery following this.

KEY POINTS

• Immediate and adequate fluid resuscitation is essential for any patient who is haemodynamically compromised following upper GI bleeding.

• Carefully evaluate the history to ensure that the initial suspicion of upper GI bleeding is correct.

• Consider the likely cause – specifically ensure that the possibility of varices is considered.

• Early upper GI endoscopy will identify the cause in most cases.

• Calculation of the Rockall score will help to categorise the risk of death or rebleeding.

• Patients at high risk should be managed in the HDU or specialist GI bleeding unit.

• Early discussion with the surgical team is essential for high-risk cases.

Further reading

BSG Endoscopy Committee. Non-variceal upper gastrointestinal haemorrhage – guidelines. *Gut* 2002; **51**(iv): iv1–6

Lau JY, Sung JJ, Lee KK *et al.* Effect of intravenous omeprazole on recurrent bleeding after endoscopic treatment of bleeding peptic ulcers. *N Engl J Med* 2000; **343**: 310–16

Rockall TA, Logan RFA, Devlin HB, Northfield TC. Incidence of and mortality from acute upper gastrointestinal haemorrhage in the United Kingdom. *BMJ* 1995; **311**: 222–6

A 60-year-old man with diarrhoea

A 60-year-old man is referred to hospital after collapsing in his bathroom. Mr Imran Khalid describes a one-week history of diarrhoea that has become gradually worse. Mr Khalid is now passing up to 15 loose, watery stools per day. This morning Mr Khalid felt light-headed while in the lavatory and passed out briefly on standing up after defaecation. Mr Khalid was reviewed by his GP who recommended hospital admission.

What challenges will this patient present?

• Diarrhoea is a common symptom, but a relatively infrequent cause for acute medical admission
• Diarrhoea has a wide variety of causes, but many of these do not usually present acutely (see Table 42)
• Most cases of acute diarrhoea are self-limiting and are managed by the patient's GP without the need for hospital involvement
• Referral to hospital may reflect a concern that the patient requires intravenous hydration because of rapid fluid loss or co-existent vomiting
• Social factors in older or immobile patients who are unable to reach a lavatory may also lead to hospital admission
• Some cases represent an exacerbation of a chronic bowel condition, such as inflammatory bowel disease
• Early consideration of infection control precautions is essential for any patient presenting with diarrhoea: gloves and apron should be worn for any direct patient contact and wherever possible the patient should be isolated in a side room away from other patients (see Box 20)

Mr Khalid is brought into the acute medical unit by the ambulance crew and placed in an observable side room close to the nurses' station. Initial assessment reveals Mr Khalid to be pale but fully conscious and breathing spontaneously with a respiratory rate of 18/min. Mr Khalid's

pulse is 120/min, regular with a thready character, and blood pressure 80/40. Mr Khalid is cool peripherally and his mucous membranes are dry with poor skin turgor and slow capillary refill. Mr Khalid is orientated and is not in pain.

What immediate management is required?

The initial diagnosis indicates that the patient is shocked, almost certainly as a result of hypovolaemia.

The following measures should be undertaken.
• Check patency of airway and apply high-flow oxygen
• Establish peripheral intravenous access with a 12- or 14-gauge cannula
• Take blood for full blood count (FBC), urea and electrolytes (U&E), liver function tests (LFT) and C-reactive protein (CRP)
• Commence intravenous infusion of fluid (e.g. normal saline 500 mL over 30 min)
   ○ recheck pulse and blood pressure every 15 min and give more as required
• Obtain an ECG
   ○ this will help to exclude a co-existent cardiac cause for shock
• Check arterial or venous blood gases
   ○ measurement of lactate and base deficit will help to identify the severity of shock; measurement of sodium and potassium level on the blood gas analyser will help guide electrolyte replacement

After infusion of 500 mL of fluid Mr Khalid's blood pressure has improved to 100/60 and his pulse has fallen to 100 beats/min. He remains cool peripherally.

Mr Khalid's ECG reveals a sinus tachycardia but no evidence of myocardial ischaemia or infarction.

Arterial blood gas (while breathing high-flow oxygen) is as follows: pH 7.34, pCO2 4.8, pO2 18.3, standard bicarbonate 20, base excess −3.4, lactate 2.5, K 3.4, Na 131.

Venous blood has been sent to the laboratory, as above, and results are awaited.

Acute Medicine: Clinical Cases Uncovered. By C. Roseveare.
Published 2009 by Blackwell Publishing, ISBN: 978-1-4051-6883-0

Table 42 Classification/causes of diarrhoea

Classification/cause	Suggestive clinical features	Comments
Infective		
Viral gastroenteritis Infective colitis	Short history Contacts also infected Usually co-existent vomiting Fever/constitutional upset	Highly infectious – ensure isolation precautions are undertaken (see Box 20)
Other bacterial enteritis (e.g. *Escherichia coli*, cholera)	History of contact with animals or recent travel; usually profuse diarrhoea and extremely unwell	Remember to consider unusual infections in patients with immunodeficiency (e.g. AIDS) and in patients returning from tropical areas
Inflammatory		
Crohn's disease	Previous episodes/long history Extraintestinal man-ifestations (see Table 43)	May cause diarrhoea because of malabsorption with small bowel disease/resection or due to colitis
Ulcerative colitis	See Table 43	
Neoplastic		
Colonic carcinoma	Usually age >40 Weight loss/appetite loss Often co-existent bleeding/anaemia	Onset of diarrhoea may be the change of bowel habit often associated with colonic carcinoma
Carcinoid syndrome	Watery diarrhoea Often long history Associated flushing	Rare – tumours secrete 5-hydroxy-indoleacetic acid, which can be identified in the urine
Drug induced		
Laxative drugs	History of laxative use Prior history of eating disorder	Laxatives may be prescribed for prior constipation or may be abused as a means of weight loss (in which case use may not be volunteered by patient)
Idiosyncratic drug reaction	Any new drug prescribed before onset of diarrhoea	Virtually any drug can cause diarrhoea in a susceptible patient; usually starts within 1 week of starting the medication
Drug toxicity	Increase in drug dosage Onset of renal/liver failure	Digoxin toxicity is one cause of this problem, particularly in older people
Metabolic		
Renal failure	May be previously documented	Usually results from markedly elevated urea; remember that diarrhoea may be the cause of the uraemia due to dehydration or sepsis
Thyrotoxicosis	Tachycardia, sweating, flushing, upper eyelid lag and lid retraction, weight loss	Not common but worth considering, particularly when the patient is markedly tachycardic and has lost weight
Other		
Irritable bowel syndrome	Usually long history Very frequent stool, especially in the morning No weight loss/bleeding Rarely wakes the patient at night May be other irritable bowel type symptoms – bloating, intermittent constipation, cramping pain, etc.	Diarrhoea probably related to increased gut motility Symptoms can be very severe/distressing, but not life threatening Patients may have had repeated admissions/investigations May be psychological factors in some patients Often worth studying previous hospital records and contacting GP prior to initiating further extensive tests
Constipation with overflow	Often elderly or history of chronic constipation prior to onset Abdominal distension/bloating Faecal impaction apparent on abdominal/rectal examination	Liquefied stool 'escapes' past the impacted stool in the colon Abdominal radiograph should help to confirm the diagnosis

Box 20 Infection control issues for patients with diarrhoea

Whenever a patient is admitted to hospital with diarrhoea, infection control should be considered unless transmissible infection can be ruled out. Viral gastroenteritis can spread rapidly through a ward and can be serious in older or immunocompromised people. Bacterial infection and *Clostridium difficile* can also be transmitted via a faeco-oral route.

Benefits of isolation need to be balanced against the fact that patients in isolation rooms may be more difficult to observe. Patients who are haemodynamically unstable, or require cardiac monitoring because of electrolyte imbalance or shock, may initially require an observation or high dependency area. In this case careful barrier precautions should be taken (gloves/apron to be worn, care with all body fluids, etc.) to minimise risks of transmission.

It should also be remembered that alcohol gel is not effective against many enteric infections. Careful hand washing with soap and warm water is essential when managing patients with suspected infective diarrhoea.

Most hospitals have written policies relating to infection control for patients with diarrhoea, which you should refer to if in doubt.

What further management is required?

• Although Mr Khalid is starting to improve, he continues to show evidence of hypovolaemia and will require more fluid
• Insertion of a urinary catheter may be helpful to monitor urine output, which gives a useful guide to the effectiveness of rehydration
• Mr Khalid's sodium and potassium are slightly low, probably reflecting electrolyte loss with the stool: intravenous potassium supplementation may be required
• Mr Khalid is mildly acidotic with a slightly elevated lactate, probably reflective of dehydration and shock; this should improve with rehydration
• Abdominal and erect chest radiographs should be requested (see below)
• As Mr Khalid's condition stabilizes, it is now important to obtain a history and conduct a more detailed clinical examination

The diarrhoea started quite abruptly one week earlier, since when Mr Khalid has been opening his bowels 10–15 times each day and three or four times every night. The stools are watery in consistency and contain a small quantity of blood. Mr Khalid has not felt like eating because of nausea and the need to open his bowels immediately after eating. He has lost 3 kg in weight over the past week.

Mr Khalid's past history includes hypertension and paroxysmal atrial fibrillation. He has no prior history of bowel disease. He had a chest infection three weeks ago for which he was treated with amoxicillin for one week; this seemed to settle. Mr Khalid's only medications are aspirin and bendroflumethiazide, which he has taken for many years. Two days before the onset of symptoms Mr Khalid had a chicken curry at a restaurant; otherwise, he has eaten the same food as his wife who has not been unwell. Mr Khalid has not travelled abroad in the past year and no other close contacts have been unwell.

Mr Khalid remains tachycardic (pulse 96 beats/min) but his blood pressure has improved after 2 L of fluid (120/70); his abdomen is generally distended and mildly tender without peritonism. Bowel sounds are active. A rectal examination reveals watery stool but no masses and no blood is seen on the glove.

A chest radiograph is normal.

An abdominal radiograph shows an empty dilated colon with loss of haustral pattern and oedema of colonic wall.

Is this a new 'acute' problem or an exacerbation of a chronic diarrhoeal illness?

• This is an important question to address when taking the history, since it will have a considerable impact on the further management of a patient presenting to hospital with diarrhoea
• Patients with inflammatory bowel disease (ulcerative colitis or Crohn's disease) frequently experience relapse and remission of their condition, which frequently results in diarrhoea. Although this will usually be manageable in an outpatient setting, a severe exacerbation may result in hospital admission
• The treatment of such patients is often complex, and early involvement of a specialist in gastroenterology is recommended

If a diagnosis of Crohn's disease or ulcerative colitis has been previously made, the patient (and GP) will usually be aware of this; if necessary, ask the patient directly.

Other clues suggesting a pre-existing problem include:
• A prior history of recurrent diarrhoea
• A long duration of symptoms (weeks or months)
• Gradual worsening of symptoms

In this case Mr Khalid and the GP are not aware of any prior history of inflammatory bowel disease. The acute onset and short history are more suggestive of a new acute cause.

What is the likely diagnosis?

• The presence of bloodstained diarrhoea is suggestive of colitis; this is supported by the radiological features showing an empty, dilated colon with thickened wall (see Box 21)

• The high stool frequency, abdominal pain, distension and tenderness, biochemical abnormalities and lactic acidosis indicate that the inflammation is severe

• The persistent tachycardia is concerning, but may reflect continued hypovolaemia; this will need to be monitored closely. There are no other features to suggest imminent perforation (see Table 44)

• The abrupt onset of symptoms without prior history of inflammatory bowel disease (IBD) is most suggestive of infection as the cause. As Mr Khalid consumed a chicken curry two days prior to the onset, organisms such as *Campylobacter* and *Salmonella* should be considered

---

Box 21 Does the patient have colitis?

• The term *colitis* implies inflammation of the colon, which can have a number of causes (see Table 43)

• Establishing whether the colon is acutely inflamed is important, as this may result in progressive dilatation and perforation of the colon. When this happens, the leakage of colonic contents into the peritoneum results in faecal peritonitis, which has a significant mortality. Appropriate treatment, careful monitoring and timely surgical intervention will usually prevent this complication

• A careful history, examination and review of investigation results should enable the clinician to identify features suggestive of colitis, categorise its severity and predict the likelihood of imminent perforation (see Table 44)

If there is deemed to be an imminent risk of colonic perforation:

• Keep the patient 'nil by mouth'
• Ensure adequate fluid resuscitation/analgesia
• Commence intravenous antibiotics: usually cefuroxime 750 mg tds and metronidazole 500 mg tds
• Contact the on-call surgical team and request early review

• The recent antibiotic course raises the possibility of *Clostridium difficile* infection

• The prior history of paroxysmal atrial fibrillation requires consideration of ischaemic colitis. Thyrotoxicosis is also a possible cause of diarrhoea in patients with atrial fibrillation

Investigation results are as follows (normal ranges in brackets):

• *haemoglobin 136, white cell count 16.4, neutrophils 11.5, platelets 446*
• *sodium 133, potassium 3.1 (3.5–5), urea 12.5 (2–6), creatinine 135 (75–125)*
• *liver function tests normal*
• *C-reactive protein 166 (<10)*
• *lactate 2.5 (0.5–1.5)*
• *thyroid function normal*

What do these blood results suggest?

• The raised white cell count and CRP are suggestive of an acute inflammatory process; this would support the clinical suspicion of infection as the likely cause, but IBD can produce similar results

• The low sodium and potassium levels probably reflect electrolyte loss with the stool

• The raised urea and creatinine probably relate to dehydration, but will require further monitoring; slight elevation of lactate reflects a degree of tissue hypoxia

• Bendroflumethiazide (a thiazide diuretic) may have exacerbated the dehydration and electrolyte abnormalities

What further management is required?

• Correct electrolyte abnormalities
  ○ continue intravenous fluid with potassium supplementation
  ○ consider checking/correcting magnesium level (hypomagnesaemia may accompany hypokalaemia in patients with diarrhoea)
  ○ omit the bendroflumethiazide until the diarrhoea settles

• Monitor renal function/acidosis
  ○ will usually correct with fluid resuscitation
  ○ severe renal failure may suggest infection with *Escherichia coli* 0157 (haemolytic-uraemic syndrome)

• Send stool for culture
  ○ will usually take 24–48 h to identify organism
  ○ ask specifically for *Clostridium difficile* toxin measurement

Table 43 Causes of colitis

Condition	Suggestive clinical features	Comments
Inflammatory bowel disease (Crohn's disease or ulcerative colitis)	Prior history (patient or GP should be aware of this) Extraintestinal manifestations: erythema nodosum, iritis, episcleritis, arthritis, sacroiliitis	Relapsing/remitting course means most patients will have had previous episode Flare-up of IBD may be precipitated by infection
Infective colitis	Abrupt onset. Prominent fever Suggestive dietary history (especially chicken, eggs) Recent travel, contact with other infected patient Stool often green in colour (due to presence of bile in stool)	
Pseudomembranous colitis (antibiotic-related colitis, *Clostridium difficile* infection)	Often older age group Profuse watery diarrhoea Usually received antibiotics in preceding 4 weeks Recent hospital stay/contact with affected patient Previous episode	May relapse following treatment
Ischaemic colitis	Older age group Usually bloody diarrhoea Associated with ischaemic heart disease, atrial fibrillation	Results from mesenteric ischaemia due to embolism or atheroma Typically large blood volume in stool, disproportionate to other clinical features
Diverticulitis	Older age group Left iliac fossa pain/tenderness, fever May be prior history of diverticular disease	Diverticular disease is common in older patients and usually asymptomatic; consider other causes May bleed profusely Toxic dilatation uncommon: perforation of diverticulum/abscess formation may occur

  ○ remember low sensitivity of stool culture (approx. 30%): negative culture does not exclude bacterial infection
• Consider antibiotic therapy
  ○ oral metronidazole or oral vancomycin for *C. difficile* infection
  ○ oral ciprofloxacin if campylobacter or salmonella suspected
  ○ intravenous cefuroxime/metronidazole if evidence of peritonism, concerns about imminent perforation or patient unable to take oral medication
• Consider intravenous steroid therapy if severe colitis and IBD cannot be excluded

• Allow oral fluids (unless high risk of perforation)
  ○ high calorie drinks should be considered
  ○ the patient will often not feel like solid food and eating often precipitates further episodes of diarrhoea

Mr Khalid has been in a side room on the ward for 24 hours. He is receiving intravenous normal saline with potassium supplementation. His repeat urea and electrolytes (U&E) on day 2 reveal resolution of the hypokalaemia and mild renal impairment. Mr Khalid's lactate is now normal. He continues to have frequent diarrhoea and remains pyrexial (38°C overnight), with pulse >100 beats/min. Blood pressure

Table 44 Clinical/radiological/biochemical and endoscopic features in colitis with indicators of severity and imminent perforation

Feature suggesting colitis	Indicator of severity	Factors suggesting perforation may be imminent
Clinical		
Diarrhoea	Higher frequency	Tenderness/peritonism
Blood in stool	Larger quantity of blood	Marked/Increasing distension
	Abdominal pain	Persistent hypotension/increasing
	Abdominal distension	tachycardia
	Hypotension/tachycardia	
Biochemical		
	Hypokalaemia, uraemia, lactic acidosis	Falling potassium; rising lactate
Radiological		
Empty colon (no stool visible)	Thickened wall; loss of haustral pattern	Dilatation of lumen (>10cm)
	Entire colon empty	
Endoscopic		
Mucosal inflammation on rigid/flexible sigmoidoscopy	More severe inflammation	

is 130/70. Mr Khalid's abdomen remains distended with mild generalised tenderness. He has been started on oral ciprofloxacin and metronidazole. Mr Khalid is taking oral fluids but has not felt like eating.

The laboratory telephones to inform you that C. difficile toxin has been identified in his stool culture.

What is the diagnosis and further treatment?

The diagnosis is likely to be pseudomembranous colitis due to *C. difficile* infection. Further monitoring/treatment should be as follows:

• Commence a 'stool chart'
  ○ this should record each stool passed, along with its consistency, colour and presence of blood. The Bristol Stool Scale (see Table 45) is often used to categorise stool consistency
  ○ reduction in stool frequency and improved consistency of stools will help to identify an improvement in Mr Khalid's condition
  ○ generally avoid antidiarrhoeal medication (e.g. loperamide/codeine phosphate) – this will artificially reduce stool frequency and impair the utility of the stool chart; it may also precipitate toxic dilatation/perforation of the colon in patients with acute colitis
• Continue regular observations (e.g. using the early warning score (EWS))

  ○ remember that if the patient has been started on steroids, features of peritonism (pain, tenderness, pyrexia) may be masked: rising pulse may be the only reliable physical sign. The EWS therefore may underestimate the severity of the illness
• Monitor U&E daily
  ○ the potassium level may continue to fall, requiring further correction
• Revise antibiotic therapy in the light of stool culture results
• Consider probiotics ('live yoghurt') for patients with *C. difficile* infection

Does Mr Khalid require endoscopic examination of the colon?

Some of the issues surrounding the need for endoscopy are discussed in Box 22.

In this case endoscopy is not required, as a clear explanation for Mr Khalid's symptoms has been identified and there is no reason to suspect any other underlying condition.

Although metronidazole is usually effective against C. difficile, in view of the lack of significant improvement in Mr Khalid's condition since admission, both the ciprofloxacin and metronidazole are stopped and he is started on oral vancomycin, 125 mg tds. Mr Khalid continues to have

Table 45 The Bristol Stool Scale

Stool type	Description	
1	Separate hard lumps, like nuts (hard to pass)	
2	Sausage shaped but lumpy	
3	Like a sausage but with cracks on the surface	
4	Like a sausage or snake; smooth and soft	
5	Soft blobs with clear-cut edges (passes easily)	
6	Fluffy pieces with ragged edges; a mushy stool	
7	Watery, no solid pieces; entirely liquid	

diarrhoea but the stool frequency gradually reduces over the next 48 hours with the resolution of the pyrexia. The stool consistency gradually becomes more solid, as documented on his stool chart. Over the next few days Mr Khalid's oral intake improves and he is able to go home after four days in hospital. His bendroflumethiazide is restarted before discharge.

Mr Khalid is advised to take live yoghurt (one or two helpings daily) over the next few weeks. He makes a full recovery, with stools returning to normal within three weeks.

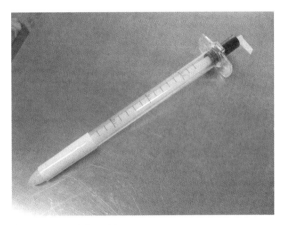

Figure 36 Rigid sigmoidoscope.

Box 22 Endoscopy for patients with acute diarrhoea

Direct visualisation of the colonic mucosa and biopsy sampling may be helpful in the early management of some patients admitted to hospital with diarrhoea. The benefits of endoscopy are as follows:
- may enable confirmation of the clinical suspicion of colitis, through direct examination of the colonic mucosa or histological analysis of biopsies
- may enable establishment of the severity and extent of the colitis
- may help to establish the cause of the inflammation
- may enable identification of other contributory factors – e.g. diverticular disease, colonic cancer.

It should be remembered, however, that in many cases endoscopic examination does not influence management, may be uncomfortable for the patient and may be hazardous. Biopsies taken in patients with acute colitis often fail to distinguish between infective and other inflammatory causes. Discussion with a gastroenterologist is often worthwhile before undertaking or requesting endoscopy.

If endoscopy is considered, three techniques may be employed.

Rigid sigmoidoscopy may be performed on the ward, although the views obtained may be very limited in patients with diarrhoea, and the procedure is often extremely uncomfortable for the patient. Biopsies may be taken using this equipment (see Fig. 36).

Flexible sigmoidoscopy is usually undertaken in the endoscopy unit; this involves a limited examination of the rectum and distal colon; better views are obtained than with rigid sigmoidoscopy and it is easier to take targeted biopsies using this technique.

Colonoscopy is generally unnecessary in the acute phase and is hazardous in patients with acute colitis, when it can result in perforation or further dilatation of the colon. Colonoscopy may be necessary after resolution of the acute problem, to exclude an underlying structural or inflammatory cause.

CASE REVIEW

This case describes a 60-year-old man who is admitted to hospital after collapsing at home following a one-week history of watery diarrhoea. This came on abruptly, two weeks after completion of a course of amoxicillin for a chest infection. Mr Imran Khalid has a past history of paroxysmal atrial fibrillation and hypertension (treated with bendroflumethiazide and aspirin) but no previous bowel disease.

On arrival in hospital Mr Khalid is pyrexial and showing signs of hypovolaemia, requiring rehydration with normal saline. Initial investigations reveal hypokalaemia, hyponatraemia and mild renal impairment with elevation of white cell count and CRP. An abdominal radiograph shows an empty, slightly dilated colon, suggestive of an acute colitis.

Given the short history it is thought that infective colitis is the most likely cause for the symptoms. Mr Khalid is isolated in a side room and commenced on oral ciprofloxacin and metronidazole. His haemodynamic and electrolyte abnormalities improve following rehydration, but his diarrhoea and pyrexia persist. The laboratory 'phones the ward to say that C diff toxin has been identified in his stool. Mr Khalid's antibiotics are changed to oral vancomycin and he shows improvement in stool frequency and consistency over the next 48 hours with full recovery within three weeks.

KEY POINTS

- Although most patients with diarrhoea can be effectively managed in the community, patients who have become dehydrated and those who are deemed at risk of colonic perforation may require urgent hospital assessment and treatment.
- A flare-up of a pre-existing diarrhoeal illness may require different management, so should be considered early in the assessment process.
- Isolation of the patient should always be considered where infection is a possible cause of diarrhoea – the need for this should be balanced against the need for close monitoring if the patient is acutely unwell.

- Initial treatment should include rehydration and correction of any electrolyte abnormality.
- Patients with suspected acute colitis will require close observation to ensure that the colon is not at risk of imminent perforation.
- Recording of stool frequency and consistency will give a guide to the patient's progress.
- *C. difficile* infection should be treated with oral metronidazole, which should be changed to oral vancomycin if the patient's condition does not improve.

Further reading

Carter MJ, Lobo AJ, Travis SPL. Guidelines for the management of inflammatory bowel disease in adults. *Gut* 2004; **53**(v): v1–16

Colleypriest B, Gordon H. Acute management of the patient with diarrhoea. *Acute Med* 2004; **3**(3): 96–102

Starr J. *Clostridium difficile* associated diarrhoea: diagnosis and treatment. *BMJ* 2005; **331**: 498–501

Case 11   A 37-year-old woman with sudden severe headache

PART 2: CASES

You are telephoned by a GP about a 37-year-old female patient he has been called to see. This morning while at work Mrs Annika Jenski described a sudden onset of severe headache. Mrs Jenski has a past history of migraine but this headache is very different. Mrs Jenski has vomited twice and the pain has now continued for 2 h with no relief from paracetamol or ibuprofen. The GP is concerned about the possibility of subarachnoid haemorrhage (SAH).

What challenges will this patient present?

• Sudden severe headache is the characteristic symptom of a SAH, usually caused by spontaneous bleeding from a cerebral 'berry' aneurysm

• SAH can be catastrophic, resulting in raised intracranial pressure, hydrocephalus, permanent cerebral damage or death

• In many cases, however, a massive bleed is preceded by a sentinal haemorrhage, a small bleed providing clinicians with a warning of what may be around the corner

• Failure to recognise this condition can have devastating consequences for the patient, with a high probability of subsequent litigation against the clinical staff involved in the original assessment

• It is crucial for clinicians to maintain a high index of suspicion for the diagnosis of SAH when assessing patients presenting to hospital with sudden, severe headache

On arrival in hospital Mrs Jenski remains in considerable pain. She is clutching her head and prefers to keep her eyes shut. However, Mrs Jenski is able to answer questions appropriately, obeys commands and opens her eyes when requested. Mrs Jenski is holding a vomit bowl and has recently vomited. Her blood pressure is 150/90 with a pulse of 100 beats/min.

Acute Medicine: Clinical Cases Uncovered. By C. Roseveare.
Published 2009 by Blackwell Publishing, ISBN: 978-1-4051-6883-0

What immediate management is required?

Mrs Jenski is breathing spontaneously and has a Glasgow Coma Score of at least 14/15 (see p. 127). Mrs Jenski should therefore be able to maintain her own airway. Blood pressure is a little high, but this may relate to the pain and distress she is experiencing.

The following management is required.

• Ensure patency of the airway and calculate the Glasgow Coma Score (GCS)

• Connect to cardiac monitor and pulse oximeter

• Apply oxygen via a facemask

• Obtain intravenous access

• Send blood for full blood count (FBC), urea and electrolytes (U&E), liver function tests (LFT), clotting screen, and group and save

• Prescribe analgesia (see below) and an intravenous antiemetic (e.g. cyclizine 50 mg, 8 hourly)

• Ask the nursing staff to undertake neurological observations (neuro obs) every 30 min (see Fig. 37)

How should the choice of analgesia be determined?

• The choice of analgesic should be determined according to the severity of the pain

• Intramuscular (IM) injections of codeine phosphate (30–60 mg 2 hourly, maximum 240 mg in 24 h) are a common choice in this situation and frequently result in a significant improvement in pain

• Stronger opiate analgesia (e.g. intravenous morphine sulphate 5–10 mg) may be required; in such cases consideration should be given to the impact this may have had on pupillary responses and the conscious level when interpreting subsequent neurological observations

After intramuscular administration of 60 mg of codeine phosphate and 50 mg of intravenous cyclizine Mrs Jenski appears more comfortable. She still prefers to lie still with her eyes shut, but says the pain is easing. Mrs Jenski's blood pressure has improved to 130/70, pulse 90 beats/min. Mrs Jenski is now able to give a full history and consent to clinical examination.

Mrs Jenski describes that she felt well this morning and went to work as usual. While walking to the bathroom Mrs Jenski experienced a sudden and very severe headache at the back of her head. The pain was of such intensity that it made her fall to her knees. Mrs Jenski has never experienced pain like it before. Shortly after the onset of the pain she vomited. The pain continued unabated until the injection Mrs Jenski was given on the ward. Mrs Jenski continues to feel nauseated. She finds that movements of her head worsen the pain, as does bright light. The pain was also worse when Mrs Jenski vomited.

Mrs Jenski describes a previous history of migraine, but this has never started abruptly, and the pain is usually focused around the front of her head on the left side. Mrs Jenski normally experiences flashing lights in her vision with her migraine, which have not occurred this time. There is no other significant past history of note and no recent history of head trauma, although she had a car accident with whiplash to her neck three months ago.

On examination Mrs Jenski is in discomfort, worsened by head movement. Her neck is slightly stiff. There is mild tenderness over the occiput and neck muscles. The remainder of her examination, including a full neurological assessment, is entirely normal.

Are the clinical features compatible with a diagnosis of subarachnoid haemorrhage?

The characteristic features of the headache of SAH are described in Table 46. Alternative diagnoses may need to be considered, but only after SAH has been excluded (see Table 47).

Mrs Jenski has mentioned a number of symptoms that should raise concern.

- Abrupt onset of pain
- Severity described as worst ever
- Worst pain at the onset
- Prolonged duration

Does the 'normal' clinical examination make SAH less likely?

Clinical examination of patients with SAH is usually entirely normal. It is unusual to find focal neurological signs on examination of patients with SAH. The history alone should be the trigger to proceed to further investigation. The following abnormalities may be found, but usually in association with a large bleed.

Table 46 Characteristic features of the headache in subarachnoid haemorrhage (SAH)

		Comments
Site	Often occipital or generalised	Localised/unilateral pain is unusual in SAH
Onset	Abrupt/explosive or rapid onset (over seconds/minutes)	Patient will usually remember what they were doing at the time of onset. Onset is usually during activity Patients classically describe pain as 'like being struck on the head'
Character	Continuous, unremitting	
Radiation	May radiate all over cranium/into neck	
Associated symptoms	Nausea/vomiting Syncope Drowsiness/irritability	Focal neurological symptoms/signs are unusual following SAH
Time course	Pain is worst at onset Usually persists over several hours	Transient headache (seconds or minutes)
Exacerbating/relieving factors	Often exacerbated by straining/vomiting, etc.	
Severity	Very severe	Often described as 'worst ever headache'

Table 47 Differential diagnosis of sudden severe headache

Condition	Clinical features/comments
Subarachnoid haemorrhage (SAH)	See text/Table 46; remember that no clinical feature will reliably distinguish SAH from any of the other conditions listed in this table; exclusion of SAH by CT and lumbar puncture (LP) is usually required before consideration of other diagnoses
Thunderclap migraine	May be clinically indistinguishable from SAH; usually young patients with past history of migraine; often unilateral; patient may describe previous episodes
Benign coital cephalgia	A form of 'thunderclap' headache occurring during sexual intercourse (often at the point of orgasm); remember that SAH during sexual intercourse is also well recognised
Cervicogenic pain	Pain originating from cervical spine may radiate to the occiput; often marked local tenderness and pain increased by movements of head; may be history of preceding neck pain/injury/whiplash
Cranial venous sinus thrombosis	Usually more gradual onset but sudden in up to 10% of patients May be history suggestive of thrombophilia (previous deep vein thrombosis/pulmonary embolism, etc.) or risk factors for thrombosis (see p. 40, Table 17) Often papilloedema and raised CSF opening pressure on LP. CT brain will often be normal unless intravenous contrast given (radiologists will usually not do this unless there is a specific request to do so)
Pituitary apoplexy	Results from infarction of, or haemorrhage into pituitary gland Often associated with a pituitary adenoma Examination may reveal hypotension, ophthalmoplegia and/or bitemporal hemianopia but may be entirely normal Often overlooked on CT. MRI scanning required for diagnosis
Carotid artery dissection	Pain is often unilateral ('hemicranial') with associated Horner's syndrome/other unilateral neurological signs May be preceding history of neck injury/trauma CT and CSF often normal: CT or MR angiography is usually required
Trigeminal neuralgia	Sudden, 'shooting' pains over face rather than scalp/head; usually transient and unilateral

- Drowsiness, agitation or confusion
- Evidence of raised intracranial pressure – hypertension, bradycardia, papilloedema
- Subhyaloid haemorrhages on fundoscopy

What further investigation is required to confirm/refute the diagnosis of SAH?

Further investigation usually requires two tests:
- CT brain scan
- Lumbar puncture (LP)

It is usual practice to undertake a CT scan of the brain for all patients where there is clinical suspicion of SAH.

The scan may show:
- Direct evidence of SAH – blood in subarachnoid spaces and/or ventricles
- Evidence of hydrocephalus – due to obstruction of cerebrospinal fluid (CSF) flow by the haematoma

- Alternative pathology to account for headache – cerebral tumours, other forms of intracranial bleeding, etc.

Mrs Jenski is transferred to the CT scanner and undergoes a CT brain scan; this is reported as normal by the on-call neuroradiologist and Mrs Jenski returns to the ward. Her headache is now much better controlled and she has not vomited again. Neurological observations have been stable and Mrs Jenski remains apyrexial. She is keen to go home and asks if the normal scan has 'excluded' a brain haemorrhage.

Does a normal CT brain scan exclude the diagnosis of SAH?

The simple answer is *no*.
- CT brain scanning is normal in up to 10% of patients following SAH

• The incidence of a false-negative scan rises with longer delays in scanning following onset of pain, and is also dependent on the experience of the interpreting radiologist
• Whenever the CT brain scan is normal, patients with suspected SAH should undergo lumbar puncture

Why undertake a lumbar puncture in suspected SAH?

The aim of LP in suspected SAH is to show evidence of blood in the cerebrospinal fluid, which is in communication with the subarachnoid space.

Evidence of recent bleeding may be indicated by:
• Microscopy showing red blood cells within the CSF
• Photochemical analysis showing breakdown products of haemoglobin (haem pigments) in the CSF

What should be considered before undertaking lumbar puncture?

• **Has the CT scan already shown the diagnosis?** Ensure an experienced radiologist has examined the images – if SAH (or an alternative diagnosis) is confirmed on CT, lumbar puncture is usually not required
• **Are there contraindications to lumbar puncture?** (see Table 48)
• **What was the time of onset of headache?** Lumbar puncture should be delayed for at least 12 h following the onset of headache to enable accurate interpretation of the haem pigment levels (see Table 49)
• **Is equipment available to measure CSF opening pressure?** Raised pressure may be an indication of an alternative diagnosis if fluid analysis is normal (e.g. cerebral venous sinus thrombosis – see Table 46)
• **Have you contacted the laboratory** to ensure that they are able to analyse the fluid on arrival? This is particularly important if the procedure is being undertaken outside normal working hours. Delayed analysis may affect the accuracy of the results, requiring the procedure to be repeated

What cerebrospinal fluid samples should be obtained?

• 0.5 mL in fluoride oxalate (or EDTA) bottle for protein/glucose measurement (not usually abnormal in case of SAH but may suggest alternative diagnosis)
• Two samples of 1 mL each (labelled 2 and 3) sent to microbiology department for cell counting and culture
• One sample (minimum 1 mL) for spectrophotometric analysis: cover immediately to protect from light and send to biochemistry department

Mrs Jenski is observed closely on the ward, with hourly neuro obs until 12 h from the onset of the symptoms, at which time your registrar undertakes a lumbar puncture. This proves to be a difficult procedure. CSF is obtained at the third attempt, and is noted to be bloodstained. The CSF opening pressure is measured at 20 cmH$_2$0. Samples are sent off as above and the results are phoned back to the ward 1 h later as follows:

• *red cell count – bottle 2, 975 rbc/mm^3; bottle 3, 450 rbc/mm^3*
• *total oxy/methaemoglobin absorbancy: 0.25 (normal range <0.023)*
• *bilirubin absorbancy: 0.076 (normal range <0.007)*

How should these CSF results be interpreted?

• A guide to interpretation of CSF results is shown in Table 49
• There are large numbers of red blood cells in bottle 2

Table 48 Contraindications to lumbar puncture (LP)

Clinical/CT evidence of raised intracranial pressure	Risk of 'coning' when cerebrospinal fluid (CSF) is removed – reduction of CSF pressure below foramen magnum causes herniation of brainstem through this foramen, resulting in brain damage/death
Reduced conscious level/cerebral irritability	Coning is more likely in this situation even in the absence of CT abnormalities
Coagulopathy/thrombocytopenia	Where LP is required, platelet/clotting abnormalities should be corrected first

Table 49 Interpretation of cerebrospinal fluid (CSF) results in suspected subarachnoid haemorrhage (SAH)

	Time from bleed to appearance in CSF	Persistence in CSF	Comments
Red blood cells	Immediate	No	Absence of red cells from CSF generally excludes SAH within previous 48 h May appear in CSF following 'traumatic' lumbar puncture – red cell count will be lower in bottle 3 than in bottle 2 in this case 'Uniform' blood staining (same number of blood cells in bottle 2 and 3) is more suggestive of SAH
Oxy/methaemoglobin	Immediate	No	May appear in CSF following traumatic LP Absence of these pigments from CSF excludes SAH within preceding 48 h
Bilirubin	12 hours	Yes	Delayed appearance in CSF means that if LP is delayed for 12 hours from onset of symptoms, presence of bilirubin in CSF indicates bleed rather than traumatic LP May persist in CSF for 2–3 weeks following bleed – therefore useful when presentation to hospital is delayed

with fewer in bottle 3, which may be a result of the 'traumatic' LP; trauma could also explain the raised level of oxy/methaemoglobin
• However, a traumatic LP could not explain the raised level of bilirubin as this takes >12 h to appear in the CSF
• The raised bilirubin level is strongly suggestive of SAH as a cause for Mrs Jenski's symptoms

If subarachnoid haemorrhage is confirmed, what further management/ treatments should be instituted?

• Ensure symptoms remain adequately controlled
• Contact on-call regional neurosurgical team
• Commence nimodipine 60 mg orally every 4 h*
• Continue regular (at least hourly) neurological observations
• Careful fluid balance – reduction in plasma volume may increase cerebral ischaemia: ensure at least 3 L of fluid daily
• Compression stockings as deep vein thrombosis (DVT) prophylaxis (avoid anticoagulants until the aneurysm has been treated)

• Prescribe regular laxative – analgesia-induced constipation is common

*Nimodipine is a calcium antagonist, which has been shown to improve outcome following SAH, probably as a result of reduced cerebral vasospasm. If the patient is unable to swallow, a nasogastric tube should be sited. Intravenous nimodipine can only be administered via a central venous cannula, and so is generally avoided.

The neurosurgical team have been contacted and are planning to arrange transfer to the neurosurgical unit within the next 24 h to arrange magnetic resonance angiography with a view to treatment of the causative aneurysm if possible. Mrs Jenski has been stable on the ward for the past 18 h, receiving oral nimodipine (60 mg 4 hrly) and codeine phosphate with paracetamol when required for pain control.

You are called back to the ward because Mrs Jenski's neurological state has deteriorated. The nurses report that her conscious level has dropped. The Glasgow Coma Score is 8/15. Mrs Jenski's blood pressure has risen to 150/100 with a pulse of 50 beats/min.

What is the likely explanation for the deterioration in conscious level following SAH?

Possible causes include:
- Rebleeding: a further SAH
- Obstructive hydrocephalus: usually due to compression of the fourth ventricle
- Cerebral vasospasm: usually occurs later
- Seizure: unwitnessed seizure may be followed by a 'post-ictal' phase
- Drug-induced, e.g. following strong opiate analgesia

Which immediate actions should be taken?

- Assess the patency of Mrs Jenski's airway
- Apply oxygen and connect to cardiac monitor
- Recheck conscious level and pupillary responses
- Contact on-call anaesthetic/ITU team
- Inform the neurosurgical team of Mrs Jenski's deterioration
- Check Mrs Jenski's drug chart to ensure no culprit drug has been administered
- Arrange urgent repeat CT brain scan: Mrs Jenski is likely to require intubation and anaesthetic supervision during this procedure as she is drowsy and may not have the protective reflexes to prevent aspiration if she vomits

Mrs Jenski is intubated and undergoes a CT brain scan, which now reveals massive subarachnoid haemorrhage, extending into the fourth ventricle and resulting in early hydrocephalus. The neurosurgical team agree to immediate transfer to the neurosurgical intensive care unit following CT. Following urgent insertion of a CSF shunt Mrs Jenski's conscious level improves, enabling extubation. Magnetic resonance angiography the following day reveals an anterior communicating artery berry aneurysm that is suitable for surgical 'clipping'. This is undertaken the following day. Following a prolonged period of neurological rehabilitation Mrs Jenski is discharged from hospital three months later.

CASE REVIEW

A 37-year-old woman has been admitted with a history of sudden onset of severe headache associated with vomiting. This is improved with analgesia and a CT brain scan is normal. However, a subsequent lumbar puncture reveals raised levels of bilirubin, suggestive of a recent subarachnoid haemorrhage, which is the likely source of the patient's symptoms. Mrs Annika Jenski is observed closely on the ward, during which a sudden deterioration in her condition occurs. Mrs Jenski is intubated by the on-call anaesthetist and a repeat CT scan reveals that she has developed obstructive hydrocephalus which requires insertion of a shunt to lower the intracranial pressure. Following this, Mrs Jenski undergoes surgical clipping of an aneurysm that is the likely cause of her bleed. Mrs Jenski makes a full recovery after a prolonged period of neurological rehabilitation.

Recognition of the suggestive symptoms of subarachnoid haemorrhage in this case ensured appropriate investigation. A normal CT brain scan does not exclude the diagnosis, as illustrated by this case. Had Mrs Jenski been allowed home following the normal scan her subsequent deterioration could not have been identified and managed as quickly. As a result the outcome might have been very different.

It should be noted that, in most cases presenting in this way, CT and LP are both normal, enabling SAH to be excluded. As indicated in Table 47, the differential diagnosis is quite wide. Many of the conditions listed are benign and would not normally require hospital treatment, so the patient may be discharged once the symptoms improve. However, care should be taken to ensure that a serious cause other than SAH has also been excluded. Where possible the patient should be given a 'positive' diagnosis before discharge from hospital care. If this is not possible, a careful discussion is required with the patient prior to discharge, particularly if the symptoms are ongoing. The patient should be reassured that SAH has been excluded, but give clear instructions both to the patient and their GP regarding further action if the symptoms continue or worsen.

KEY POINTS

- Sudden severe headache is the hallmark of SAH.
- All patients presenting with suspected SAH should undergo a CT brain scan as soon as possible after admission.
- A normal CT brain scan does not exclude SAH.
- When the CT is normal a LP should be undertaken.

- LP should be delayed for >12 h following the onset of symptoms.
- Following confirmation of SAH, early discussion with a neurosurgical team is required.
- Consider alternative explanations for the headache when SAH has been excluded.

Further reading

Davenport R. Acute headache in the emergency department. *J Neurol Neurosurg Psychiatry* 2002; **72**(ii): ii33–7

Edlow JA, Caplan LR. Primary care: avoiding pitfalls in the diagnosis of subarachnoid hemorrhage. *N Engl J Med* 2000; **342**(1): 29–36

Hill S, Pinton A. Cerebrospinal fluid analysis in suspected subarachnoid haemorrhage. *Acute Med* 2006; **5**(1): 17–19

van Gijn J, Rinkel GJE. Subarachnoid haemorrhage: diagnosis, causes and management. *Brain* 2001; **124**: 249–78

Case 12 A 21-year-old man presenting following a seizure

You are called by a nurse at the university health centre regarding a 21-year-old male student who has been brought into the health centre having collapsed on the street outside. According to witnesses at the scene Josef Malek fell to the ground and started shaking violently. This lasted approximately 5 min, during which time Mr Malek was apparently unconscious. Mr Malek was also incontinent of urine and bit his tongue. After cessation of the shaking, Mr Malek remained unconscious for around 20 min, following which he has gradually become more alert. Mr Malek is now drowsy and confused, but responding to questions. There are no apparent injuries. The nurse has no other information about Mr Malek, but his mother has been contacted and will come directly to the hospital.

What challenges will this patient present?

• The witness's description of unconsciousness, associated with shaking, tongue-biting and urinary incontinence followed by gradual recovery is strongly suggestive of a *generalised tonic–clonic seizure (grand mal* seizure*)*
• In some cases the diagnosis is clear-cut but the differential diagnosis in Table 50 should be considered, particularly if a good witness account is not available
• Generalised seizure can occur as a result of other medical conditions – an underlying cause should always be considered (see Table 51)
• Management will be different if the patient has a prior history of seizure or a previous diagnosis of epilepsy. A history should always be sought from any available source if the patient is unable to provide this themselves
• Prolonged seizure (*status epilepticus*) is a life-threatening medical emergency. Recurrent seizures are also common in the early stages – the patient will need to be observed closely following arrival in hospital
• Following a seizure the post-ictal phase may result in prolonged drowsiness, confusion, agitation or aggression; this may complicate assessment of the patient

You are fast-bleeped by the nurse on the medical admissions ward. Shortly after Mr Malek's arrival on the ward he started shaking violently and became unconscious once more. You attend immediately and observe that there is generalised rigidity with muscular shaking of all limbs. The nurse reports that this has been ongoing for approximately 2 min. Mr Malek's eyes are closed and he is not responding to verbal commands. Mr Malek's breathing is noisy, with harsh gurgling sounds emanating from his airway. There is some blood coming from his mouth. Mr Malek is in bed with cotsides and does not appear to be in danger of injury at present.

What immediate management is required?

• Protect the airway
  ○ try to get Mr Malek onto his side or into the recovery position
  ○ listen to the breathing to detect if the airway may be obstructed by secretions or blood (as in this case – possibly from biting of the tongue)
  ○ rigidity of the jaw may make standard airway techniques impossible (e.g. chin-lift/jaw thrust)
  ○ insertion of a nasopharyngeal airway may be a useful adjunct to airway management and will allow suction of secretions
  ○ if the breathing remains noisy or gurgling, call for the assistance of an anaesthetist
• Apply high-flow oxygen (e.g. 15 L/min via a non-rebreath mask) and record oxygen saturation
• Obtain intravenous access
• Check pulse and blood pressure
• Check capillary blood glucose, to exclude hypoglycaemia as a cause for seizure
  ○ administer 25–50 mL of 50% glucose intravenously if the patient is hypoglycaemic

Acute Medicine: Clinical Cases Uncovered. By C. Roseveare.
Published 2009 by Blackwell Publishing, ISBN: 978-1-4051-6883-0

Table 50 Differential diagnosis for patients with suspected seizure

Syncope	Much more common than epilepsy; caused by transient cerebral hypoperfusion; may be preceded by nausea, light-headedness, blurred vision, sweating; patient becomes pale and sweaty; collapses to the floor; there may be associated shaking (myoclonic jerks) and even urinary incontinence; recovery is much faster than with seizure; there is no post-ictal phase; tongue biting is generally not a feature
Migraine	Preceded by visual aura; there may be altered state of consciousness; migraine headache very similar to the post-ictal headache
TGA	No true seizure activity; thought to be due to cerebral vasospasm; characterised by marked retro- and anterograde amnesia, lasting less than 24 h; full recovery and good prognosis
Sleep disorders	Narcolepsy – disorder of REM sleep; uncontrollable urges to sleep; can occur at inappropriate times
	Cataplexy – sudden decrease in voluntary muscle tone; often in response to strong or sudden change in emotion
	Sleep paralysis – the feeling of being awake but unable to move
Non-epileptiform seizures/dissociative seizures/pseudoseizure	May be misdiagnosed epilepsy or occur concurrently; corneal reflexes preserved during seizure; resistance to eye opening often a feature; can be very difficult to diagnose

REM, rapid eye movement; TGA, transient global amnesia.

Table 51 Underlying causes for seizure

Epilepsy	New diagnosis
	Poor compliance with medication
	Exposure to a trigger
	Lowered seizure threshold (concurrent illness or metabolic disturbance)
Infection	Meningitis
	Encephalitis
	Hyperthermia
Metabolic disturbance	Hypoglycaemia
	Hepatic encephalopathy
	Uraemia
	Hypomagnesaemia
	Hypocalcaemia
	Hyponatraemia
Drugs	Alcohol withdrawal
	Alcohol intoxication
	Recreational drugs
	Benzodiazepine withdrawal
Intracerebral	Previous stroke
	Acute severe stroke
	Subdural haematoma
	Subarachnoid haemorrhage
	Tumours
	Benign
	Malignant (primary or secondary)

○ consider intravenous vitamin B prior to administration of glucose if there is a possible history of malnutrition or alcohol excess to avoid precipitating Wernicke's encephalopathy (see p. 155)
- Ensure that Mr Malek is protected from potential injury – metal bars on the cotsides of beds should be covered with soft pillows

Following insertion of a nasopharyngeal airway and suction of bloodstained secretions, the gurgling inspiratory noises have ceased. Oxygen saturation is recording 98% with high-flow oxygen with a pulse of 100 beats/min. The blood pressure is difficult to obtain because of continued muscular activity, but the radial pulse is clearly palpable. The blood glucose recording is 6.3 mg/L. After 5 min seizure activity is continuing.

Should the seizure be terminated with drugs?

- Most seizures are self-terminating; however, prolonged seizure can be life-threatening, particularly if there is compromise to the airway
- Most clinicians will treat seizure that persists for >5 min, although treatment should not be delayed if the airway is thought to be obstructed or if the patient's oxygen saturation is falling
- Status epilepticus is usually defined as a seizure lasting >30 min or multiple seizures occurring without recovery

between; this patient's second seizure occurred fairly soon after the initial episode, and it is unclear whether there was full recovery between the attacks

• Most hospitals will have a local protocol or guideline for the management of seizure and status epilepticus

• Intravenous lorazepam (1–2 mg by intravenous bolus) is the usual drug of choice for initial management of non-terminating seizure; further doses up to a maximum of 8 mg can be given if required

• Diazepam can be used as an alternative to lorazepam and can be given rectally if intravenous access cannot be obtained

Mr Malek is given 2 mg of intravenous lorazepam. The seizure appears to stop, but within 5 min Mr Malek has started fitting again without recovering consciousness. Mr Malek is given two further 1 mg boluses of lorazepam with no effect.

What further management is required?

The patient is progressing to status epilepticus in view of the prolonged and recurrent seizure activity, which is not responding to conventional therapy. The following actions are necessary.

• **Call for senior help** – an anaesthetist may be required to assist with airway management; transfer to intensive care will be necessary if the seizure activity does not cease

• **Commence an intravenous infusion of phenytoin** (assuming the patient is not already taking this drug) – an initial infusion of 18 mg/kg (maximum 1 g) diluted in 100 mL of normal saline over 20 min

• **Obtain an arterial blood gas sample** – this will enable assessment of the degree of metabolic acidosis, which is a common consequence of prolonged seizure

• **Send venous blood** for full blood count, electrolytes, liver function, calcium, glucose, C-reactive protein and blood culture (if any suspicion of sepsis)

• **Commence cardiac monitoring** (phenytoin can result in cardiac arrhythmias)

A phenytoin infusion is started and the seizure ceases after approximately 5 min. Mr Malek is now drowsy, mumbling, disorientated and confused. The nasopharyngeal airway is still in situ and does not appear obstructed. Inspection of Mr Malek's tongue reveals an abrasion along one side that is not bleeding. There is no other apparent injury. Mr Malek's blood pressure is 160/80 mmHg, his pulse 100 beats/min.

The monitor appears to show sinus tachycardia. Oxygen saturation is 99% on high-flow oxygen with respiratory rate 14 breaths/min.

Arterial blood gases (while breathing 15 L/min O_2) are as follows: pH 7.19, pCO_2 6.5, pO_2 25.6, HCO_3 16.5, base excess –6.5, lactate 4.7, Na 136, K 4.7.

What are the next steps in his management?

• Formal assessment of conscious level using the Glasgow Coma Score (GCS, see p. 127):

  ○ if the GCS is <8 Mr Malek's airway is still likely to be in danger, as he may aspirate secretions or vomit; endotracheal intubation may be required

• Regular neurological observations ('neuro obs') every 15–30 min (see p. 131)

  ○ his conscious level will be impaired as a result of the 'post-ictal' state and the sedative drugs he has received

  ○ speed of recovery is variable but a gradual improvement of conscious level should be expected

  ○ any significant deterioration in conscious level (usually defined as a two-point reduction in the GCS) should be taken seriously, as it may suggest sinister intracranial pathology as a cause of the original seizure (see Table 51) or ongoing non-convulsive seizure activity

• Commence a seizure chart, ensuring documentation of any further convulsive seizure activity

• Obtain an ECG and request a chest radiograph

• Repeat the arterial blood gas to ensure improvement of acid base disturbance:

  ○ rapid recovery of lactic acidosis is usual following discontinuation of seizure

• Obtain a full history from any available source; this may include:

  ○ witnesses at the scene of the original episode

  ○ staff at the health centre to which he was initially brought

  ○ the ambulance crew who brought him to hospital

  ○ Mr Malek's friends and relatives

  ○ Mr Malek's GP

  ○ Mr Malek's hospital records

• Conduct a full examination including detailed neurological assessment

Specific issues to consider during the history and examination are summarised in Table 52.

Mr Malek's mother has now arrived on the ward. She reports that her son is 23 years old and has no serious past

Table 52 Points to consider on history and examination following admission with seizure

History

Previous history of seizures

A family history of seizures

Any history of head injury in the past

History of headaches or focal neurology (suggestive of space-occupying lesion)

Any specific triggers (flashing lights, loud noises, alcohol-intoxication, sleep deprivation, fevers, menstruation in female patients)

Drugs (ask about illicit drugs)

Previous stroke

Examination

Assess for signs of infection – particularly evidence of meningitis

Rash, neck stiffness, photophobia should all prompt early senior input

Features of chronic liver disease

Spider naevi, palmar erythema, jaundice, ascites, etc.

External evidence of head injury

Bruising, scalp tenderness, abrasions, cuts, etc.

Evidence of other injury

Shoulder dislocation or limb fracture should be actively sought

Detailed neurological assessment

Look for evidence of focal neurological abnormality

Remember that post-ictal paralysis following seizure can be focal/unilateral (Todd's paralysis) – this can be mistaken for stroke (see Case 14)

Bilateral upgoing plantar responses can also be seen as a post-ictal phenomenon

Look for needle track marks suggestive of illicit drug use

Pinpoint pupils may suggest opiate usage

Dilated, sluggishly reactive pupils may suggest anticholinergic drug overdose

medical history. There is no documented personal or family history of epilepsy and Mr Malek takes no regular medication. Six months earlier Mr Malek had an episode where he apparently 'fainted' while alone at home. He woke up on the floor without any clear explanation, and no obvious injury. Mr Malek was tired for the rest of the day, but chose not to visit the doctor despite his mother's concerns. Mr Malek has not reported any headaches or other neurological symptoms recently and there is no history of head injury.

Mr Malek is a student at the university and lives in a shared house with friends. He is currently undertaking his exams, for which he had been working very hard. Mr Malek's mother has been concerned that he has not been sleeping properly in recent weeks. She thinks he drinks around 15 pints of beer and smokes 10 cigarettes per week. As far as she is aware Mr Malek does not take illicit drugs. He has a driving licence but does not own a car at present.

Mr Malek's university friends report that he complained of feeling generally unwell this morning and did not attend lectures. They think he was planning on visiting the university health centre this morning.

On examination Mr Malek's GCS remains at 13/15. He is disorientated in time and place, and his eyes open in response to command. Mr Malek has a mild pyrexia (37.5°C) and there are some coarse crepitations at the base of his right lung. The abrasion on his tongue is not bleeding. There are no external signs of injury and Mr Malek is not in pain on movement of his limbs. There is no neck stiffness or photophobia and no petechial rash. The remainder of Mr Malek's examination is unremarkable.

The results of initial investigations are as follows:
- Hb 14.5, white cell count 15.4, platelets 268
- Na 137, K 4.5, urea 3.5, creatinine 67
- liver function tests/calcium/magnesium normal
- urinalysis: clear
- ECG: sinus tachycardia – otherwise normal
- chest radiograph – mild right basal shadowing; otherwise normal
- repeat arterial blood gas (while breathing room air):
pH 7.36, pCO$_2$ 4.6, pO$_2$ 10.5, HCO$_3$ 21, base excess –2.1, lactate 1.9

What do the history, examination and investigations suggest?

• The history suggests a primary generalised seizure; although there is no prior history of epilepsy, the unwitnessed episode six months ago may have been a previous seizure

• There is no clear precipitant, although sleep deprivation is a possible trigger

• Mild pyrexia and elevation of the white cell count suggest the possibility of underlying infection, which is also supported by Mr Malek feeling unwell on the morning of admission; however, all of these features can also be seen as a direct consequence of a seizure in the absence of infection. Patients often report non-specific symptoms in the lead-up to a seizure (termed an 'aura')

• The chest radiograph abnormality, mild hypoxia and right basal crackles may reflect pre-existing pulmonary infection, or aspiration of secretions/vomit during the seizure

Does Mr Malek require an urgent brain scan?

Urgent CT or magnetic resonance brain scanning should always be considered in the following situations.

• Where there has been any suspicion of recent head injury (prior to or during the seizure)

• Where there is focal neurological deficit on examination

• Where there have been neurological symptoms in the lead-up to admission

• Where there is any suspicion of meningitis:

  ○ in this case a lumbar puncture will also be required if the scan is normal

  ○ if meningococcal disease is considered possible, remember that intravenous antibiotics should be administered without delay (e.g. cefotaxime 2 g, 4 hrly)

• Where there is prolonged seizure (>30 min) or prolonged unconsciousness that is not improving following discontinuation of the seizure – in such cases the patient will often require general anaesthesia, intubation and ventilation for the purposes of transfer and imaging

Over the next few hours Mr Malek's condition gradually recovers. The drowsiness resolves. Mr Malek remains breathless on mild exertion and desaturates to 95% when his oxygen is removed. He is reviewed by the chest physiotherapist and following her treatment he expectorates some green sputum. Mr Malek starts oral co-amoxyclav (625 mg three times daily) on the presumption that he has pneumonia, possibly related to aspiration. He is able to confirm his mother's history with no further additions. He admits that he was incontinent during the episode six months ago; with hindsight he thinks that this

was probably a similar, albeit less prolonged, attack to that which he experienced this morning.

It is decided that urgent CT brain scanning is not required. Mr Malek's mother asks if he will start medication to prevent this problem from recurring.

Should Mr Malek start regular anti-epileptic drug therapy?

This issue is complex and there are no clear-cut answers. Treatment will reduce the risk of recurrent episodes, but does not affect the long-term prognosis. Decisions regarding treatment are often more complex in young women, where there in the risk of fetal abnormality with some drugs should the patient become pregnant. Some drugs also interact with the oral contraceptive pill.

It is often worth discussing treatment with a neurologist or epilepsy specialist if your hospital has one. Following a single, isolated seizure without any of the features listed below, the decision to start anti-epileptic drug therapy can usually be deferred until outpatient review.

Regular anti-epileptic drug therapy should be considered where there is:

• Evidence of more than one episode

• Structural intracranial disease (e.g. tumour, stroke or head injury)

• A prolonged seizure or status epilepticus resulting in admission

Given that this episode was prolonged and probably represents a second seizure, Mr Malek starts taking regular oral sodium valproate following discussion with the on-call neurology registrar. Mr Malek continues with the oral co-amoxyclav, and the following morning his breathing is much improved. Mr Malek's chest now sounds clear and he has had no further episodes of seizure. He is keen to go home.

For how long should the patient be kept in hospital?

• Following a first hospital attendance with seizure a patient should usually be observed for a minimum of 12 h, or until there is full neurological recovery; in cases of prolonged seizure the post-ictal phase may last for much longer

• If there are complicating factors such as infection, injury or aspiration these should be addressed prior to discharge from hospital

• If a patient lives alone a more prolonged period of inpatient observation may be required

What else do you need to consider prior to discharge?

- **Driving restrictions:**

   The DVLA has strict guidelines on driving for patients who have experienced a seizure. Up-to-date advice can be found on their website (www.dvla.gov.uk). The main points to remember are:
   - following a seizure, patients are obliged to inform the DVLA; they should not drive a car or motorbike until the DVLA advises them to do so
   - the medical team caring for the patient should inform the patient of this obligation; the patient should also be advised that failure to comply with this advice will almost certainly invalidate their car insurance
   - most patients will not be able to drive any vehicle for a minimum of one year from the seizure
   - the medical team is not required to inform the DVLA directly unless there is reason to believe that the patient is continuing to drive
- **Employment, hobbies and other activities:**
   - the patient should be advised to avoid activities that might put them at risk should a further seizure occur. Patients who work in the building industry may have to discuss health and safety implications with their employer
   - patients should also be advised not to take baths when alone in a house, as drowning incidents have been reported
- **Follow-up:**
   - most patients who have experienced a seizure should be referred to a neurologist for follow-up after discharge from hospital. This will enable the organisation and review of brain imaging tests (e.g. CT or MRI scan). Many hospitals will run a specific *first seizure clinic* from which these investigations can be coordinated
   - an electroencephalogram (EEG) is often useful to classify the nature of the seizure disorder and to define the need for ongoing treatment
   - depending on local practices it may be helpful to book these investigations at the time of the patient's discharge from hospital so that they can be undertaken prior to specialist neurology review
   - follow-up will also enable those who go on to receive a diagnosis of epilepsy to be offered the psychological support they may require and for their families to be educated in epilepsy; there may be an epilepsy nurse specialist who is able to provide advice and support following discharge

Mr Malek is discharged from hospital and is prescribed sodium valproate 200 mg twice daily, increasing to 400 mg twice daily after one week; an outpatient cerebral MRI scan and EEG are booked to be carried out prior to follow-up in the hospital's first seizure clinic. Arrangements are also made for Mr Malek to be contacted by the hospital's epilepsy nurse specialist one week after discharge. He is advised to contact the DVLA and not to drive until their advice is received.

CASE REVIEW

In this case a 23-year-old student is referred to hospital after collapsing in the street outside the university health centre. The description from witnesses at the scene suggests Mr Josef Malek has experienced a generalised tonic–clonic seizure. Although Mr Malek appears to recover from the initial event, a further seizure occurs shortly after his arrival in hospital. His airway is initially compromised by bloodstained secretions coming from an abrasion on his tongue; however, this is cleared with suction and the insertion of a nasopharyngeal airway.

Despite a total of 4 mg of intravenous lorazepam, the seizure continues, requiring the administration of a phenytoin infusion. This results in termination of the seizure, following which Mr Malek makes a gradual recovery. Further history obtained initially from his mother suggests a prior unwitnessed seizure six months earlier, on which basis Mr Malek starts taking sodium valproate 200 mg twice daily. Clinical examination and a chest radiograph reveal right basal consolidation. Mr Malek is treated with chest physiotherapy and oral co-amoxyclav and makes a rapid recovery.

On discharge from hospital 24 h later Mr Malek is referred to the first seizure clinic and an epilepsy nurse specialist, with arrangements made to have an EEG and

Continued

cerebral MRI prior to this appointment. Mr Malek is advised to contact the DVLA and not to drive pending their advice.

Management of seizure in the context of previous 'known' epilepsy differs from the management of a first seizure. In this situation it is always important to establish whether the patient is already under the care of a neurologist and to clarify the usual pattern of seizure control. In some cases there is a clear explanation for the deterioration in seizure control, such as a change in medication, poor compliance with treatment or reduced drug absorption because of vomiting or diarrhoea. Intercurrent illness, particularly sepsis, may also influence seizure control.

It is important to remember that non-epileptic attacks (pseudoseizures) can affect patients with a prior history of epilepsy. Up to 25% of patients who require intubation for seizure are subsequently labelled as having had pseudoseizure. Distinction of such episodes from 'true'

seizures can be very difficult. Measurement of serum prolactin (usually elevated following a true seizure) can be helpful in some cases, if measured within an hour of presentation; in cases of severe difficulty, obtaining a prolonged EEG recording may be diagnostic – absence of epileptiform activity in the trace during a witnessed seizure strongly suggests pseudoseizure.

Older people admitted following a seizure are much more likely to have a structural brain abnormality causing the seizure. Seizure is a recognised presentation of cerebral tumours and CT brain scanning should always be undertaken as soon as possible. Given that 50% of cerebral tumours represent metastases from distant sites, the history, examination and investigations should include careful consideration of a source of primary tumour; breast examination is mandatory in female patients and careful inspection of the skin should be undertaken for evidence of skin tumours.

KEY POINTS

- Generalised tonic–clonic seizure is a potentially life-threatening medical emergency.
- Initial management of seizure should concentrate on protection of the patient's airway and ensuring that they are not in danger of injury during the attack.
- When a seizure is prolonged (>5 min) or where the airway is deemed to be in danger, termination of seizure is required; an intravenous benzodiazepine (e.g. lorazepam) is the usual first drug of choice.

- Phenytoin infusion may be helpful if the lorazepam fails to terminate the seizure.
- Following cessation of seizure activity, a careful history should be obtained, focusing on possible underlying causes for the seizure and any prior similar episodes.

Further reading

Commission on Classification and Terminology of the International League against Epilepsy. *Epilepsia* 1981; **22**: 489

Francis P, Baker GA. Non-epileptic attack disorder (NEAD): a comprehensive review. *Seizure* 1999; **8**(1): 53–61

Pohlmann-Eden B *et al.* The first seizure and its management in adults and children. *BMJ* 2006; **332**: 339–42

Shorvon S. The management of status epilepticus. *J Neurol Neurosurg Psychiatry* 2001; **70**(2): 1122–7

Walker M. Status epilepticus: an evidence based guide. *BMJ* 2005; **33**: 673–7

PART 2: CASES

The emergency department has contacted you regarding a 22-year-old man who has been brought in by his friends. Andy Jennings is apparently normally fit and well, with no known medical problems. Mr Jennings was last seen the previous evening when he was reported as being well; however, his friends became concerned when Mr Jennings did not appear for breakfast, at which point they entered his room and found him unresponsive on the bed.

What challenges will this patient present?

• The unconscious or comatose patient will always require urgent assessment
• The differential diagnosis is vast (see Table 53)
• The available history is often poor, necessitating the physician to make key judgements on the basis of limited information

Upon your arrival, Mr Jennings is lying on his side. Respiratory effort is poor with a rate of 5 breaths/min, and he has harsh upper airway sounds. Mr Jennings is centrally and peripherally cyanosed with unrecordable oxygen saturation; blood pressure is 80/55 mmHg.

What immediate management is required?

The ABC approach should be used as follows
• Airway: obstruction is a major concern for any patient with reduced conscious level. Airway management should include:
  ○ appropriate positioning of patient (on his side or in the recovery position)
  ○ chin lift or jaw thrust manoeuvres
  ○ insertion of Guedel or nasopharyngeal airway if tolerated
  ○ suction to remove upper airway secretions or vomit
  ○ removal of loose false teeth or other potential obstructing objects from the mouth
• Breathing:
  ○ apply oxygen (e.g. 15 L via non-rebreath mask)
  ○ recheck respiratory rate
  ○ check oxygen saturation: if the pulse oximeter is not able to record a figure due to poor peripheral circulation obtain an arterial blood gas sample
• Circulation:
  ○ recheck the pulse and blood pressure
  ○ insert an intravenous cannula and infuse fluid if hypotensive or evidence of shock (see Case 8)

Vomit and secretions are sucked from Mr Jennings' mouth and upper airway, following which his breathing is less noisy. A Guedel airway is inserted, which Mr Jennings tolerates without difficulty. High-flow oxygen is applied and 1000 mL of normal saline is infused rapidly via a peripheral cannula. His blood pressure now measures 100/60 and his pulse oximeter reading is 99%. His respiratory rate remains low at 7 breaths/min.

Arterial blood gas analysis reveals pH 7.32, pCO_2 7.6, pO_2 19.5, base excess −1.2, lactate 1.8.

• The blood gases indicate a respiratory acidosis that probably relates to poor respiratory drive
• Mr Jennings is oxygenating adequately with supplemental oxygen applied and the normal lactate suggests adequate tissue perfusion at present. This will need to be monitored closely
• It is now important to assess Mr Jennings' conscious level more thoroughly (often termed 'D' – for 'disability' – in the ABCDE approach, see p. 7)

Acute Medicine: Clinical Cases Uncovered. By C. Roseveare.
Published 2009 by Blackwell Publishing, ISBN: 978-1-4051-6883-0

Table 53 Causes of impaired conscious state

Cause	Clinical features
Cerebral pathology	
Ischaemic stroke/Intracerebral haemorrhage	More common in older patients; if patient is deeply unconscious, ischaemic stroke is unlikely; brainstem haemorrhage is a possible explanation for sudden loss of consciousness: this may mimic the signs of opiate toxicity (pinpoint pupils, respiratory depression)
Subarachnoid haemorrhage	Usually a large bleed, or complicated by obstructive hydrocephalus if the patient is comatose so should be visible on CT scan; lumbar puncture is required to completely exclude subarachnoid haemorrhage, but may be hazardous in the context of reduced conscious level
Extradural haematoma	Extradural, usually follows soon after documented head injury; sudden deterioration in consciousness with pupillary inequality
Subdural haematoma	More common in older patients – head injury may have been apparently trivial and occurred several weeks prior to admission. Drowsiness often gradual in onset and conscious level may fluctuate
Post ictal	In known epileptic or following first seizure; if seizure unwitnessed may be difficult to diagnose; look for signs of unexplained bruising (suggestive of seizure), incontinence, tongue biting
Intracranial tumours	These generally do not cause acute deterioration in conscious level unless there has been associated bleeding, or there is a rapidly rising intracranial pressure, e.g. due to obstructive hydrocephalus
Respiratory disease	
Hypercapnia and carbon dioxide narcosis	see Case 6; remember raised CO_2 (due to respiratory depression) may be the consequence rather than the cause of reduced conscious level
Carbon monoxide poisoning	Faulty gas equipment, especially boilers, and smoke inhalation are the most common reasons for this
Severe hypoxia	May also cause seizure; look for underlying cause of hypoxia
Sepsis	
Meningitis/encephalitis	The 'classic' presentation with headache, photophobia, and neck stiffness is often absent. Reduced conscious level may be the only sign of intracranial sepsis
Systemic	Non-neurological infection can also result in reduced conscious level, e.g. urinary sepsis in the elderly, meningococcal septicaemia without meningitis
Metabolic	
Hypoglycaemia Chronic liver disease Hypothermia	Usually patients on insulin or oral hypoglycaemics; sometimes taken as a deliberate overdose. Also occurs in patients with liver disease. True 'fasting hypoglycaemia' is very uncommon
Hyponatraemia	Acute or severe hyponatraemia may result in seizure or reduced conscious level
Uraemia	Other features to suggest this are a history of renal disease, hiccupping and pruritus
Hepatic encephalopathy	Usually evidence of chronic liver disease (jaundice, spider naevi, ascites, etc.); onset usually gradual

Table 53 *Continued*

Cause	Clinical features
Pharmacological	
Opiates	May be as a result of illicit, or prescribed, drug usage; pinpoint pupils and respiratory depression for opiate toxicity
Benzodiazepines	Following benzodiazepine overdose patients often simply appear 'deeply asleep' – pulse, blood pressure and pupils are usually unaffected due to the wide 'therapeutic index' of these drugs (i.e. the large difference between the therapeutic and toxic dose)
Alcohol	Can result in impaired consciousness alone, or commonly in conjunction with other drugs (see also Case 16)
Any drug with sedative properties	e.g. antiepileptic medication, antidepressant drugs – obtain a full drug history from the patient and anyone else in the patient's household; some drug levels may be measured in the laboratory

How should Mr Jennings' conscious level be assessed?

- The simplest method of assessment of conscious level is the AVPU score:
  - ○ **alert**
  - ○ response to **voice**
  - ○ response to **pain**
  - ○ **unresponsive**
- A more accurate assessment of level of consciousness can be obtained using the Glasgow Coma Scale (GCS) (see Table 54)
- Use of the GCS will enable *quantification* of the level of consciousness
  - ○ a score of <8 usually implies that the patient will not have the protective reflexes to prevent aspiration of vomit or secretions; in this situation urgent measures to improve the conscious level should be undertaken where possible; if this is not possible immediate anaesthetic support should be sought to enable formal protection of the airway by the insertion of an endotracheal tube
  - ○ indications for early anaesthetic/critical care team involvement are listed in Table 55

Mr Jennings withdraws from painful stimuli, opens his eyes in response to pain and makes incomprehensible sounds, giving a total GCS of 8 (E, 2; V, 2; M, 4) and AVPU rating of P. Mr Jennings is starting to cough on the Guedel airway, which is removed and replaced by a nasopharyngeal airway.

Table 54 The Glasgow Coma Score

Eye opening	Score
Spontaneously	4
To speech	3
To painful stimulus	2
No response	1

Best verbal response	
Orientated	5
Disorientated	4
Inappropriate words	3
Incomprehensible sounds	2
No response	1

Best motor response	
Obeys verbal commands	6
Localises painful stimuli	5
Withdrawal from pain	4
Flexion to pain	3
Extension to pain	2
No response	1

Table 55 Findings that may suggest the need for early involvement from anaesthetic/critical care team for an unconscious patient

Glasgow Coma Score <8

Inability to maintain adequate airway

Ongoing hypoxia despite airway adjuncts and oxygen therapy

Persistent vomiting

Agitation resulting in a risk of injury to the patient

Persistent seizure

The need to transfer the patient for a computed tomography brain scan

Is there a reversible cause of Mr Jennings' reduced conscious level?

Having addressed ABC and D, exposure of the patient (E) is required to address this question.

Although the causes of reduced consciousness are numerous (Table 53), there is a small number of conditions where immediate action can make a huge difference to the patient's outcome.

• **Hypoglycaemia**: reversible with administration of glucose

• **Opiate or benzodiazepine overdose**: see Boxes 23 and 24

• **Meningococcal septicaemia/meningitis**: early administration of antibiotics will dramatically improve mortality

• **Head injury/trauma**: particularly if there is a potential of co-existent neck trauma

What further actions are required?

• **Measure capillary blood glucose**: if <3 administer intravenous glucose (e.g. 25–50 mL 50% glucose); a rapid improvement in conscious level usually follows. Remember that capillary readings can be inaccurate in the context of hypoglycaemia – if there is clinical suspicion of hypoglycaemia (see Table 56) empirical administration of glucose should be considered even if the glucometer reads a normal level. Most blood gas analysers will also provide a more accurate glucose level. The mnemonic ABCDEFG (airway, breathing, circulation, don't ever forget glucose) may serve as a useful reminder!

• **Check size of pupils**: if pupils are both small (pinpoint pupils) an opiate overdose is a strong possibility (see Box 23). Administer naloxone 400 µg as intravenous bolus – as with hypoglycaemia an immediate response is

---

Box 23 Opiate toxicity

Clinical features
• reduced conscious level
• pinpoint pupils
• respiratory depression

Treatment of suspected opiate toxicity

If opiate toxicity is suspected then give naloxone 400 µg i.v./i.m. immediately. This dose may be repeated up to five times if necessary; however, recovery is often virtually instantaneous. The half-life of naloxone is much shorter than most opiates and therefore infusions of naloxone, sometimes for up to 48 h, may be required to prevent a relapse of consciousness. When giving an infusion, it is normal to start it at approximately two-thirds of the dose required to achieve an improvement in conscious state. For example:

• 3 × naloxone 400 µg vials (1200 µg) are given and the patient wakes up
• the patient subsequently deteriorates and you wish to start an infusion
• 2/3 of 1200 µg = 800 µg, therefore start infusion at 800 µg/h
• to make the infusion, dilute 4 mg (10 vials) in 20 mL of normal saline or 5% glucose
• the rate can then be calculated and adjusted accordingly (in this case 4 mL/h)

---

likely if the diagnosis is correct; however, the long duration of action of some opiate drugs in comparison with naloxone means that further bolus doses are likely to be required, followed by an infusion in some cases

• **Look closely for a petechial rash** (see Plate 5) suggestive of meningococcal disease in the context of reduced conscious level; a fever or history of rapidly progressive infective symptoms preceding onset of coma should also raise the suspicion of this condition. Administer a large dose of intravenous antibiotic (e.g. benzlypenicillin 2.4 g or cefotaxime 2 g) if there is any possibility of this

• **Search for bruises/injuries and try to obtain a history of possible trauma prior to collapse:** unequal pupils, particularly if one is large and unresponsive, may suggest raised intracranial pressure (e.g. from intracranial bleed). If trauma is possible, ensure a hard neck collar is applied until neck injury can be excluded

• **Look for evidence of needle 'track marks'** over the antecubital fossae or evidence of other injection sites, suggestive of intravenous drug abuse (particularly opiates)

Table 56 Suggested investigations for an unconscious patient

Test	Rationale	Comments
FBC	Raised WCC, low platelets in sepsis	Incidental findings, e.g. anaemia, may require further investigation
U&E, calcium	Hyponatraemia may cause seizure or reduced consciousness; hypercalcaemia may cause seizure	Underlying cause may require further investigation
LFT	Evidence of chronic liver disease – may suggest hepatic encephalopathy as cause for unconsciousness	Remember blood-borne hepatitis (B and C) in patients with history of drug abuse
Clotting	Risk of intracranial haemorrhage if abnormal Abnormality may reflect chronic liver disease	If very abnormal consider possibility of undisclosed paracetamol overdose (or use of anticoagulant drugs) (see Case 21)
Paracetamol level	May have taken overdose (see Case 21)	Interpretation will depend on timing of consumption. Remember possibility of overdose of paracetamol/opiate combination (e.g. co-codamol) in patients with evidence of opiate toxicity
Other drug level	Many drugs can be measured on blood tests; particularly useful for antiepileptic drugs (e.g. phenytoin, carbamazepine)	Take an 'extra' plain blood sample and send to the lab; if further history comes to light about possible drug consumption this may be useful
Glucose	More accurate than capillary measurements	Incidental raised levels will need to be repeated after recovery. If insulin overdose is suspected, take a sample at the time of hypoglycaemia for measurement of insulin and c-peptide level
Alcohol level	Quantification of alcohol level may help to determine if this is the cause for unconsciousness	Rarely alters management, unless very high levels in which case dialysis may be required
Urine toxicology screen	Many drugs may be measured in urine	Usually takes >24 h for result to be available so little value in acute setting; however, can be useful in retrospect to identify cause of unconsciousness; also useful if possibility of administration of drug by a third party without knowledge of the patient
ECG	Arrhythmias due to drug use; evidence of myocardial ischaemia, pericarditis or recent MI	Myocardial ischaemia is associated with cocaine use
Chest radiograph	Evidence of aspiration Incidental findings	
CT brain scan	Evidence of intracranial pathology	See text
Lumbar puncture	Evidence of meningitis or subarachnoid haemorrhage	Always perform CT brain prior to LP and remember that CT does not exclude raised intracranial pressure: in the context of reduced consciousness LP can be hazardous and should be carefully considered with advice of senior colleagues

CT, computed tomography; FBC, full blood count; LFT, liver function test; LP, lumbar puncture; U&E, urea and electrolytes; WCC, white cell count.

PART 2: CASES

Box 24 Benzodiazepine toxicity/overdose

This can occur either as a result of an act of deliberate self-harm or secondary to medical administration.

Benzodiazepines can result in flaccidity, ataxia/dysarthria, hypotension, respiratory depression and coma; however, this is usually only seen when there is significant toxicity, and most cases of benzodiazepine toxicity can be managed conservatively. If there is significant respiratory compromise then the benzodiazepine can be reversed.

Treatment

Flumazenil 100–200 µg i.v. should be given immediately by slow intravenous injection, and this may be repeated if there is a positive response

Flumazenil is a specific benzodiazepine antagonist

Like naloxone it has a very short half-life, and therefore repeated administration or infusion may be required

Note that *care must be taken* with flumazenil as it can sometimes precipitate seizures, particularly in patients who are on long-term benzodiazepines, those who have also taken tricyclic antidepressants or those who already suffer with seizures/epilepsy

It should generally *not be given* to patients who have taken mixed or unknown substances in overdose, or those who have been given benzodiazepines to terminate seizure activity

---

• **Look for evidence of chronic liver disease** (spider naevi, palmar erythema, gynaecomastia, jaundice, ascites, testicular atrophy)

• **Smell the patient's breath** for alcohol or ketones

• **Start a neuro observation chart** (see Fig. 37): this will enable recording of the level of consciousness and other clues to Mr Jennings' neurological status, and for these to be followed over time by different members of staff

Blood glucose is measured at 5.2 mmol/L and you can find no signs of intravenous drug abuse. Mr Jennings' respiratory effort remains extremely poor, and he has bilateral pin-point pupils.

The respiratory examination is unremarkable; there is no evidence of a rash or fever and no sign of bruising or injury. The history you have been given, suggesting that Mr Jennings was found on his bed, is not supportive of head injury or other trauma immediately before the onset of symptoms.

There is no evidence of chronic liver disease and Mr Jennings does not smell of alcohol.

The clinical picture is suggestive of opiate toxicity.

How can we get a collateral history?

The paucity of background information that usually accompanies the unconscious patient can make decision making more difficult, so use all available resources to your advantage.

The potential sources of information that should be explored are listed on p. 160. It will be particularly important to establish whether Mr Jennings could have access to prescribed opiate drugs, or is a known addict.

Specific questions to ask will include:

• Is there a history of previous drug (or alcohol) abuse?

• Does the patient or a family member receive prescribed opiate drugs?

• Were any drugs/empty medication packets found at the scene, or was there any evidence at the scene of drug abuse (syringes, needles, etc.)?

• Has he been unwell in the lead-up to the collapse: febrile illness, recent headaches, etc.?

• Is there a recent history of depression or past history of suicide attempts?

• Is there any past history of seizure?

The ambulance crew has already left, but did not report finding any medication packages or drugs at the scene. You telephone Mr Jennings' GP, who informs you that he has no pre-existing medical conditions, is on no regular medication, and does not regularly attend the practice. You question his friends, who report no recent illness, head injury or previous seizure. However, they are evasive in their responses to questions about drug usage and hint that Mr Jennings may have tried smoking heroin recently.

You administer naloxone 400 µg by intravenous bolus and review his response. Within 40 s of giving the naloxone you notice a marked improvement in Mr Jennings' conscious state. He spontaneously opens his eyes and tries to sit up in bed. You calculate his GCS to be 13/15. You reassure Mr Jennings that everything is under control and he appears to understand; however, within 5 min his GCS has fallen again to 8/15. The nurse then approaches you, asking whether, in light of his fluctuating GCS, he requires an urgent CT brain scan.

Do we need to perform an urgent computed tomography (CT) brain scan?

• A CT brain scan should always be considered for patients with reduced conscious level where no clear-cut cause has been identified

• Remember that one cause does not preclude another; for example, a patient may have taken a large dose of

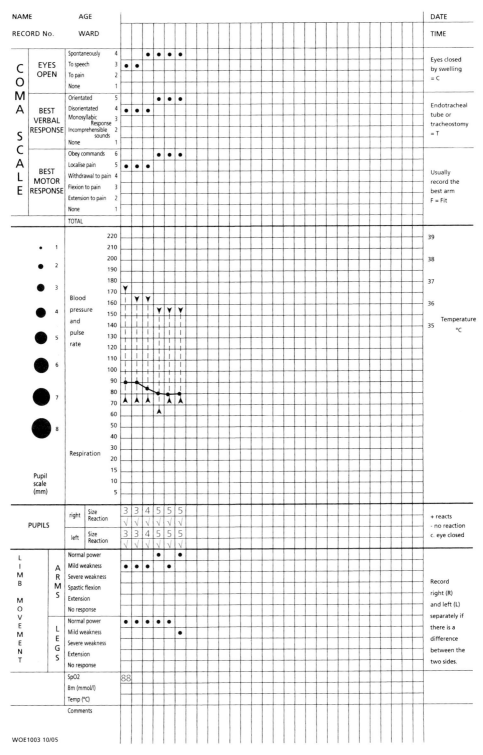

Figure 37 Neurological observations chart: recordings should usually be undertaken at 30-min intervals.

opiate to relieve a headache due to raised intracranial pressure, or may have sustained a head injury following a seizure

• It should be remembered that there may be risks in transfer of an unconscious patient to the CT scanner: if the airway is likely to be at risk (e.g. GCS <8) an anaesthetist should accompany the patient to the scanner. Often the patient is anaesthetised and formally intubated for the purposes of the scan

There are, however, some caveats to CT imaging to be aware of.

• A normal CT brain scan does not completely exclude subarachnoid haemorrhage (SAH) – see Case 11

• A normal CT brain scan cannot completely exclude raised intracranial pressure (ICP). Keep this diagnosis in mind if there are other clinical features suggestive of raised ICP, e.g. nausea and vomiting, papilloedema, impaired GCS, false localising signs such as sixth cranial nerve palsy, and bradycardia with hypertension

• A normal CT brain scan may not exclude an early ischaemic stroke.

• CT imaging may be required to exclude contraindications to lumbar puncture, if this is deemed necessary

You review the situation clinically and feel that in light of Mr Jennings' initial good response to naloxone, the likelihood of an intracerebral lesion causing his impaired conscious state would be low, and that a CT scan at the present time is not indicated. You decide to persevere with naloxone therapy and give Mr Jennings a repeat stat dose of 400 μg, which has the same affect as previously; therefore, you commence him on an i.v. infusion of naloxone to run for the next 24 h. Mr Jennings maintains his GCS at 14/15 with the naloxone infusion, his airway is protected and his blood pressure and oxygen saturations are now 110/75 and 97% respectively.

You note that Mr Jennings desaturates to 90% on removal of the oxygen. Examination of his chest reveals crackles at the right base.

What other investigations and treatment are required urgently?

• Further investigations for an unconscious patient and their rationale are summarised in Table 56

• It is particularly important to consider measuring the blood paracetamol level in this situation. Many paracetamol/opiate combination drugs are available,

some of which can be purchased without prescription. Interpretation of the paracetamol level will be difficult unless Mr Jennings is able to tell you at precisely what time he took any medication. If there is a suspicion of drug overdose in this setting it is advisable to start treatment with *N*-acetyl cysteine if any paracetamol is detected on blood testing (see Case 21). Monitoring of liver function and blood clotting over the next 24–48 h will determine the need to continue this, along with discussions with Mr Jennings as his condition improves

Investigations reveal normal haemoglobin with a raised white cell count (17.5, neutrophils 12.7). Electrolytes and renal function are normal. His alanine transaminase (ALT) is slightly raised at 65 with otherwise normal liver function tests (LFT). Blood clotting is normal and paracetamol is not detected in the blood.

An ECG shows sinus tachycardia, but no other abnormality.

A chest radiograph reveals right basal shadowing (see Fig. 38).

What further treatment is required?

• The clinical and radiological features suggest that Mr Jennings has right basal pneumonia. This may have been caused by aspiration of vomit or stomach contents while unconscious: this probably explains the desaturation when oxygen is removed

• Ensure that Mr Jennings is nursed in a semi-recumbent position (i.e. sitting up in bed) and that his

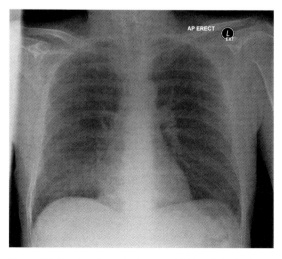

Figure 38 Chest radiograph showing right basal shadowing.

conscious level is maintained at a level where he will continue to protect his airway and cough effectively
• Chest physiotherapy may be helpful if Mr Jennings will comply with this
• Mr Jennings should be started on intravenous antibiotics (e.g. co-amoxyclav 1.2 g i.v. tds)
• Regular treatment with saline nebules (e.g. 5 mL 4–6 hourly) and humidified oxygen will help Mr Jennings to expectorate
• The respiratory rate and oxygen saturation should be monitored closely
• Consider deep vein thrombosis (DVT) prophylaxis (e.g. subcutaneous enoxaparin 40 mg od)

Four hours later you are asked to review Mr Jennings by the nursing staff as he is now becoming increasingly agitated and demanding to leave. Mr Jennings is declining further medical observations and has disconnected the naloxone infusion around 15 min ago. When you arrive on the ward you find Mr Jennings sitting on the edge of his bed packing his belongings; the security staff are in close proximity but have not attempted to restrain him. You note that Mr Jennings' pupils are once again small.

Why has Mr Jennings become agitated and should he be prevented from leaving?

Mr Jennings is free to leave hospital against medical advice unless:
1 He is deemed to lack the mental capacity to understand the implications of this decision
2 He has a mental illness requiring further assessment or treatment that is likely to put him or others at risk.

If the patient is deemed to lack capacity he can be detained and treated if the doctor treating him believes this to be in his best interests.

If he has a mental illness requiring treatment, he can be detained under the Mental Health Act. This requires the completion of formal paperwork and the options for treatment are more limited. This is dealt with in more detail in Case 21.

In determining whether Mr Jennings should be detained, it is important to consider the cause for his agitation. In this case consider the following:

• **Drug (or alcohol) withdrawal** – the effects of naloxone in reversing the opiate can lead to a violent withdrawal reaction; sweating and tachycardia may be present
• **Hypoxia** – sometimes a vicious circle ensues: the patient refuses oxygen because of their agitation, leading to worsening hypoxia
• **Hypoglycaemia** – particularly in patients with liver disease or diabetes
• **Sepsis** – in this case relating to the pneumonia
• **Previously undiagnosed intracranial pathology** – e.g. subdural haematoma

With a security guard nearby you talk to Mr Jennings, who now admits to having taken an expensive 'hit' of heroin earlier that day. Mr Jennings denies being depressed or having suicidal thoughts. He does not have a history of mental illness. He says that he is not an addict but occasionally uses heroin as well as other drugs. Mr Jennings usually smokes it but today injected for the first time. Mr Jennings appears to understand your questions and does not appear to lack capacity.

You explain to Mr Jennings the reason for your concern and the need for him to stay in hospital for treatment of the pneumonia. In addition, the duration of action of the heroin is such that he would probably collapse again shortly after leaving hospital. You agree to reduce the infusion rate of the naloxone to reduce the symptoms of withdrawal.

Mr Jennings agrees to stay to allow treatment and restart the naloxone.

While you are talking to Mr Jennings you note that he is becoming increasingly drowsy; his respiratory rate is slowing again with pinpoint pupils. You help Mr Jennings to lie back down on his bed and reconnect the naloxone infusion at a slightly lower rate than before, aiming to maintain his respiratory rate >10 breaths/min. You reapply his oxygen, which produces a saturation of 97%.

Mr Jennings is weaned off the infusion over the next 24 h. Mr Jennings makes a good recovery from the pneumonia, changing to oral antibiotics after 24 h and he leaves hospital the following day.

Mr Jennings is given the contact numbers for the drug and alcohol advisory services on discharge.

CASE REVIEW

A 22-year-old man is brought into hospital by ambulance after friends found him unconscious at home. Mr Andy Jennings' airway is initially compromised by secretions that are cleared with suction. His respiratory rate is reduced and blood pressure is low. Mr Jennings is also noted to have bilateral pinpoint pupils. The initial GCS is measured at 8/15. Blood gases reveal a mild respiratory alkalosis with a normal blood glucose. A limited history is available from his GP, although his friends report the possibility of opiate use in the recent past.

Mr Jennings is given oxygen, intravenous fluids and naloxone, following which his conscious level improves dramatically, although this improvement is temporary. A provisional diagnosis of opiate toxicity is made and Mr Jennings starts a naloxone infusion, maintaining his GCS at 14/15, although he continues to desaturate on removal of oxygen. A CT brain scan is not deemed to be necessary, given the marked change in conscious level after administration of naloxone.

Further examination reveals evidence of consolidation at the base of his right lung, which is confirmed on a chest radiograph. Mr Jennings starts intravenous antibiotics, with a presumptive diagnosis of pneumonia probably due to aspiration.

After transfer to the ward, Mr Jennings becomes agitated and wishes to leave the hospital. He is assessed as being mentally competent and there is no evidence of mental illness or suicidal ideation, but he agrees to stay voluntarily after an explanation of the reasons for his detention in hospital. Mr Jennings makes an uneventful recovery, having been weaned off the naloxone after 24 h.

This case summarises some of the diagnostic and practical issues regarding the investigation of a young, unconscious patient. For older patients the differential diagnosis may be different, with a higher incidence of intracranial pathology, spontaneous intracranial bleeding, subdural haematoma, etc. These patients will therefore almost always require CT brain scanning. It should be remembered that opiate toxicity can also occur in older people, although the circumstances are usually somewhat different (see Box 25).

Box 25 It is not only intravenous drug abusers who are at risk of opiate toxicity!

An 83-year-old woman was admitted to hospital having been found, unconscious, by her son. She was known to suffer with hypertension for which she was treated with ramipril, and also had mild chronic renal impairment. She had tripped and fallen onto her chest one week previously for which she had consulted her GP regarding analgesia. The GP had prescribed her codeine phosphate 60 mg po to be taken as required, up to a maximum of 240 mg per day. This had produced a good analgesic effect. Her son had noted her to be confused and uncharacteristically drowsy the previous evening. He had visited her this morning and found her lying, unconscious, on the floor.

On arrival her airway was patent, she was warm and well perfused but making poor respiratory effort. Glasgow coma score was 5/15. Blood sugar was normal; however arterial blood gas analysis revealed a respiratory acidosis with a $paCO_2$ of 9 kPa. Her creatinine was also significantly elevated at 343 mmol/L and a chest radiograph revealed two rib fractures.

Urgent CT brain was undertaken, which was reported as normal and she was started on non-invasive ventilation with a presumptive diagnosis of pulmonary contusion, leading to hypercapnoea and impaired conscious level.

Twenty-four hours later there was no improvement in the acidosis, conscious state, or respiratory effort despite escalation of the non-invasive ventilation. Repeat examination revealed bilateral pin-point pupils. After an intravenous 400 µg bolus of naloxone, her conscious level improved markedly. She required a naloxone infusion, but within 40 min had a normal pH, pCO_2, and her GCS improved to 15/15 with no further requirement for non-invasive ventilation. She made a full recovery and was discharged home 48 h later.

Opiate toxicity should always be considered as a cause for reduced conscious level, particularly when elderly patients with renal impairment have been recently prescribed analgesic drugs. Renal elimination of opiate drugs may be further reduced if drowsiness results in poor fluid intake and worsening renal impairment. Always examine the pupils and consider a therapeutic trial of naloxone – an immediate improvement in conscious level may be considered diagnostic and may save further unnecessary investigation.

KEY POINTS

- Airway management is the most important aspect of initial management for an unconscious patient.
- Easily reversible causes, particularly drug overdose and hypoglycaemia, should be actively sought.
- A good collateral history can often reveal the diagnosis; use all available resources to obtain this.
- If you do send your patient for a CT scan, ensure that there are appropriate nursing, medical, anaesthetic and resuscitation facilities available for the transfer.
- Use of naloxone may result in symptoms of opiate withdrawal for patients who are regular users.

Further reading

Booth SA, Leary TS. Coma – emergency management of the unconscious patient. *J Acute Med* 2004; **3**(1): 9–16

Hoffman RS, Goldfrank LR. The poisoned patient with altered consciousness: controversies in the use of a 'coma cocktail'. *JAMA* 1995; **274**(7): 562–9

Sprigings D, Chambers J. The unconscious patient. In: *Acute medicine: a practical guide to the management of medical emergencies*, 4th edition. Blackwell Publishing, Oxford, 2008

Case 14 A 64-year-old man presenting with unilateral weakness

You are telephoned by a GP to refer a 64-year-old man whom he was called to see this morning. Mr Philip Nuss's daughter found him collapsed on the floor when she visited at 9 am, and was unable to get him up. She called the GP who noted that Mr Nuss had lost all power in the right side of his body and was unable to speak or comprehend simple commands. The GP believes that Mr Nuss may have been on the floor for most of the night. He has a long history of hypertension and tablet-controlled diabetes.

What challenges will this patient present?

• Acute onset of hemiparesis (unilateral weakness) or hemiplegia (complete loss of power on one side) usually implies that the patient has had a stroke, although there are several other important causes to consider (see Table 57)

• Stroke is a common cause of hospital admission, particularly in older people

• Stroke is classified either as ischaemic, caused by reduced blood flow to an area of the brain, or haemorrhagic, caused by an intracerebral bleed

• Distinguishing between ischaemic and haemorrhagic stroke is essential as prevention of recurrence will be very different for the two groups

• In some cases of ischaemic stroke, early treatment with a thrombolytic drug to break down the blood clot occluding a cerebral blood vessel may be justified; neurosurgery may be possible for certain cases of intracerebral bleeding

• In this case the fact that Mr Nuss cannot speak (dysphasia) will cause difficulties in obtaining a history; hopefully Mr Nuss's daughter and GP will be able to provide the necessary background

• The possibility of Mr Nuss being on the floor overnight and history of use of oral hypoglycaemic drugs should

raise concerns about co-existent hypothermia and hypoglycaemia

On arrival Mr Nuss appears cool and drowsy. His tympanic temperature reads 36.8°C. Blood pressure is 190/100; Mr Nuss's pulse is 100 beats/min and noted to be irregularly irregular; oxygen saturation is 94% while breathing room air. Mr Nuss's Glasgow Coma Score is difficult to assess because of his difficulty speaking and apparent lack of comprehension; however, Mr Nuss's eyes are open and he appears to be moving the limbs on the left side normally. The right side of his mouth is drooping and his right arm and leg are flaccid with no detectable muscle power. Capillary blood glucose reads 2.5 m/L.

What immediate management is required?

• Confirm patency of the airway and administer oxygen

• Obtain intravenous access and administer 25 mL 50% glucose:

  ○ although hypoglycaemia usually results in drowsiness and coma rather than focal neurological deficit, an unwitnessed seizure precipitated by hypoglycaemia can result in unilateral paralysis (Todd's paralysis); correction of hypoglycaemia occasionally results in resolution of apparent 'stroke'

• Ensure the patient is kept nil by mouth – the severity of Mr Nuss's weakness is likely to have resulted in impairment of his ability to swallow safely; aspiration of food or oral fluid can have serious consequences

• Obtain an ECG and request a chest radiograph

• Send venous blood for full blood count, urea and electrolytes (U&E), liver function tests (LFT), erythrocyte sedimentation rate (ESR), lipids and blood glucose

Is Mr Nuss a potential candidate for thrombolytic therapy if ischaemic stroke is confirmed?

The criteria for thrombolytic therapy are shown in

Acute Medicine: Clinical Cases Uncovered. By C. Roseveare.
Published 2009 by Blackwell Publishing, ISBN: 978-1-4051-6883-0

Table 57 Causes of unilateral weakness

Cause	Clinical features	Comments
Ischaemic stroke	Abrupt onset Usually painless Risk factors for atheromatous disease Current or past atrial fibrillation	In young patients consider underlying causes such as vasculitis, thrombophilia or carotid artery dissection
Haemorrhagic stroke	History of hypertension Headache preceding onset History of recent head injury, or evidence of recent trauma may indicate traumatic intracranial bleeding (subdural/extradural)	Much less common than ischaemic stroke Traumatic haemorrhage (e.g. subdural/extradural) usually causes global weakness/reduced conscious level, but can occasionally present with hemiparesis
Hemiplegic migraine	Usually prior history of migraine – rarely diagnosed in patients aged >40 Headache and visual symptoms are usual (but not universal)	Usually a diagnosis of exclusion – detailed cerebral imaging (usually MRI scanning) is required to exclude vascular cause
Seizure with Todd's paralysis	May be prior history of witnessed seizure or history of epilepsy Other associated symptoms/signs to suggest unwitnessed seizure (tongue biting, incontinence, injury) Spontaneous recovery over a few hours is usual	Consider treatable causes of seizure, such as hypoglycaemia, electrolyte imbalances, etc. (see Case 12)
Cerebral tumour	Onset usually more gradual unless haemorrhage has occurred within a tumour Prior history of headache, malaise, weight loss, etc. Symptoms of distant primary tumour (or prior history of cancer elsewhere)	If suspected a contrast-enhanced CT scan may be required for diagnosis: this will need to be discussed with the radiologist; the radiologist will want to know if the patient has renal failure and whether they are taking metformin
Cerebral abscess	Symptoms suggestive of infection (fever, malaise) usually precede onset of weakness May be symptoms/signs of distant site of infection	Consider endocarditis as a distant site of infection; contrast-enhanced CT may be required (see above)
Multiple sclerosis	Usually prior episodes of weakness – diagnosis may have been confirmed previously. First episode may be misdiagnosed as stroke	Symptoms more commonly bilateral; MRI scan will be required for diagnosis
Spinal cord lesion	Absence of cranial nerve symptoms/signs or dysphasia and no hemianopia	Symptoms more commonly bilateral; may be unilateral weakness with contralateral sensory symptoms/signs
LMN lesion	Symptoms confined to one limb or region; reduced or absent reflexes LMN VIIth nerve palsy results in weakness of eye closure as well as drooping of the mouth; upper motor neurone palsy affects only the mouth	Generalised peripheral neuropathic disease (e.g. Guillain–Barré syndrome) rarely mistaken for 'stroke'

LMN, lower motor neurone.

Box 26. Although not all hospitals in the UK currently offer thrombolysis for stroke, if thrombolysis is available and the patient fulfils the criteria, speed is essential. Only early intervention has been shown to produce significant benefit. Rapid clinical assessment and cerebral CT scanning will be required in these cases.

Box 26 Thrombolysis for acute ischaemic stroke

The recombinant tissue plasminogen activator alteplase (Actilyse) has been licensed in the UK for the treatment of acute ischaemic stroke since 2003. However, only a small proportion (2%) of patients presenting to hospital with stroke fulfil the criteria for this treatment.

The principle surrounds the ability of the thrombolytic to break down the clot occluding the cerebral blood vessel, resulting in restoration of blood flow to that area. Given the devastating consequences of stroke, prevention of brain injury in this way could have major implications. However, the treatment is associated with a significant risk of primary intracerebral haemorrhage (approximately 1 in 30), which itself may prove fatal. Given that the benefit is only seen if treatment is given early, to offset this risk the drug must be given within 3 h of the onset of symptoms. During this time the patient must be transported to hospital and the diagnosis confirmed by CT scanning. Many hospitals do not have the facilities to provide CT scanning quickly enough for such patients.

Inclusion and exclusion criteria are summarised below.

Inclusion criteria for thrombolysis
Onset of symptoms within 3 h of drug administration
Haemorrhage excluded by cerebral imaging
Patient aged >18 years
Neurological deficit lasting >30 min and not rapidly improving

Exclusion criteria for thrombolysis
Very large infarct on CT scan
Seizure at onset of symptoms
Blood pressure >110 diastolic; >185 systolic
Patient on warfarin or receiving heparin in preceding 48 h
Previous stroke within 3 months
Glucose <2.8 or >22
Platelets <100
Previous cerebral or subarachnoid haemorrhage
Recent gastrointestinal bleed, surgery, pancreatitis or pericarditis

---

• In this case the onset of weakness is not clearly defined, but is likely to be greater than 3 h from Mr Nuss's arrival in hospital. Thrombolysis is therefore not an option

Following administration of intravenous 50% glucose the blood sugar increases to 11.7 m/L, but there is no change in Mr Nuss's clinical condition. Oxygen saturation is now reading 99% with Mr Nuss breathing 15 L of oxygen via a non-rebreath mask.

An ECG shows atrial fibrillation with a ventricular rate of 100 beats/min; there is left ventricular hypertrophy consistent with long-standing hypertension.

A chest radiograph is unremarkable.

Mr Nuss's daughter has now arrived on the ward and is asking to speak to you.

What further information should be sought from the history and examination?

• Although Mr Nuss's daughter is requesting information from you, it is important to use this opportunity to acquire as much history as can be obtained. As the patient is apparently unable to communicate, other sources should be sought including:
  ○ the patient's family
  ○ the patient's general practitioner
  ○ previous hospital records
• Important features in the history are summarised in Table 57
• Risk factors for cerebrovascular disease should be sought and clearly documented (Table 58)
• Examination should concentrate on confirming the distribution and severity of any weakness, and identifying if there are any precipitating factors

Table 58 Risk factors for atheromatous cerebrovascular disease

Hypertension
Hyperlipidaemia
Diabetes mellitus
Obesity
Family history of ischaemic stroke or ischaemic heart disease
Cigarette smoking

Mr Nuss's daughter reports that he has been widowed for the past four years and currently lives alone. She had spoken to Mr Nuss on the phone at 7 pm last night, at which time he reported feeling tired and that he was going to bed early; however, Mr Nuss had no other complaints at that time. He has recently recovered from a flu-like illness, but has no other recent illness. When she arrived at Mr Nuss's house this morning she found him on the floor of his living room, still wearing the clothes he was wearing the previous day. She noted the right-sided weakness and that Mr Nuss was unable to communicate. The GP was called and he arranged admission by ambulance. There is no history of recent head injury and Mr Nuss has not complained of headaches or other neurological symptoms recently.

Mr Nuss was diagnosed with diabetes 10 years ago and has been treated with gliclazide 80 mg twice daily for the past eight years. He has been on amlodipine 5 mg daily for the past 15 years. Three years ago Mr Nuss had an episode of transient speech loss, lasting approximately 3 h. He was seen by his GP, who diagnosed a transient ischaemic attack (TIA) and commenced aspirin 75 mg daily. Mr Nuss underwent a carotid Doppler scan, which showed no significant stenosis. An ECG at that time was reportedly normal. The aspirin was discontinued one year ago because Mr Nuss developed a peptic ulcer. Mr Nuss has not had any gastrointestinal symptoms since the drug was stopped.

He manages independently and his daughter visits regularly. Mr Nuss smoked 20 cigarettes a day until 10 years ago and drinks small quantities of alcohol. He drives a car and is right handed.

On examination Mr Nuss has a dense right hemiplegia. There is no evidence of a recent head injury or bruising to suggest a seizure. Mr Nuss's gaze is diverted to the left and he appears to be unaware of his right-hand side. Reflexes are increased on the right and his right plantar response is extensor (upgoing). Mr Nuss is unable to speak or follow simple commands. Pulse is 100 beats/min and irregularly irregular. The blood pressure remains elevated at 200/110. Heart sounds are normal and there are no murmurs; there are no carotid bruits.

What is the likely diagnosis based on the history and examination findings?

• **Acute ischaemic stroke** is the most likely cause of Mr Nuss's symptoms. The clinical features are suggestive of a left-sided total anterior circulation infarct (TACI) (see Table 59). The left hemisphere is usually the *dominant* hemisphere (particularly in right-handed patients),

Table 59 Classification of ischaemic stroke

1. Total anterior circulation infarction (TACI)
All three of:
(a) dense hemiplegia
(b) homonymous hemianopia
(c) higher cerebral function disturbance, i.e. dysphasia, visuospatial disturbance, agnosia
2. Partial anterior circulation infarction (PACI)
Any two of the above or isolated monoparesis
3. Lacunar infarction (LACI)
Pure motor stroke
Pure sensory stroke
Sensory/motor stroke
Ataxic hemiparesis – ataxia same side as weakness
Note: no hemianopia, no cortical deficit with at least two out of arm, leg or face involved and with the whole limb involved
4. Posterior circulation infarction (POCI)
Cranial nerve palsies with opposite side sensory and/ or motor deficits
Bilateral simultaneous sensory and/or motor loss
Dysconjugate eye movements
Cerebellar dysfunction without ipsilateral weakness
Isolated hemianopia or cortical blindness

which houses the areas of the brain responsible for speech and understanding (Broca's and Wernicke's areas)

Risk factors for ischaemic cerebrovascular disease in this case include:

- previous diabetes and hypertension
- history of cigarette smoking
- previous TIA

Alternatively this could be an *embolic* stroke as a result of Mr Nuss's atrial fibrillation (see Box 27)

• **Intracerebral haemorrhage (ICH)** is less likely than ischaemia; patients with chronic hypertension can develop *Charcot–Bouchard* aneurysms, which can rupture leading to ICH; however, this condition is much less common than ischaemic stroke, even in patients with hypertension

• **Intracranial tumour:** on occasions a bleed into a pre-existing tumour can result in sudden onset of weakness, although the onset of symptoms is usually much more gradual. Preceding headache and malaise is common in this situation

• **Seizure with Todd's paralysis:** given that the episode probably happened the previous evening, some recovery would have been expected by now. There has been no improvement in Mr Nuss's condition since administra-

---

Box 27 Atrial fibrillation and acute ischaemic stroke

Patients with atrial fibrillation are at risk of acute cardioembolic stroke.

The uncoordinated contraction of the atrium results in failure of extrusion of blood from the left atrial appendage. This can result in the development of thrombus within the left atrium, which can embolise into the systemic circulation. If the embolism travels into the cerebral vessels, this can result in ischaemic stroke.

Large-scale audits have demonstrated that the stroke risk can be reduced by anticoagulation therapy with warfarin. This treatment can reduce the overall yearly risk of cerebral embolism from around 3% to 1%. Patients who are at particular risk of stroke include those with pre-existing hypertension, dilated atrium on echocardiogram or left ventricular failure. Previous ischaemic stroke, or transient ischaemic attack, is a risk factor for the development of further embolic events in patients with atrial fibrillation. Treatment with warfarin will reduce the risks of recurrent stroke in this situation.

The benefits of warfarin should be weighed up against the risks of bleeding with this drug. Risks will be increased in patients with a history of previous bleeding, unexplained anaemia and falls. Close monitoring is also required with regular blood testing – patients who comply poorly with monitoring are also at higher risk of bleeding.

The decision on whether to treat a patient with warfarin following a stroke in the context of atrial fibrillation is never straightforward. If the stroke is already severe and disabling, with limited recovery it can be argued that prevention of a further stroke may not alter the patient's long-term outcome or quality of life. Decisions should be taken on an individual basis, taking into consideration the views of the patient (where possible) and those of their carers. The decision can also be reviewed following discharge from hospital, in the light of the patient's progress.

---

tion of glucose, so hypoglycaemia is unlikely to have been the primary cause

Mr Nuss's daughter is told that her father has almost certainly has a stroke affecting the left side of his brain, which controls the right-hand side of his body, speech and comprehension. Given that it is likely that Mr Nuss has been affected for over 12 h already with no apparent improvement, the prognosis is poor. There are no specific measures that have been shown to improve the outcome at this stage, although some spontaneous improvement may occur. The daughter asks if Mr Nuss will be having a CT brain scan.

Should a CT brain scan be undertaken?

• CT brain scanning is almost always required following suspected stroke

• The scan will help to define whether the stroke is ischaemic or haemorrhagic, which will guide further treatment and investigation

• For patients in atrial fibrillation this is particularly important, as they may be considered for anticoagulation with warfarin if haemorrhage is excluded

• CT will also enable exclusion of intracranial tumour as the cause for the patient's symptoms

• In some cases the severity of the patient's symptoms or co-morbidities may suggest that CT will not influence the patient's outcome

When should the CT scan be undertaken?

• Ideally CT scanning should be undertaken as soon as possible after presentation

• In practice, a delay of up to 48 h before the CT scan will not usually influence the patient's outcome; even if the patient has had a haemorrhagic stroke, there is no evidence that starting aspirin before the CT findings are known adversely affects prognosis

• A delay of >48 h may make distinction between ischaemia and haemorrhage difficult as the appearances on CT can be very similar after this period: MRI scanning may be more helpful in distinguishing the appearances after 48 h, although the availability of this test may be even more limited

• An urgent CT brain scan is necessary in the following situations:

 ◦ a patient presenting within 3 h of the initial episode – to enable identification of those suitable for thrombolysis

 ◦ the possibility of a head injury precipitating the initial collapse

 ◦ a severe headache at the time of onset of weakness

 ◦ deterioration of conscious level following presentation – to exclude a surgically remediable haemorrhage or obstructive hydrocephalus

 ◦ prior anticoagulation treatment – particularly if the

patient has a metal prosthetic heart valve that requires ongoing anticoagulation treatment

○ predominance of 'posterior fossa' symptoms (e.g. cerebellar or occipital symptoms) – posterior fossa haemorrhage is more likely to be amenable to surgical intervention

A CT scan is arranged within 48 h of Mr Nuss's admission. The medical student attached to your team asks you whether you will undertake carotid Doppler investigation. You praise him for his enthusiasm and suggest he goes to the library to look this up (while you reach for your copy of Acute medicine: clinical cases uncovered*).*

Should a carotid Doppler scan be undertaken in this case?

• Some of the issues around the need for carotid Doppler scanning are summarised in Box 28

• In Mr Nuss's case, given that there is a dense hemiplegia it is unlikely that urgent carotid artery surgery would be considered at this stage, even if a significant stenosis were diagnosed

---

Box 28 Stroke and carotid artery disease

Patients with carotid artery stenosis may be at risk of embolic stroke due to thrombus formation within the stenosed vessel. Patients with significant stenosis (70–99%) are at particularly high risk. For this group carotid endarterectomy may be beneficial in preventing *recurrent* stroke where there has been a previous transient ischaemic attack (TIA) or partial stroke affecting the anterior cerebral circulation.

Carotid stenosis can be diagnosed by Doppler ultrasound scanning of the vessels. Although this is a simple and non-invasive test, it is important to consider whether the patient's treatment will be affected by the outcome.

Therefore, before requesting carotid Doppler, consider the following:
• Would the patient be well enough to undergo carotid endarterectomy?
• Has the patient had a confirmed anterior circulation TIA or partial ischaemic stroke?

Patients whose stroke is haemorrhagic, affecting the entire anterior circulation territory (TACI), or in the posterior circulation territory (POCI) should not normally undergo carotid Doppler.

• Confirmation of cerebral infarction would also normally be required prior to consideration of carotid surgery

• At present there is no indication for a carotid Doppler scan

• If Mr Nuss's condition improves over the next few days, and assuming ischaemic stroke is confirmed, the decision can be reviewed

What management is recommended while awaiting a CT scan?

• **Keep the patient nil by mouth** until formal assessment of swallowing can be undertaken. In Mr Nuss's case swallowing is unlikely to be safe given the dense hemiplegia

• **Administer intravenous fluid and consider insertion of a nasogastric (NG) tube** – nutrition is important and Mr Nuss has almost certainly gone without food for some time before admission. He is also likely to be relatively dehydrated

• **Continue to apply oxygen by mask** – maintain oxygen saturation >95%

• **Monitor cardiac rhythm** – Mr Nuss's atrial fibrillation may require rate control; if the rate is persistently >100 beats/min administer digoxin 500 μg intravenously (or via NG tube)

• **Control blood glucose using dextrose/insulin infusion**

• **Insert a urinary catheter or apply a convene** – the patient is likely to be incontinent of urine

• **Commence aspirin 75 mg daily (via NG tube)** – although Mr Nuss has not had a CT brain scan to exclude haemorrhage, most clinicians will prescribe aspirin in this situation, since there is no evidence that it adversely affects the outcome even in those patients who are subsequently diagnosed with cerebral haemorrhage

• **Commence lipid-lowering therapy** (e.g. simvastatin 20 mg daily) – even in the context of normal lipid levels, treatment with a statin may reduce recurrent ischaemic episodes. The decision whether to continue this in the longer term will need to be reviewed in the light of Mr Nuss's progress

• **Apply thromboembolic disease (TED) stockings** – prophylactic heparin is not recommended in this situation

Mr Nuss is referred to the hospital's stroke unit, although there are currently no beds available. He is therefore kept in a monitored bed within the acute medical unit.

Over the next 12 h there is slight improvement in Mr Nuss's condition. He appears to be following commands and his gaze is no longer diverted to the left. However, there is no recovery in the power on Mr Nuss's right side and he remains aphasic. Swallow assessment confirms that he cannot swallow safely, and a feeding regimen is commenced via a NG tube. Mr Nuss remains in atrial fibrillation at an average rate of 110 beats/min and is therefore given two 'loading' doses of digoxin 500 μg intravenously, followed by 125 μg daily via the NG tube. Mr Nuss also starts aspirin 75 mg daily and simvastatin 20 mg daily via the NG tube.

His blood pressure remains elevated at 190/110.

The CT brain scan confirms that Nr Nuss has an infarct affecting the middle cerebral artery territory on the left, with extensive ischaemia in the left cerebral hemisphere (see Fig. 39)

The admission blood results are as follows:
- *haemoglobin 166, white cell count 12.7, platelets 280*
- *Na 133, K 3.7, urea 9.6, creatinine 120*
- *glucose 10.7 (after administration of initial bolus of 50% glucose)*

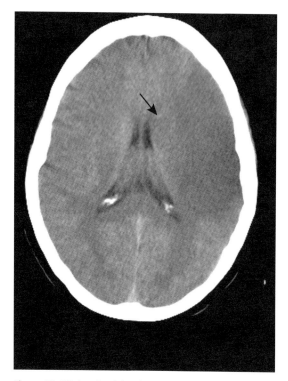

Figure 39 CT showing infarction in the left middle cerebral artery territory (arrow)

- *liver function tests normal*
- *total cholesterol 6.8 mg/L.*

Should the high blood pressure be treated?

- Although hypertension is a risk factor for the development of cerebrovascular disease, active lowering of blood pressure in the early stages following a stroke is not normally recommended
  - following a stroke *cerebral autoregulation* of the blood flow can be affected, such that lowering blood pressure may reduce the cerebral blood flow
  - around an area of infarction there is usually an area of brain tissue where the blood supply is reduced ('watershed' area)
  - lowering the cerebral blood flow can reduce blood supply to this area, resulting in 'extension' of the stroke ('watershed infarction')
- The usual practice is to administer the patient's 'normal' antihypertensive medication, where possible, but not to attempt more aggressive lowering of blood pressure unless the blood pressure is dangerously high (e.g. diastolic >120 mmHg or systolic >200 mmHg)
- After approximately two weeks a more active approach to blood pressure lowering is usually undertaken, using combinations of angiotensin-converting enzyme (ACE) inhibitors and thiazide diuretics, which have been shown to improve the long-term prognosis following stroke

Mr Nuss's amlodipine is restarted and he continues on aspirin and digoxin. His heart rate stabilises at 80–90 beats/min and his blood pressure comes down slightly to 170/90. Mr Nuss is transferred to the hospital's stroke unit for further treatment and rehabilitation.

Two weeks after admission Mr Nuss is started on a combination of perindopril and a thiazide; he is also given warfarin as prophylaxis against a further embolic stroke in view of his atrial fibrillation. The digoxin is continued for rate control.

Mr Nuss spends a further two months in hospital, during which time a percutaneous gastrostomy feeding tube is inserted as he remains unable to swallow safely. Mr Nuss is able to follow some commands, but there is no significant recovery of speech or the power on his right-hand side and he remains heavily dependent on nursing care. Mr Nuss is discharged to a nursing home with little expectation of further significant recovery.

CASE REVIEW

A 64-year-old man with a past history of hypertension and tablet-controlled diabetes is referred to hospital after being found collapsed by his daughter. Mr Philip Nuss is unable to move his right arm or leg and is also apparently unable to communicate or comprehend commands. An examination reveals right-sided hemiplegia with right-sided sensory inattention, brisk reflexes and an upgoing plantar response. He also has a right upper motor neurone VIIth cranial nerve palsy. He is noted to be in atrial fibrillation, which is confirmed by an ECG.

Although Mr Nuss is hypoglycaemic on arrival in hospital, administration of intravenous glucose does not alter his neurological status. Mr Nuss is commenced on intravenous fluid and kept nil by mouth.

A TACI is felt to be the most likely cause for Mr Nuss's symptoms but the duration of symptoms exceeds the 3 h time window for thrombolysis to be of benefit. Supportive therapy is instituted pending a CT brain scan, which confirms that he has had a large middle cerebral artery ischaemic stroke. Mr Nuss is unable to swallow safely, and an NG tube is therefore inserted for administration of nutrition and medication. Mr Nuss is treated initially with aspirin and simvastatin. The aspirin is subsequently changed to warfarin, in view of his co-existent atrial fibrillation.

Although there is minor improvement in Mr Nuss's degree of comprehension and sensory inattention, there is no significant recovery of power in the limbs of the right-hand side. Mr Nuss's ability to swallow does not return, and a percutaneous gastrostomy tube is inserted to replace the NG tube for long-term feeding. Mr Nuss remains heavily dependent on nursing care and is discharged from hospital to a nursing home after three months of inpatient care.

This case demonstrates the potentially devastating consequences of acute ischaemic stroke. Apart from the small subgroup of patients who derive benefit from thrombolysis, the management of ischaemic stroke is mainly centred upon supportive care and prevention of recurrence while waiting for any spontaneous recovery to occur. Patients presenting to hospital following a small stroke may undergo a dramatic and rapid recovery; if this is total and occurs within 24 h, the attack is often termed a TIA. For these patients it is essential to address any reversible risk factors, thereby minimising the risk of recurrence. This will include blood pressure and diabetic control, lipid-lowering therapy, diagnosis and management of carotid artery disease, antiplatelet therapy and anticoagulation in patients with atrial fibrillation. Occasionally an acute ischaemic stroke is a reflection of another underlying process, such as vasculitis, thrombophilia or dissection of the carotid or vertebral arteries. These conditions should always be considered when a stroke occurs in the absence of apparent risk factors, particularly in younger patients.

Unfortunately, only approximately 5% of patients who present to hospital with dense, persisting hemiplegia will regain their independence. Given this poor prognosis it may be appropriate to consider whether a patient should be resuscitated in the event of cardiopulmonary arrest. Sensitive discussions with the patient's family should enable clinicians to establish what the patient's view of this would have been, and will therefore assist in this decision.

KEY POINTS

- Acute hemiparesis is usually caused by stroke – which is either ischaemic or haemorrhagic.
- Patients presenting to hospital immediately after the onset of symptoms should be referred for rapid investigation, since early diagnosis of ischaemic stroke may enable thrombolysis.
- History and examination should enable identification of risk factors for stroke and exclude alternative explanations for the symptoms.
- If the patient does not meet the criteria for thrombolysis, initial treatment is mainly supportive.

- A CT brain scan within 48 h of the onset of symptoms will enable differentiation of ischaemic and haemorrhagic stroke and exclusion of tumour as the cause of the patient's symptoms.
- Patients with atrial fibrillation should be considered for anticoagulation with warfarin if a haemorrhagic stroke is excluded.
- Long-term management will include modification of risk factors for cerebrovascular disease, including control of high blood pressure and lowering of cholesterol.

Further reading

Adams HP, del Zoppo G, Alberts MJ *et al.* Guidelines for the early management of adults with ischemic stroke: a guideline from the American Heart Association/ American Stroke Association Stroke Council, Clinical Cardiology Council, Cardiovascular Radiology and Intervention Council, and the Atherosclerotic Peripheral Vascular Disease and Quality of Care Outcomes in Research Interdisciplinary Working Groups. *Stroke* 2007; **38**: 1655–711

Khaja AM, Grotta JC. Established treatments for acute ischaemic stroke. *Lancet* 2007; **369**: 319–30

Warlow C. Therapeutic thrombolysis for acute ischaemic stroke. *BMJ* 2003; **326**: 233–4

A 60-year-old man presenting following a blackout

PART 2: CASES

A 60-year-old man is referred to hospital after experiencing three episodes of loss of consciousness over the previous four days. During one of these attacks Mr Nagai was noted to shake violently. He had a myocardial infarction three years ago, but has been well since then. Mr Nagai takes ramipril 5 mg and bendroflumethiazide 2.5 mg daily for hypertension, as well as aspirin and simvastatin. He recovered fully between the episodes and currently feels well. His GP feels that he requires urgent assessment in hospital in order that a serious cause can be excluded.

What challenges will this patient present?

• Transient loss of consciousness (TLOC) has many causes, most of which can be grouped under the umbrellas of either *syncope* or *seizure*
• Syncope results from reduction in cerebral blood flow whereas seizure is an electrical phenomenon resulting from the paroxysmal discharge of cerebral neurones
• Distinguishing syncope from seizure is an essential part of the initial evaluation of a patient admitted with TLOC
• Assuming Mr Nagai does not require immediate resuscitation on arrival in hospital, a careful history will be required to determine the likely cause
• If syncope is the likely cause, attention should be given to determining whether this has a cardiac origin

On arrival in hospital, Mr Nagai is alert and orientated and appears well. Initial observations reveal a pulse of 60 beats/min with blood pressure 140/70, a respiratory rate of 14 breaths/min and oxygen saturation 99% while breathing room air. Blood glucose is 4.7 mmol/L.

Acute Medicine: Clinical Cases Uncovered. By C. Roseveare.
Published 2009 by Blackwell Publishing, ISBN: 978-1-4051-6883-0

What initial management is required?

• A careful history, preferably from both the patient and a witness, will help to establish the type of 'attack' that the patient has experienced (see Table 60)
• A key question to ask the patient is: 'Do you remember falling?' – this will help to determine whether loss of consciousness was the *cause* of the patient's collapse, or occurred as a *result* of a head injury sustained at the time of a fall
• Specific information that should be sought from the patient or a witness to the attack should include:
  ○ speed of onset of symptoms: (abrupt or gradual?)
  ○ skin colour during attack (pale or flushed?)
  ○ total duration of loss of consciousness
  ○ movements and breathing pattern during attack: any witnessed convulsion and its duration?
  ○ body tone: floppy or rigid?
  ○ speed of recovery after attack: any post-ictal phase?

Mr Nagai describes three episodes over the past 48 h. Each occurred without warning, while seated. Mr Nagai remembers feeling hot and 'light-headed' prior to the onset on each occasion but has no other recollection of the event. When Mr Nagai came round after the events he felt light-headed, cold and sweaty for a few minutes, but was back to normal within a few minutes. He had not been incontinent during the attacks and he had not sustained any injury or tongue biting.

Mr Nagai's wife witnessed each of the attacks. On each occasion he appeared 'vacant' momentarily and then went very pale, following which his eyes rolled back and he slumped forwards. On one occasion Mr Nagai's body appeared to shake violently for a few seconds. He appeared to be very floppy, and his skin felt cold and clammy to touch. Each of the attacks lasted no more than 5 min, at the end of which he 'came round' fairly abruptly, talking coherently and asking what happened, although he remained pale and sweaty for a further 5–10 min.

Table 60 Common causes of transient loss of consciousness (LOC) with key historical features

Cause	Historical features	Comments
Syncope	Pallor prior to and during episode Patient feels cold to touch and 'floppy' Brief duration Rapid recovery	See Table 62 for further information regarding the specific causes of syncope
Seizure	Aura prior to collapse Prolonged unconsciousness Slow recovery	Non-convulsive seizures (petit mal or complex partial seizures) may cause LOC without shaking
Hypoglycaemia	Usually a history of diabetes treated with tablets/insulin Pallor, intense sweating and cold skin Rapid recovery with administration of glucose	Contrary to popular belief, hypoglycaemia due to fasting in the absence of insulin or oral hypoglycaemic therapy is extremely rare
Vertebrobasilar insufficiency	Episodes occur on extension of neck Often history of cervical spine arthritis Often accompanied by nausea/vertigo	Occurs because of a reduction of blood flow through vertebral arteries, causing brainstem ischaemia; other forms of transient ischaemic attack (TIA) do not cause loss of consciousness
Hyperventilation	Usually brief Rapid recovery Paraethesia noted around mouth, in fingers, toes, etc., before or after episode Patient or witness may notice rapid respiratory rate Other adrenergic symptoms – dry mouth, forceful/rapid heartbeat, sweating	Anxiety regarding the cause of the attacks may result in a vicious circle, increasing the frequency of attacks

Are the episodes caused by syncope, seizure or some other cause?

In Mr Nagai's case the history is strongly suggestive of *syncope* as the likely cause. The main pointers are:
• Pallor, floppiness and cold peripherae during the attack
• Absence of tongue biting, injury or incontinence
• Short duration and rapid recovery

Why did the patient 'shake violently' during one of the attacks?

Violent shaking is often considered pathognomonic of seizure; however, shaking may also be seen following episodes of syncope, probably due to cerebral hypoxia during the episode. This phenomenon is often termed *syncopal seizure* – it is crucial to distinguish this from *true seizure*, which carries very different implications for further investigation, employment and driving. Features that are suggestive of a true seizure are listed in Table 61.

• In this case the shaking is likely to have resulted from syncope rather than 'true' seizure, for the reasons described above.

Since Mr Nagai's myocardial infarction three years ago, he has experienced occasional bouts of chest pain, but none in the past six months, and there have been no episodes of loss of consciousness prior to this. Mr Nagai does not experience palpitations, although he has noticed slight breathlessness on exertion over the past year. Mr Nagai's GP recently increased his ramipril from 2.5 mg to 5 mg daily for hypertension and commenced bendroflumethiazide 2.5 mg daily.

An examination reveals a pulse of 55 beats/min, regular, with blood pressure 140/70; a soft systolic murmur is noted, but no other abnormality is detected.

An ECG shows evidence of a previous inferior myocardial infarct (Q-waves in leads II, III and AVF) but no other abnormality – see Fig. 40.

Table 61 Features distinguishing true seizure from seizure caused by syncope

	True seizure	Syncopal seizure
Prodrome	May be a repetitive aura, e.g. an odd smell, abdominal discomfort	Patient feels light-headed, hot, flushed
Convulsion	Shaking usually starts at onset of loss of consciousness (LOC) Prolonged shaking Tongue biting Incontinence	Brief shaking, often after onset of LOC Tongue biting/incontinence are uncommon
Recovery	Prolonged post-ictal phase: sometimes several hours of drowsiness/ confusion	Usually full recovery within a few minutes

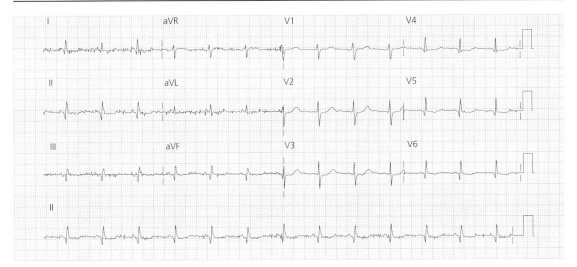

Figure 40 ECG on admission: Q-waves are visible in the inferior leads (II, III and AVF) and also in leads V5 and V6, indicating a previous inferolateral myocardial infarction. The irregularity in the baseline (particularly in leads I and AVL) is artefactual (possibly due to patient movement); this obscures the P-waves, but these are clearly visible in the chest leads (V1–V6); the PR interval is normal (approx 0.16 s) and all P-waves are followed by a QRS complex indicating that the patient is in sinus rhythm with no evidence of heart block.

What is the likely cause for Mr Nagai's syncope?

• Causes of syncope, along with important historical features, are listed in Table 62

• Although it may be of interest to postulate different causes of benign syncope, the most crucial aspect of this phase of Mr Nagai's initial management is to determine whether these attacks are likely to represent *cardiac* syncope. This will help to determine whether Mr Nagai needs to be kept in hospital for further management or treatment, or whether further investigation can be undertaken as an outpatient.

• If cardiac syncope is deemed likely, inpatient investigation is usually required. Most other causes can be managed in an outpatient setting. Many hospitals have a specialist syncope clinic, which will enable appropriate investigations and follow-up to be undertaken

• Specific features that may suggest cardiac syncope are listed in Table 63

• Mr Nagai's prior cardiac history, systolic murmur and age should raise the suspicion of cardiac syncope. However, there are no diagnostic features on the ECG

• The recent increase in Mr Nagai's antihypertensive medication might be an alternative explanation for his symptoms, although there is no postural element in the history

Mr Nagai is admitted into an observation bed on the hospital's acute medical unit and connected to a cardiac monitor with the facility to record any arrhythmia.

Table 62 Causes of syncope

Cause	Historical features	Comments
Cardiac		
Bradyarrhythmia	May be history of ischaemic heart disease (IHD), previous arrhythmia Use of beta-blocker, calcium antagonists or antiarrhythmic drugs No postural relationship	Sinus node disease or atrioventricular conduction defects are the usual cause of bradyarrhythmia resulting is syncope
Tachyarrhythmia	May be history of IHD, previous arrhythmia Patient may notice palpitation prior to collapse May be family history of collapse/sudden death in some inherited syndromes	Ventricular arrhythmia is more common in patients with IHD Rapid supraventricular tachycardia (SVT) may also be responsible for syncope
Myocardial infarction/ischaemia	Chest pain prior to onset Ongoing hypotension Symptoms/signs of heart failure Exertional syncope may occur with severe myocardial ischaemia	Syncope usually suggests cardiogenic shock or co-existent arrhythmia
Pulmonary embolism	Usually acute shortness of breath Pleuritic chest pain prior to onset of collapse (not consistent in massive pulmonary embolism, PE) Risk factors for PE (see Case 2)	Syncope occurs due to loss of cardiac output from obstruction of main pulmonary trunk, or hypoxia
Aortic stenosis	History of aortic valve disease/heart murmur Syncope typically occurs with exertion due to outflow obstruction Clinical signs of aortic stenosis: heaving apex, slow rising pulse, ejection systolic murmur, low pulse pressure	Aortic valve disease also associated with tachy- and bradyarrhythmias
Neurally mediated syncope		
Simple faint (vasovagal syncope)	Prodrome – patient feels hot, nauseated, light-headed Posture – usually upright Precipitant – e.g. unexpected event, pain, needles, etc. Rapid recovery – usually 20–30 s only	No implication for driving if the diagnosis can be made with confidence; remember the 'three Ps' (prodrome, posture, precipitant) Tilt table testing may be helpful in the diagnosis
Carotid sinus syncope	Usually older patients Collapse may occur with wearing tight collar	Diagnosis is made by performing carotid sinus massage under strictly controlled conditions with cardiac monitoring, usually in a syncope clinic
Situational syncope	Cough syncope – brought on by coughing Post-prandial syncope – after meals Micturition syncope – during urination	A careful history should provide the diagnosis
Postural hypotension		
Hypovolaemia	History suggestive of dehydration or blood loss	Cause of dehydration (e.g. diarrhoea, diuretic use, poor fluid intake during warm weather) Blood loss – gastrointestinal bleeding, etc.
Autonomic failure	History of diabetes, chronic alcohol excess Parkinson's disease	Often clear history of recurrent collapse on rising

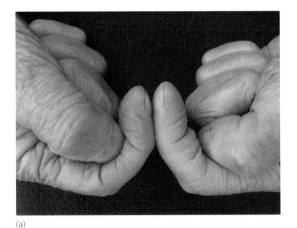

(a)

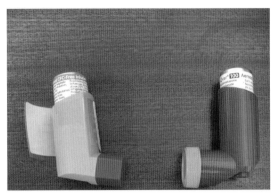

Plate 2 Metered dose inhalers.

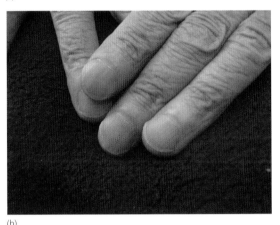

(b)

Plate 1 Finger nail clubbing. Note the loss of nail fold angle (a) and increased curvature of the nail with swelling of the nail bed (b).

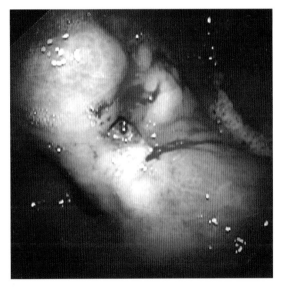

Plate 3 Gastric ulcer with stigmata of recent haemorrhage: this ulcer is sited on the incisura of the stomach just above the pylorus on the lesser curve. The pylorus can be seen below and to the left of the ulcer. In the centre of the ulcer is a small, fresh blood clot, which is likely to be overlying a blood vessel that has recently bled; there is also some fresh blood oozing from the ulcer edge. The mucosa adjacent to the ulcer is pale as a result of local injection of adrenaline, leading to vasoconstriction. Diathermy of the vessel in the ulcer base may also be effective.

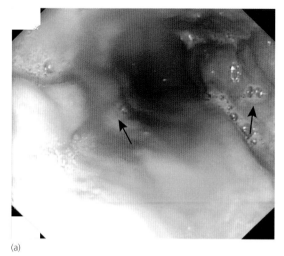

(a)

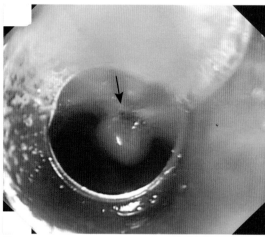

(b)

Plate 4 (a) Oesophageal varices – two cords of varices are shown (arrows) (b) Oesophageal varix following application of a 'band' (arrow).

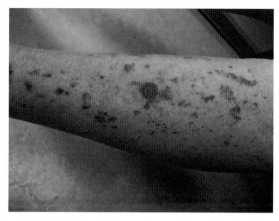

Plate 5 Petechial rash. The purple areas do not blanch with local pressure. Causes include thrombocytopenia, abnormal blood clotting and vasculitis. If the patient is acutely unwell or the rash is spreading rapidly this rash is highly suspicious of meningococcal septicaemia.

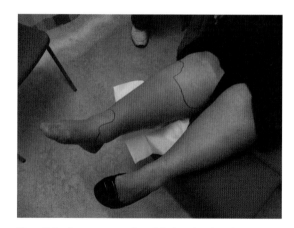

Plate 6 Erythematous, swollen right leg showing clear demarcation, typical of cellulitis. The extent of the erythema has been marked with a black pen – this is often helpful in determining whether the cellulitis is progressing or receding following initiation of treatment. If the patient remains unwell or the erythema extends beyond the line, it may be necessary to change the antibiotic or commence intravenous treatment. Sequential monitoring of the C-reactive protein may also be helpful in determining response to treatment.

Table 63 Features suggesting a high risk of cardiac syncope

Age >50 years

Co-existent cardiac-type chest pain

Known coronary artery disease or cardiac failure

Valvular heart disease (especially aortic valve disease)

Previous arrhythmia (tachy- or bradyarrhythmia)

ECG abnormalities (see below)

Family history of sudden death

Presence of a cardiac device (pacemaker or implanted cardiac defibrillator)

ECG abnormalities which are *suggestive* of a cardiac cause for syncope

Bifascicular or trifascicular block

Mobitz type I second-degree heart block

Asymptomatic bradycardia <50 beats/min

Pre-excited QRS complexes ('delta' wave or short PR interval)

Evidence of myocardial ischaemia (ST segment change or T-wave inversion)

ECG abnormalities which are *diagnostic* of a cardiac cause for syncope

Sinus bradycardia <40 beats/min

Symptomatic sinus pause >3 s

Mobitz type II second-degree heart block

Third-degree heart block

Rapid supraventricular/ventricular tachycardia

Pacemaker malfunction with pauses >3 s

What further investigations are required?

Further investigations should include:

• **Full blood count**: anaemia or acute bleed might be responsible for syncope

• **Urea, electrolytes, calcium and serum magnesium**: electrolyte abnormalities, particularly hypokalaemia and hypomagnesaemia, may be responsible for arrhythmias; diuretic treatment is the commonest cause

• **Thyroid function tests (TFT)**: bradyarrhythmias due to hypothyroidism; tachyarrhythmia due to thyrotoxicosis

• **Chest radiograph**: may identify co-existent pathology;

if there is a pacemaker *in situ*, the position/integrity of wires may be assessed

• **Echocardiography**: in selected cases, particularly those with heart murmurs or clinical evidence suggestive of cardiac failure – this may identify valvular abnormalities (particularly aortic stenosis) and enable assessment of left ventricular function

Initial investigation reveals serum potassium of 3.1 mmol/L (normal 3.7–6.3 mmol/L); renal function and other blood tests are all normal, including thyroid function. A chest radiograph reveals mild cardiomegaly but is otherwise normal. Echocardiogram shows mild mitral regurgitation with mild systolic dysfunction.

What further monitoring/treatment is required?

• **Continuous cardiac monitoring** on the ward is essential following the decision to admit the patient. It is essential not to miss the opportunity to record the cardiac rhythm during a subsequent attack. If previous episodes have happened only while the patient has been ambulant, it may not be possible to record this using a rigid bedside monitor. Some wards have the facility for 'telemetry' whereby the patient may be mobile around the ward while still connected to a cardiac monitor. Alternatively a portable recording device (24 h tape) may be applied while the patient is still an inpatient to ensure that any episodes are captured

• **Correct haematological/biochemical abnormalities** (e.g. anaemia, electrolyte imbalances or thyroid dysfunction): these may require further investigation. In this case the low potassium level is likely to be drug induced (bendroflumethiazide is a thiazide diuretic, which can result in renal potassium loss); if this drug needs to be continued, regular monitoring and potassium supplementation may be required

In most cases, specific treatment cannot be started until the diagnosis is absolutely clear. Tachyarrhythmias may require anti-arrhythmic drugs, but these will tend to exacerbate bradyarrhythmia; the latter may require a pacemaker.

Mr Nagai starts taking oral potassium supplement tablets and is observed on the ward, undergoing continuous telemetry recording for 48 h. During this period Mr Nagai has no further episodes of syncope and there are no documented arrhythmias on the cardiac monitor. Mr Nagai is fully mobile on the ward with no apparent restriction to his activity.

How long should the patient be kept in hospital?

Often the patient will have no further episodes while on the ward, and a decision needs to be taken regarding the required length of hospital stay. This will vary depending on the clinical scenario; sometimes other factors, such as the patient's home circumstances or co-existing illnesses, may influence the duration of hospital stay.

• Unless a serious underlying cause has been identified during the above investigation, it is rarely justified to keep the patient in hospital if they have gone 48 h without a witnessed event

• Further investigation, such as 24 h cardiac monitoring, can usually be arranged on an outpatient basis following discharge

• Many hospitals run specialist syncope clinics, which can facilitate the further investigation of patients with suspected syncope, including the provision of more complex tests for neurally mediated syncope

What are the implications for driving and employment?

It is vital to consider the implications of the events leading to admission on the patient's driving and future employment.

Although commonly forgotten by hospital doctors, advice on driving is an essential component of discharge information for patients admitted following a blackout.

Whether or not the patient drives a car should be documented in their notes at the time of the initial clerking: this is a vital component of the social history. Similarly the nature of their work, any relevant hobbies or pastimes should be sought and documented carefully. Prior to discharge the medical team should review this information in the light of subsequent events.

The DVLA guidance following loss of consciousness is complex, but can be found on the DVLA website (www. DVLA.gov). In practice there is always an implication for driving unless the medical team are confident that the collapse represented a simple faint. Advice given to the patient should be documented carefully in their medical notes. It is the patient's responsibility to ensure that they inform the DVLA and cease driving, but the doctor is required to advise the patient to do this. Failure to do so could result in litigation against the doctor if a car accident results from a further attack while driving. In this case Mr Nagai should be advised not to drive until further investigations into the possibility of a cardiac cause have been completed.

What should Mr Nagai do if the problem recurs?

Assuming no diagnosis has been made, but a serious (i.e. cardiac) cause cannot be excluded, Mr Nagai must be advised to return immediately to hospital if the episodes continue. Confirming a diagnosis may be a challenge, particularly if episodes are infrequent. Repeated admissions to hospital and 24 h cardiac monitoring may be necessary.

In some cases, simple advice may reduce the frequency of attacks; for example, patients with postural hypotension should be advised to avoid rising immediately from a sitting to a standing position; patients with postprandial syncope should be advised to avoid large meals; reducing diuretic medication during hot weather may reduce a tendency to dehydration and hypovolaemia.

Following discharge Mr Nagai undergoes a series of three 24 h cardiac monitor sessions that have been arranged as outpatient investigations. The first two are normal; during the third tape Mr Nagai experiences an episode of syncope lasting approximately 5 min. Analysis of the tape reveals an episode of complete heart block with ventricular response rate 30 beats/min (Fig. 41). Mr Nagai is re-admitted to hospital on that day and undergoes insertion of a permanent pacemaker, which results in complete resolution of all attacks.

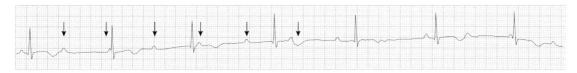

Figure 41 Rhythm strip showing complete heart block (CHB): by laying a sheet of paper alongside the rhythm strip, marking the P-waves and moving the sheet along, it becomes clear that, while the P-waves are occurring at regular intervals, they are not in any way associated with the QRS complexes. Some occur immediately after the QRS complexes, some are 'hidden' within the T-wave (arrows). This dissociation is pathognomonic of CHB. The QRS complexes are of narrow calibre and occur at a rate of around 50 beats/min, indicating that this rhythm arises in the atrioventricular node (nodal escape rhythm). Ventricular escape rhythms produce broad complexes (see p. 57) and tend to be slower.

CASE REVIEW

A 60-year-old man with a past history of hypertension and ischaemic heart disease was referred to hospital after experiencing three blackouts. During one of these episodes, Mr Nagai was noted to shake violently. However, the history obtained from his wife who had witnessed the events was suggestive of syncope. Mr Nagai was noted to be mildly hypokalaemic, which was probably due to the recent addition of bendroflumethiazide for treatment of hypertension. An ECG revealed evidence of an old inferior myocardial infarction, but no significant arrhythmia. In view of his prior cardiac history Mr Nagai was considered to be at high risk of a cardiac cause for the syncope and was therefore admitted onto the ward for cardiac monitoring for 48 h. When no further episodes occurred during this period, Mr Nagai was allowed home, having been given advice not to drive pending further investigation. Mr Nagai underwent 24 h cardiac monitoring on three occasions, on the third of which he had an episode of syncope coinciding with a period of complete heart block on the monitor. Mr Nagai was re-admitted and underwent insertion of a permanent pacemaker, following which no further episodes occurred.

KEY POINTS

- Most cases of transient loss of consciousness requiring hospital admission occur as a result of syncope or seizure.
- Early distinction of syncope and seizure is essential since this will determine what further observation, investigation and treatment are required.
- If syncope is deemed the likely cause of the episodes, features suggestive of a cardiac source should be sought.

- Patients at high risk of cardiac syncope should be admitted to hospital for further investigation and monitoring.
- Prior to discharge all patients should be given advice regarding driving, the potential implications for their employment and what to do if the episodes recur.
- Bradycardia resulting in syncope may require insertion of a permanent pacemaker.

Further reading

Brignole M (Chairperson), Alboni P. Benditt D *et al.* Guidelines on management (diagnosis and treatment) of syncope – update 2004. *Europace* 2004; **6**: 467–537

Gammage MD. Temporary cardiac pacing. *Heart* 2000; **83**: 715–20

Kenny RA (ed). *Syncope in the older patient.* Chapman and Hall, London, 1996

Mangrum MJ, DiMarco JP. The evaluation and management of bradycardia. *New Engl J Med* 2000; **342**: 703–9

Reed MJ, Gray A. Collapse query cause: the management of adult syncope in the emergency department. *Emerg Med J* 2006; **23**: 589–94

Case 16) A 45-year-old man with acute confusion

A 45-year-old man is brought to hospital having become acutely confused. Mr Desmond Parsons' friends who arrived with him reported that he has had a long history of heavy alcohol consumption dating back 10 years since the breakdown of his marriage. Mr Parsons had an attempted 'detox' last year, which was arranged by his GP, but only remained abstinent for a few weeks. Since this morning Mr Parsons has been behaving strangely and appears disorientated, not recognising his friends and becoming increasingly agitated and unsteady on his feet. Mr Parsons' friends called the GP, who has requested urgent hospital admission for further investigation and treatment. According to the GP Mr Parsons has had at least one grand mal seizure in the past, but has been poorly compliant with medication.

What challenges will this patient present?

The acutely confused patient with alcohol dependence presents a number of challenges to the admitting clinician.

- The differential diagnosis for the cause of the confusion is broad
- The patient may present difficulties in assessment, monitoring and investigation due to lack of cooperation
- There may be ongoing issues related to alcohol withdrawal

On arrival in the hospital Mr Parsons is clearly extremely agitated. He is being verbally abusive to the ambulance staff and attempting to climb off their trolley. There is evidence of bruising over Mr Parsons' chest and upper limbs, but no sign of head injury. He does not smell of alcohol, but there is a smell of stale urine, which suggests he may have been incontinent. Mr Parsons appears flushed and tremulous and is very unsteady when he attempts to walk, requiring support from two members of staff.

Acute Medicine: Clinical Cases Uncovered. By C. Roseveare.
Published 2009 by Blackwell Publishing, ISBN: 978-1-4051-6883-0

Initial observations reveal a pulse of 120 beats/min, regular, which is of good volume and palpable radially. It is not possible to obtain Mr Parsons' blood pressure, temperature or pulse oximetry reading because of poor compliance, but he does not appear cyanosed.

What immediate management is required?

- Assessment of airway, breathing and circulation, as far as is possible
- Try to calm Mr Parsons down and establish a rapport:
  - move to a quiet, well-lit area of the ward/emergency department
  - avoid physical restraint if possible
- Contact the hospital security department in case Mr Parsons becomes aggressive or attempts to leave
- Sedation is likely to be required as Mr Parsons may endanger himself or hospital staff. Use incremental doses of benzodiazepine (e.g. lorazepam 1–4 mg i.m./i.v. or diazepam 5–20 mg i.v.)
- Establish intravenous access
- Administer intravenous thiamine (e.g. Pabrinex) – see below
- Check capillary blood glucose and correct hypoglycaemia (preferably *after* administration of thiamine)
- Send blood for full blood count (FBC), urea and electrolytes (U&E), liver function tests (LFT), clotting profile, group and save
- ECG (once Mr Parsons is compliant/appropriately sedated)
- Chest radiograph

With the assistance of two nurses a cannula is inserted. Mr Parsons' aggressive behaviour continues, preventing adequate clinical assessment, which is deemed to constitute a risk to the patient. Mr Parsons is given 2 mg of lorazepam intravenously, following which he is much calmer and more compliant. Bloods, ECG and chest radiograph are obtained.

Further history from Mr Parsons' friends reveals that he was behaving normally the previous evening, although he had been drinking very heavily yesterday. Mr Parsons vomited at least once overnight. They are not aware of any previous similar episodes. Mr Parsons has had a few falls over the last week, apparently related to alcohol intoxication, although they are not aware of any specific head injury. They are not aware of any other drug use and do not think that he would have taken a drug overdose. Mr Parsons does not take any prescribed medication.

On examination there is no evidence of chronic liver disease. Mr Parsons has a mild pyrexia (37.8°C) and there is bruising noted over his trunk and upper limbs, possibly related to restraint by the security staff. There is no specific evidence to suggest head trauma. There are coarse crackles at the base of Mr Parsons' right lung. Abdominal examination is unremarkable, and the limited neurological assessment possible within the constraints of his compliance reveals no focal abnormality. There is no obvious ataxia and eye movements appear normal. Fundi are not clearly seen.

A chest radiograph reveals right basal shadowing (Fig. 42). An ECG is normal. Bloods reveal an elevated neutrophil count, with low platelet count; electrolytes, liver function, clotting and blood glucose are normal.

What is the likely cause of the confusion?

The differential diagnosis of confusion in a patient with a history of alcohol abuse is broad. The main causes are summarised in Table 64, along with features that may help in the diagnosis.

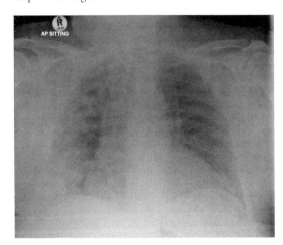

Figure 42 Chest radiograph.

In this case, possibilities include:
- **Acute alcohol withdrawal**: despite the apparent history of ongoing alcohol consumption this remains a strong possibility; the combination of tremor, confusion and tachycardia are consistent with delirium tremens
- **Unwitnessed seizure overnight, with post-ictal confusion**: the prior history of seizure raises this possibility; incontinence and bruising may support this diagnosis; alcohol withdrawal may have precipitated a seizure
- **Chest sepsis, possibly related to aspiration**: Mr Parsons vomited after heavy alcohol consumption and now has clinical and radiological signs consistent with right basal pneumonia, the commonest site for aspiration
- **Head injury with intracranial bleeding**: bruising and history of recent falls, which could have resulted in subdural haematoma, particularly in view of the low platelet count (not uncommon in patients with a history of alcohol excess)
- **Wernicke's encephalopathy:** despite the normal eye movements and absence of ataxia this cannot be discounted (see below)

Should Mr Parsons undergo a CT brain scan?

Intracranial bleeding should always be considered and is hard to exclude without cranial imaging. In practice, CT scanning requires the patient to lie still and physical restraint during the scan is not practical. Heavy sedation constitutes respiratory risks, and general anaesthesia is therefore usually recommended when an acutely agitated patient requires a scan. Clearly this adds risks of its own that need to be weighed against the benefits of the scan.

A CT brain scan should *always* be considered in the following circumstances:
- Where there is evidence of *focal* neurological deficit
- Following significant head injury
- Where no alternative explanation for the confusion can be identified (remembering that one identifiable cause does not preclude co-existent intracranial pathology)
- Where the patient's conscious level has deteriorated following arrival in hospital without alternative explanation (e.g. administration of sedative drugs)

In Mr Parsons' case a CT brain scan is not requested. Although Mr Parsons is calmer following administration of the lorazepam it is felt that he would not readily comply with the investigation and an alternative explanation for the

Table 64 Differential diagnosis of confusion in an alcoholic patient

Diagnosis	Clinical features	Comments
Alcohol/drug related		
Alcohol intoxication	Breath smells of alcohol History of recent heavy alcohol consumption/ empty bottles, etc.	May co-exist with other causes of confusion; does not preclude a more serious underlying cause
Drug overdose	Recent depression, suicidal intent or letter Empty bottles/packets found at scene History of recreational drug use, needle track marks Pinpoint pupils suggest opiate use	May be recreational or suicidal; high incidence of depression in association with alcohol dependence
Alcohol withdrawal	Recent discontinuation or reduction in intake Marked tremor/sweating Hallucinations (tactile, auditory or visual)	May co-exist with other causes of confusion
Wernicke's encephalopathy	Classic triad of confusion, ataxia and diplopia in only 10% of cases; 70% have confusion alone	Caused by cerebral thiamine deficiency – may be precipitated by co-existent illness, alcohol withdrawal, seizure, treatment of hypoglycaemia. May co-exist with other causes of confusion
Intracranial pathology		
Post-ictal confusion	Confusion occurs as initial drowsiness improves May be evidence of recent seizure – injury, tongue biting, incontinence Often history of previous seizures	Seizures may result from acute alcohol withdrawal; often unwitnessed – patient is found in post-ictal state May also accompany other illness – e.g. following head injury, sepsis, hypoglycaemia
Head injury/intracranial bleeding	History of fall/evidence of injury, bruising, etc. Focal neurological deficit in presence of extradural haematoma Fluctuating consciousness in subdural haematoma	Recurrent falls/injury are common – often unwitnessed/unreported Risk of intracranial bleeding exacerbated by blood clotting and platelet abnormalities
Other intracranial pathology	Focal neurological deficits in case of stroke/ intracerebral tumour	
Metabolic		
Sepsis	Symptoms/signs of infection: cough/sputum/ lung signs – consider possible aspiration following vomit Odour of infected urine Look for skin rashes/infections Abscesses at sites of needle injections if co-existent i.v. drug use	Fever may be absent, especially if patient has chronic liver disease Fever may accompany alcohol withdrawal without infection Consider unusual infections, if patient has risk factors for HIV
Hepatic encephalopathy	Other evidence (or history) of chronic liver disease: spider naevi, palmar erythema, jaundice, ascites Liver flap ('asterixis')	May be precipitated by other illness, especially sepsis, gastrointestinal bleeding
Hypoglycaemia	Sweating, pallor; often prior episodes History of diabetes requiring insulin or oral hypoglycaemic agents (may result from alcohol-induced chronic pancreatitis)	Often reactive hypoglycaemia due to impaired hepatic gluconeogenesis Give intravenous vitamin B before correction if possible

confusion (pneumonia) has been identified. It is decided to treat Mr Parsons' pneumonia, wait and observe his progress on the ward.

What further treatment is required?

• **Ensure adequate hydration:** Mr Parsons is likely to be in fluid deficit, given the diuretic effect of the recent alcohol. Intravenous fluids may be required. A urinary catheter may be helpful in determining fluid balance, in addition to regular pulse and blood pressure measurement

• **Ensure adequate oxygenation:** the possible aspiration pneumonia may result in hypoxaemia, and depression of the respiratory rate by sedative drugs will exacerbate this. Administer high-flow oxygen and measure arterial blood gases. Hypoxaemia despite high-flow oxygen or rising CO_2 suggestive of ventilatory failure should trigger involvement of the critical care team as mechanical ventilation may be required

• **Ensure adequate sedation:** when alcohol withdrawal is the likely cause of confusion, sedation using benzodiazepines or chlordiazepoxide is mandatory. Lorazepam (1–2 mg as required) or intravenous diazepam (10–20 mg) may be required initially. However, where possible an oral reducing regimen of diazepam or chlordiazepoxide should be prescribed. This will also reduce the risk of alcohol withdrawal seizures. The dose may have to be tailored to the individual's requirements. A typical reducing regimen of chlordiazepoxide is given in Table 65. Higher doses (e.g. 60 mg orally) may be required initially.

When agitation is thought to be due to another medical or cerebral condition, use of sedation needs to be weighed up against its potential effects on the circulatory and respiratory system. If the patient is too agitated to enable hydration, oxygenation and monitoring to be continued then further small increments of lorazepam (1–2 mg i.v. or i.m.) may be required. Lorazepam may also be required for treatment of seizures

• **Intravenous thiamine:** patients who drink excessive alcohol are frequently nutritionally deficient because of inadequate food intake as well as impaired vitamin absorption from the gut. Wernicke's encephalopathy is caused by cerebral thiamine deficiency, and should be considered for any alcoholic patient presenting with confusion. Even if an alternative explanation for confusion is diagnosed, the physiological stress of illness may increase the brain's thiamine requirement, precipitating this condition. Failure to treat may result in *Korsakoff's*

Table 65 Typical reducing regimen for chlordiazepoxide

	Day 1	Day 2	Day 3	Day 4	Day 5
9 am	20 mg	20 mg	10 mg	10 mg	
1 pm	20 mg	10 mg	10 mg		
5 pm	20 mg	10 mg	10 mg		
9 pm	20 mg	20 mg	10 mg	10 mg	10 mg

The dose will need to be titrated to individual requirements: many patients will require a higher starting dose (e.g. 30 mg 4 times daily), while others will require more gradual tapering of the dose. It is usually advisable to prescribe an additional as required dose of 10–20 mg, which the nurses can administer if symptoms of withdrawal are not controlled.

psychosis, where short-term memory is permanently damaged. High doses of intravenous thiamine are required to cross the blood–brain barrier; administration is by infusion of one or two pairs of vials, three times daily

• **Antibiotics:** in Mr Parsons' case there is clear justification for antibiotic treatment, given the clinical and radiogical signs of pneumonia. Often the features are less clear-cut, but it can be difficult to exclude sepsis as a cause for confusion, since the clinical features (pyrexia, tachycardia, etc.) may overlap with those of alcohol withdrawal. Use of broad-spectrum antibiotics to cover chest, urinary and abdominal causes of sepsis is advisable (e.g. co-amoxyclav 1.2 g i.v. tds, or cefuroxime 750 mg i.v. tds).

Where intracranial infection or bacterial meningitis is suspected it is important to ensure the antibiotic used is given in doses high enough to cross the blood–brain barrier (e.g. cefotaxime 2 g 4 hourly)

• **Other:** in cases where other specific abnormalities have been identified these will need to be addressed. Electrolyte imbalances such as hypokalaemia or hypercalcaemia can be corrected. Co-existent depressive illness is common in patients with alcohol dependency and drug overdose should always be considered.

What further monitoring is required?

• Continuous pulse oximetry
• Measurement of pulse, blood pressure and respiratory rate at least hourly
• Hourly urine measurement (if catheter *in situ*)

• Regular blood glucose testing: may develop hypoglycaemia
• Neurological observations (neuro obs) every 30–60 min: including assessment of conscious level using the Glasgow Coma Score (see p. 127)
• Documentation of any seizure activity

Interpretation of all of these parameters may be compounded by poor patient compliance and the influence of sedative drugs. An experienced nurse will often make subjective judgements about a patient that go beyond the parameters of the observation chart. Good communication between medical and nursing staff in this situation is crucial.

Mr Parsons is observed on the ward, where he remains agitated, requiring several further doses of lorazepam. Mr Parsons is treated with intravenous co-amoxyclav 1.2 g tds, along with intravenous thiamine (one pair of vials tds) and a reducing regimen of chlordiazepoxide. After 24 h Mr Parsons' condition has not improved and the nurses feel that he is becoming more confused, although his observations are unchanged. Later that day Mr Parsons has a witnessed grand mal seizure, following which he becomes deeply unconscious with a depressed respiratory rate. Mr Parsons is intubated and ventilated and undergoes a CT brain scan, which reveals a large subdural haematoma (see Fig. 43), which is likely to have been present for around three days. With hindsight this is the likely cause of his initial

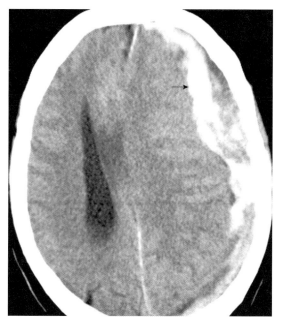

Figure 43 CT brain scan showing large left subdural haematoma (arrow).

presentation. Mr Parsons is transferred to the regional neurosurgical unit and undergoes evacuation of the haematoma, following which he makes a full recovery. He is discharged from hospital after 10 days, having declined help with his alcohol problem.

CASE REVIEW

A 45-year-old man with a documented history of alcohol dependency is brought to hospital after his friends found him in a confused and agitated state. On arrival, Mr Parsons' level of agitation compromises the initial assessment, but he is noted to be tachycardic with bruising over his face and upper limbs. Following sedation with lorazepam, an examination reveals crepitations at the base of his right lung with radiographic evidence of right basal consolidation. Mr Parsons is treated with intravenous antibiotics, fluid, vitamin B and a reducing regimen of chlordiazepoxide. While observing Mr Parsons on the ward his condition deteriorates, with reduction in his conscious level and a grand mal seizure. After intubation, Mr Parsons undergoes CT scanning of his brain, which reveals evidence of a recent subdural haematoma. Mr Parsons undergoes surgical evacuation of the haematoma and makes an uneventful recovery, although he declines offers of help with his alcohol dependency.

KEY POINTS

- Patients with alcohol dependency present difficult challenges to the admitting clinician.
- Agitation may need to be controlled with sedative drugs in order to enable clinical assessment to take place.
- Confusion in an alcohol-dependent patient requires a wide differential diagnosis

- Several conditions may co-exist to account for confusion; identification of one explanation for the confusion does not preclude the presence of other, potentially serious causes.
- CT brain scanning should always be considered, although heavy sedation and intubation may be required.

Further reading

Kosten TR, O'Connor PG. Management of drug and alcohol withdrawal. *New Engl J Med 2003;* **348**: 1786–95

Sprigings D, Chambers JB. Alcohol-related problems in acute medicine. In: *Acute medicine: a practical guide to the management of medical emergencies,* 4th edition. Blackwell Publishing, Oxford, 2008

PART 2: CASES

Case 17 An 81-year-old woman with acute confusion

A GP refers to you an 81-year-old woman whom he has been called to see. Mrs Miller normally lives in warden-controlled accommodation, but this morning she was found wandering in the garden in her dressing gown. Mrs Miller normally has some mild memory disturbance, but today appears very confused and disorientated, which is unusual for her. Mrs Miller has also been incontinent of urine. He feels this represents a toxic confusional state and would like you to admit Mrs Miller for further investigation and treatment.

What challenges will this patient present?

• Acute confusion (also termed delirium or toxic confusional state) is a common cause of hospital admission for older people

• In many cases there is a readily reversible cause that enables the patient to return home after a period of hospital treatment

• The differential diagnosis is broad (see Table 66), and difficulties in obtaining a clear history from the patient will present challenges to the admitting medical team

• In cases where there is a degree of underlying cognitive impairment (dementia), it may be difficult to determine how much of the problem is acute and therefore reversible

• Close communication with relatives, carers and community teams will be necessary at the time of admission and discharge

Mrs Miller is brought onto the ward on an ambulance trolley. She is clearly distressed and agitated. The ambulance crew transfer Mrs Miller onto a hospital bed, but she immediately tries to climb off. Mrs Miller is shouting out repeatedly and pushes the nursing staff away when they try to perform baseline observations. Mrs Miller has already pulled out the cannula that the ambulance crew managed

to insert. Mrs Miller looks pale, but not cyanosed, and her respiratory rate is not increased, with no obvious stridor or wheeze.

What immediate management is required?

• Mrs Miller's airway and breathing do not appear to be compromised; attempt to measure the oxygen saturation if Mrs Miller will wear a pulse oximeter and ask whether the ambulance crew managed to record this en route. If Mrs Miller is hypoxic this may be exacerbating her confusion

• Try to calm Mrs Miller and establish a rapport; a family member or other familiar face may be helpful in this situation

• Re-attempt to obtain information about pulse and blood pressure, to exclude shock as a cause for Mrs Miller's confusion (see Case 8)

• Ensure Mrs Miller is in a well-lit, observable area of the ward

Despite attempts to calm Mrs Miller she remains extremely agitated and confused; without a nurse continually at the bedside, she attempts to climb out, and is very unsteady on her legs with a risk of falling. When one of the nursing staff attempts to help her back into bed Mrs Miller kicks her firmly. Mrs Miller's daughter has now arrived but the situation does not improve despite her best efforts.

Should Mrs Miller be sedated to enable further assessment and treatment?

When considering this question it is important to consider the following:

• Is there a clear reversible cause that can be identified and treated to resolve Mrs Miller's confusion? For example, hypoxia, hypovolaemia, pain, urinary retention, etc.

• Have all reasonable attempts been made to improve Mrs Miller's confusion by non-pharmacological means?

Acute Medicine: Clinical Cases Uncovered. By C. Roseveare.
Published 2009 by Blackwell Publishing, ISBN: 978-1-4051-6883-0

Table 66 Causes of acute confusional state

Cause	Clinical clues	Comments
Infections Urinary Respiratory Meningitis/encephalitis (or any other)	May be fever or specific symptoms/signs related to the infection site	Focal symptoms/signs often absent; remember that bacteriuria is common in asymptomatic elderly female patients
Cardiovascular Myocardial infarction (MI) Cardiac failure	History of ischaemic heart disease; physical signs of heart failure	MI is often 'silent' in elderly patients; ECG should always be taken on arrival even in the absence of chest pain
Respiratory Hypoxia Pulmonary embolism	History of chronic lung disease; central cyanosis risk factors for PE (see Case 2)	If pulse oximetry is difficult to obtain due to poor trace or non-compliance, review blood gases
Metabolic Dehydration/hyponatraemia/hypercalcaemia/hypoglycaemia/renal failure Hyper/hypothyroidism	History of diuretic use or treatment for diabetes; diarrhoea or vomiting Dry mucous membranes and increased skin turgor suggest dehydration Bone pain, constipation, polyuria may suggest hypercalcaemia	Always check electrolytes and calcium; clinical clues may be absent Thyroid disease may be difficult to diagnose clinically – always consider thyroid function tests if not recently checked
Drug induced Opiate analgesics Sedatives Antidepressant Digoxin toxicity Overdose of any drug	Careful drug history – enquire about any new drug prior to onset of symptoms Pinpoint pupils suggest opiate excess; gastrointestinal upset in digoxin toxicity	Confusion may lead to inappropriate dosing – check dates of prescription and verify quantities of tablets
Withdrawal phenomena Alcohol Antidepressant Benzodiazepine	Enquire about alcohol consumption; 'empties' around patient's house Smell for alcohol on breath	Patients may be very secretive about drinking – even family may be unaware
Cerebral Cerebrovascular event Intracranial bleed Subdural/subarachnoid tumour	Risk factors for cerebrovascular disease Recent head injury Evidence of trauma Focal neurological signs	Full neurological examination may be difficult if patient is confused; reassessment may be required. Request regular 'neuro obs' if subdural is suspected
Other Constipation Pain Urinary retention	Faecal loading may be apparent clinically; may feel enlarged bladder – otherwise bedside bladder scan will enable estimation of residual urine	Remember that elderly patients with faecal impaction can present with diarrhoea due to 'overflow': always perform a rectal examination if possible

• Does Mrs Miller's behaviour constitute a risk to herself or to others on the ward?
• Does this risk outweigh the potential risks of sedation in an older person?

Box 29 summarises a suggested approach to consideration and delivery of sedation in this situation. Particular attention should be paid to the need for close monitoring after sedation has been delivered.

PART 2: CASES

Box 29 Suggested strategy for sedation in elderly patients with confusion

Possible reasons for urgent sedation

Severe agitation

Physical aggression to patients or staff

Significant risk of harm to self

Prolonged overactivity with risk of exhaustion

Determined attempts to abscond that have not been contained by other measures (in an incompetent patient)

Drug administration

Intravenous lorazepam: 25–30 µg/kg by slow injection into a large vein

or

Intravenous midazolam: 1.5 mg over 30 s with further doses of 0.5–1 mg at 2-min intervals until sedation is achieved

Monitoring and management

- Baseline pulse, respiratory rate, blood pressure, oxygen saturation
- Observations immediately after administration and then every 15 min for the first hour and then hourly for 12 h
- Cardiopulmonary resuscitation facilities should be available
- Flumazenil should be instantly available for oversedation
- Nurses should inform doctor if: pulse <50 or >110 beats/min, respiratory rate <10 or >20 breaths/min, systolic BP <100 mmHg, diastolic BP >110 mmHg, oxygen saturation <90%, temperature >38°C, sedation prolonged greater than expected
- One-to-one nursing
- Adequate pressure relief
- Hydration (i.v. or s.c.)
- Consider prescription of regular oral medication, e.g. 0.5 mg qds of lorazepam once patient has woken

---

- In this case the confusion is so severe that further diagnostic assessment is not possible
- In addition, Mrs Miller's behaviour now constitutes a risk of injury to herself
- Mrs Miller is also being physically aggressive towards staff members

Mrs Miller is given 0.5 mg of lorazepam i.m. Following this she seems much calmer and will allow baseline observations to be undertaken. Mrs Miller's pulse is 100 beats/min and irregularly irregular with a blood pressure of

130/70. Her oral temperature is 37.8°C. Oxygen saturation reads 94% on room air, and improves to 97% when Mrs Miller is given 2 L/min oxygen via a nasal cannula.

Mrs Miller is unable to give a history and the GP's letter gives very little background information.

How can a further history be obtained in Mrs Miller's case?

As indicated in Table 66 the differential diagnosis in this setting is broad. Obtaining a history is essential. Consider the following.

- **Telephone the GP**: obtain full details of Mrs Miller's recent and past medical history, medication list and any allergies. If the GP has undertaken any recent investigations that may not be accessible via the hospital data system, the results of these should also be sought. Find out if the community social work team or elderly mental health team have been involved in Mrs Miller's care in the past (and contact them if so)
- **Speak to Mrs Miller's daughter** (and any other relatives who may be available): find out if this is an isolated incident or whether it represents a regular pattern; if the problem has occurred in the past, what was the diagnosis and outcome at that time? Establish whether Mrs Miller's memory has been deteriorating recently and whether there has been any progressive change in her level of confusion (cognitive state). Ask if Mrs Miller is known to drink alcohol or smoke, and whether there are any empty alcohol bottles in the property
- **Speak to the warden** of Mrs Miller's accommodation
- **Access hospital records** and recent blood test results from the hospital database
- **Examine any medication packaging** that Mrs Miller has brought in with her: calculate from the dates of prescription and numbers of remaining tablets whether the patient may have been non-compliant with these and/or taken too many. The latter may have been deliberate or accidental

The GP is contacted and notes from his records that one of his partners saw Mrs Miller the previous week on a home visit; the warden had called to say that Mrs Miller was a little more confused than normal and had fallen in her flat. Mrs Miller was complaining of low back pain following the fall. The GP had commented that her urine had smelt offensive and there were white cells and nitrites on urinalysis; he had made a diagnosis of a urinary tract infection and prescribed Mrs Miller trimethoprim 200 mg twice daily, along with co-dydramol (paracetamol with dihydrocodeine) for the pain. The community matron had visited the next day and thought Mrs Miller seemed better and was coping adequately.

Mrs Miller has a past history of atrial fibrillation. She had several transient ischaemic attacks (TIAs) the previous year and started taking warfarin. Mrs Miller has mild cardiac failure and hypertension. She smoked 20 cigarettes per day until the age of 80. There is no known history of alcohol excess.

Mrs Miller's normal medication comprises warfarin 3 mg daily, digoxin 125 μg daily, ramipril 2.5 mg daily, furosemide 40 mg daily. From examination of the packaging it appears that Mrs Miller's dosing has been appropriate.

According to her daughter her confusion and memory disturbance have been getting gradually worse over the past year. Mrs Miller has also had a tendency to get constipated and complains of various aches and pains. Her appetite has never been good, but had deteriorated in the past three months and Mrs Miller's daughter thinks she has lost some weight. Mrs Miller has had a number of falls but generally copes well. Her daughter had suggested that she would be better off in a residential home earlier this year, but she was very reluctant to move from her warden-controlled flat. Mrs Miller's daughter visits most days and does her shopping. Otherwise she copes independently. This episode is completely out of character. Mrs Miller has never been incontinent. After the GP visited last week the daughter noted a dry cough and thought her mother appeared a bit flushed.

How can the degree of confusion be 'quantified'?

Quantification of confusion is usually achieved by use of a mental test scoring. This will help to assess the patient's progress, which can be particularly useful if there is underlying cognitive impairment. The commonest score used in acute medical practice is the Abbreviated Mental Test Score (AMTS), which gives a score out of 10 (see Box 30). In acute confusional states, disorientation (particularly for time) is almost invariable.

Mrs Miller's AMTS is 3/10. She is disorientated in time, place and person, but remembers her date of birth, name of the monarch and her age.

What diagnoses should be considered on the basis of the history?

- **Urinary tract infection**: this is a common cause of toxic confusional state and urinalysis showed leucocytes and nitrites last week. However, this finding is common

---

> **Box 30 Abbreviated Mental Test Score (AMTS)**
>
> **Score 1 point for each fully correct answer**
> Patient's age
> Date of birth (month and year sufficient)
> Time (to nearest hour)
> Year
> Name of hospital
> Recognition of two persons (e.g. doctor and nurse)
> Year of First (or Second) World War
> Name of present monarch
> Count backwards from 20 to 1
> Recall 'imaginary address', e.g. 20 West Street, Bathgate (ask the patient to repeat back to ensure they have understood)

in women of this age who frequently have asymptomatic bacteriuria

- **Respiratory tract infection**: viral or bacterial upper or lower respiratory tract infection is also a common cause of acute confusion in older people. Mrs Miller's daughter noted that her mother had a dry cough
- **Drug-induced confusion:** opiate drugs (e.g. codeine/morphine) can be responsible for confusion in older patients; remember to check for pinpoint pupils (see Case 13). The excretion of digoxin may be unpredictable in older people, particularly if renal function has deteriorated; symptoms of digoxin toxicity are often non-specific and can include acute confusion
- **Intracranial bleed**: particularly subdural haematoma, given that Mrs Miller has been falling recently and may have sustained a head injury. The fact that she is taking warfarin may have increased the risk of bleeding
- **Ischaemic stroke**: Mrs Miller has had previous TIAs and is in atrial fibrillation: although warfarin will reduce the risk of embolic stroke it does not eliminate this possibility
- **Dehydration or electrolyte imbalance**: Mrs Miller takes the diuretic furosemide, which may result in hyponatraemia or hypokalaemia; her fluid intake may have been poor and fever from recent infection may have resulted in excess loss through sweating. Hypercalcaemia may also be exacerbated by dehydration
- **Constipation**: although this may occur as a consequence of other systemic illness, constipation itself can precipitate confusion in older people
- **Malignancy**: Mrs Miller has been going downhill for a while; she is an ex-smoker and has been losing weight. Cancer is common in this age group and the presentation

is often non-specific. Malignancy may precipitate infection, result in electrolyte imbalances or produce cerebral metastases

Although the history has highlighted these possible causes, there are many other potential explanations; careful clinical examination is now required, although this may be limited due to poor cooperation.

Examination reveals a fast, irregular pulse of 110 beats/min with blood pressure 130/70. Mrs Miller's mucous membranes are dry and her skin turgor is increased, suggesting dehydration. There are no cardiac murmurs. Respiratory examination is difficult as Mrs Miller will not comply with instructions to take deep breaths, but there are no gross abnormalities. Abdominal examination reveals some faecal loading in the left iliac fossa but no abnormal masses. A rectal examination reveals hard faeces in the rectum. Mrs Miller appears to be tender over her lumbar spine.

Central nervous system examination is limited because of poor cooperation. Mrs Miller appears to be moving all limbs equally. There is no facial asymmetry and all reflexes are brisk but equal. The plantars are downgoing. Her pupils are 4 mm in diameter, equal and reactive. Fundoscopy is not possible. Urinalysis reveals 2+ leucocytes and 1+ nitrites.

What initial investigations are required?

A suggested list of initial investigations for patients with acute confusion is given in Table 67. Given the limitations of the history and examination in this situation, as well as the non-specific presentation of many of the causes of acute confusion, it is often necessary to request a wide range of tests before any conclusions can be reached.

In view of her recent falls, anticoagulant drug use and lumbar spine pain, a CT brain scan and lumbar spine X-ray are also requested.

Table 67 Initial investigation for a confused elderly patient

Investigation	Justification
Full blood count	Raised white cell count in infection
	Severe anaemia may cause confusion
	Raised mean corpuscular volume may suggest B12 deficiency or alcohol abuse
Urea and electrolytes	Hyponatraemia and uraemia are relatively common causes of confusion
Liver function tests	Raised transaminases in alcohol abuse
	Hepatic encephalopathy
Blood clotting	If taking anticoagulant drugs or evidence of liver disease
	Higher likelihood of intracranial bleeding if clotting abnormal
C-reactive protein/ESR	Usually raised in infective or inflammatory disorders
Thyroid function tests	Hypo- or hyperthyroidism
Calcium	Hypercalcaemia (or less commonly hypocalcaemia) may cause confusion
Glucose	Hypoglycaemia or undiagnosed diabetes
Troponin I or T	Silent myocardial infarction
Vitamin B12 and folate	Deficiency may cause confusion
Arterial blood gas	Hypoxia or hypercapnia may cause confusion
	Lactic acidosis may suggest sepsis
Chest radiograph	Pneumonia, lung tumour or cardiac failure
ECG	Silent myocardial infarction, arrhythmias, heart block, etc.
Urinalysis and urine culture	Urinary tract infection is a common cause of confusion in the elderly
Drug levels where appropriate (e.g. digoxin)	To exclude toxicity or accidental/deliberate overdose

Mrs Miller's results are as follows:

- *haemoglobin 98, white blood cells 12.8, neutrophils 9.8, platelets 108, mean corpuscular volume 88*
- *international normalised ratio (INR) 2.7*
- *Na 120, K 3.8, urea 15.7, creatinine 160*
- *protein 78, albumin 32, bilirubin 14, alkaline phosphatase 190, alanine transaminase 50*
- *glucose 6.7*
- *'corrected' calcium 3.45 (normal 2.15–2.65)*
- *C-reactive protein 70, erythrocyte sedimentation rate (ESR) 105*
- *digoxin level 1.1*
- *thyroid function normal*
- *chest radiograph: possible bulky left hilum*
- *ECG: atrial fibrillation; no other abnormality*
- *CT brain: generalised cerebral atrophy with several areas of low attenuation consistent with old infarcts. No evidence of subdural or intracranial haematoma and no evidence of new ischaemic stroke*
- *Lumbar spine radiograph: recent crush fracture of third lumbar vertebra*
- *Blood and urine culture sent (results awaited)*

How should these results be interpreted?

The INR is within the desirable therapeutic range (usually 2–3 for patients with atrial fibrillation) and Mrs Miller is not digoxin toxic. However, there are a number of abnormalities.

- **Hyponatraemia and renal impairment**: this could relate to diuretic use or could be caused by some other underlying condition; the elevated urea is disproportionate to the creatinine, suggesting an element of dehydration. Comparison with old results, if available, may be helpful. If similar values pre-date the onset of confusion they may be of less importance
- **Hypercalcaemia**: the calcium level is significantly elevated and this may be responsible for the confusion and other symptoms Mrs Miller has recently described. The cause for the hypercalcaemia should be carefully considered (see Table 68) – an underlying condition causing hypercalcaemia may have contributed to Mrs Miller's current symptoms
- **Normocytic anaemia**: this is quite a common finding in patients of this age, and may reflect underlying chronic inflammatory disease
- **Raised inflammatory markers**: there is a limited number of conditions which result in an ESR >100 (see Case 20). Although infection remains a possible explana-

Table 68 Causes of hypercalcaemia

Malignancies	
Solid organ tumours	Bronchial carcinoma
	Renal cell carcinoma
	Bone metastases (e.g. from breast, prostate, lung, etc)
Haematological malignancies	Myeloma
	Lymphoma
Endocrine	
Primary hyperparathyroidism	
Tertiary hyperparathyroidism	
Thyrotoxicosis	
Phaeochromocytoma	
Adrenal failure	
Drug induced	
Calcium supplements	
Milk-alkali syndrome	
Thiazide diuretics	
Other	
Sarcoidosis	
Paget's disease with immobility	
Familial hypocalciuric hypercalcaemia	

tion, it would be unusual for a 'simple' urinary or respiratory tract infection to produce this level of elevation
- **Abnormal chest radiograph**: non-specific abnormalities may be difficult to interpret; the bulky hilum may suggest malignancy or lymph node enlargement or may be a normal variant. Comparison with old radiographs is mandatory if these are available
- **Crush fracture of lumbar vertebra**: this may have resulted from a recent fall and is probably responsible for Mrs Miller's pain

Review of the hospital pathology database reveals that Mrs Miller's electrolytes were checked one month earlier; at that time her urea was 10.7 and creatinine 136 with sodium 130. A chest radiograph undertaken three months ago is very similar to the current imaging.

What is the likely diagnosis and how should she now be managed?

- The combination of raised ESR, normocytic anaemia, hypercalcamia and renal impairment is particularly suggestive of *myeloma*
- Myeloma can also result in weakening of bones, which may have resulted in the recent vertebral fracture

• Hypercalcaemia is probably the main cause of Mrs Miller's confusion; however, this may have been exacerbated by the effects of dehydration, back pain, constipation and recent infection

Further management should be as follows.

• **Commence rehydration:** caution will be needed to avoid fluid overload, in view of Mrs Miller's previous cardiac failure. Normal saline will be the fluid of choice. Give 500 mL over 3–4 h and reassess her fluid status. Aim for 3–4 L over 24 h but be prepared to adjust the infusion rate according to Mrs Miller's clinical condition. Supplement potassium (3 g per litre of fluid) in view of initial hypokalaemia

• **Omit diuretics and angiotensin-converting enzyme (ACE) inhibitor from the drug chart:** these may contribute to the dehydration, but will probably need to be reinstituted prior to discharge

• **Monitor urine output:** this will give a guide to fluid requirements; a urinary catheter may be required if Mrs Miller is incontinent, but should be removed at the earliest opportunity in view of the potential to precipitate or prolong infection

• **Withhold antibiotics while awaiting culture results:** although it is often tempting to initiate broad-spectrum antibiotic treatment, in this case there is no good evidence of infection. Older people in hospital are at high risk of *Clostridium difficile* infection following antibiotic use (see Case 10). If Mrs Miller's condition deteriorates or evidence of infection develops, appropriate therapy can be initiated

• **Send 'myeloma screen':** this comprises blood for protein electrophoresis, looking for monoclonal elevation of immunoglobulins, and urine for Bence Jones protein

• **Recheck electrolytes and calcium after 24 hours' rehydration:** hypercalcaemia is often exacerbated by dehydration and may significantly improve simply with fluid; otherwise, further correction may be required

• **Commence laxative treatment:** constipation should be addressed early as faecal impaction may delay recovery. A regular osmotic laxative such as magnesium hydroxide should be prescribed. This may take several days to have an effect; use of a phosphate enema should be considered if faecal impaction is suspected

After 24 h of intravenous fluid treatment Mrs Miller's condition is much improved. AMTS is now 6/10, although her daughter feels Mrs Miller is still more confused than normal.

Further investigation results are as follows:
• *Na 133, K 4.1, urea 12.5, creatinine 145*
• *calcium 3.12*
• *immunoglobulins: raised IgG*
• *protein electrophoresis: monoclonal paraprotein band identified*
• *urine/blood culture: no growth*

The initial diagnosis of myeloma has been confirmed; this is the likely cause of Mrs Miller's hypercalcaemia, and probably also accounts for the raised ESR, renal impairment and anaemia. Rehydration has improved the hypercalcaemia and electrolyte imbalance, but Mrs Miller remains more confused than normal and her calcium level is still significantly elevated.

How can the hypercalcaemia be corrected?

• Use of the osteoclast inhibitor pamidronate will result in further lowering of the calcium level

• This is administered intravenously by infusion, and is less effective if the patient has not been adequately rehydrated

• An infusion of 60–90 mg should correct the hypercalcaemia

Mrs Miller is given 60 mg of pamidronate by infusion and continues to receive intravenous fluid for a further 24 h. Mrs Miller's confusion is noted to be much improved (AMTS 8/10), which her daughter confirms represents her 'normal self'. The next day her calcium level is 2.65.

Mrs Miller is referred to the haematology team, who plan to review her on the haematology day unit for discussion about further treatment of her myeloma, and consider the need for bone marrow biopsy.

Mrs Miller is reviewed by the physiotherapist who remains concerned about her poor mobility. The physiotherapist feels that she needs a period of inpatient rehabilitation to recover from the effects of the crush fracture of her lumbar vertebra. Mrs Miller is transferred to the rehabilitation ward for further mobilisation and treatment.

CASE REVIEW

An 81-year-old woman has been referred to hospital after becoming acutely confused. Mrs Miller is acutely agitated on arrival in hospital, and is deemed to be at risk of injury. She is therefore sedated with lorazepam, which also allows more detailed assessment of her condition. Mrs Miller is not able to give a history, but communication with her GP and daughter reveals that she has been becoming more confused over the past few months, and had a significant fall in her warden-controlled flat one week earlier. The GP diagnosed a urinary tract infection and prescribed trimethoprim, along with codeine and paracetamol for analgesia. Although Mrs Miller initially improved, her condition has now acutely deteriorated resulting in admission to hospital. Examination reveals AMTS of 3/10; Mrs Miller appears dehydrated and there is lumbar spine tenderness. There are no focal neurological signs.

Initial investigations reveal moderate renal impairment with hyponatraemia and significant hypercalcaemia. Mrs Miller also has a normocytic anaemia and raised ESR. There is a crush fracture of L3.

Mrs Miller's diuretics are withheld and she is given intravenous normal saline. Mrs Miller's confusion reduces over the next 24 h with improvement in her renal function and electrolytes. However, her calcium remains elevated and her daughter reports that she is not yet back to her normal self. Subsequent investigation shows a monoclonal elevation of immunoglobulin, suggestive of myeloma. Mrs Miller is given intravenous pamidronate, which resolves the hypercalcaemia and results in resolution of the confusion. She is referred to the haematologists for further investigation and treatment of her myeloma, and subsequently is transferred to the rehabilitation ward to enable full recovery from her lumbar crush fracture prior to discharge back to her warden-controlled accommodation.

This case illustrates the complex thought processes that are often required when assessing older people with confusion. The differential diagnosis is often wide, and the causes of confusion may be multiple. In this case Mrs Miller's confusion may have resulted from a combination of dehydration, hyponatraemia, hypercalcaemia, pain, constipation and codeine. A methodical approach is required, ensuring that all relevant information is obtained from any available source, particularly when no history is available from the patient, as in this case. Extensive investigation is often required before any firm conclusions can be reached.

KEY POINTS

- Acute confusion is a common cause of admission in older people.
- Although infection is the commonest cause, there are many other causes that need to be considered.
- If a history is not available from the patient, other sources of information such as the patient's GP, family or carers should be sought.
- Sedation may be required if the patient is severely agitated, but the benefits should be weighed up against the potential cardiovascular and respiratory risks.
- If no clear cause is apparent from the history or examination, a wide range of investigations including blood tests, radiographs and cross-sectional imaging may be required.
- Interpretation of investigations should, where possible, take account of previous results.

Further reading

Berenson J. Treatment of hypercalcaemia of malignancy with bisphosphonates. *Semin Oncol* 2002; **29**(21): 12–18

British Geriatric Society. Guidelines for the prevention, diagnosis and management of delirium in older people in hospital (2005). http://www.bgs.org.uk/Publications/Clinical%20Guidelines/clinical_1-2_fulldelirium.htm

Spice C, Bacon M. Delirium (acute toxic confusion) in the elderly. *CPD J Acute Med* 2003; **2**(1): 19–24

Case 18 A 25-year-old woman with acute hyperglycaemia

You are contacted by a GP regarding a 25-year-old female patient whom he has just seen in his surgery. Miss Maria Kappel has been feeling unwell for the past three weeks with excessive thirst and increased urinary frequency, associated with 7 kg of weight loss. For the past two days Miss Kappel has been vomiting. This morning her mother was concerned because Miss Kappel appeared drowsy and confused. Urinalysis in the GP's surgery revealed 4+ glucose and 3+ ketones. The capillary blood glucose reading was 25 mmol/L. Miss Kappel's breathing is deep and sighing and her breath smells sweet.

Miss Kappel has no prior history of diabetes or other medical problems.

What challenges will this patient present?

• The history of thirst (polydipsia) and urinary frequency (polyuria) is suggestive of a new diagnosis of diabetes mellitus, which is supported by the raised capillary glucose level

• The patient's young age, recent weight loss and short duration of symptoms suggest that this is likely to be Type 1 diabetes, for which Miss Kappel will require treatment with insulin

• The onset of vomiting, drowsiness and confusion in association with significant ketonuria suggests the development of diabetic ketoacidosis (DKA)

• The sweet-smelling breath (often described as 'like pear-drops') is also suggestive of a raised ketone level and the deep sighing respiratory pattern (*Kussmaul breathing*) suggests a metabolic acidosis

• DKA is a life-threatening complication of Type 1 diabetes, which (as in this case) can be the presenting symptom of newly diagnosed diabetes

• Miss Kappel will require immediate review and initia-

tion of treatment, with close monitoring following her arrival in hospital; in many cases the patient may require transfer to a high dependency unit

• Sometimes the onset of DKA is precipitated by another medical condition (see Table 69); underlying causes will need to be considered and treated as appropriate

Miss Kappel is brought into the ward by ambulance. During her transit into hospital Miss Kappel has become more drowsy. Her airway is maintained, with oxygen saturation of 99% on room air, but her breathing is rapid, with a Kussmaul respiratory pattern. Miss Kappel's pulse is 110 beats/min with blood pressure 90/40. Her hands feel cool to touch and the capillary refill time is increased at 3 seconds. Miss Kappel's mucous membranes are dry and there is increased skin turgor. The capillary blood glucose continues to read 25 mmol/L.

What immediate management is required?

• Confirm patency of the airway and apply an oxygen mask

• Assess conscious level using the Glasgow Coma Scale (GCS) (see p. 127)

  ◦ if the score is <8, or falls by 2 points or more, contact the on-call anaesthetic specialist registrar immediately, as the patient is likely to require intubation and transfer to intensive care

  ◦ commence a neurological observation (neuro obs) chart (see p. 131) and ensure this is recorded every 15 min, initially

• Establish peripheral intravenous access

• Obtain venous blood for a full blood count (FBC), urea and electrolytes (U&E), amylase, liver function tests (LFT), glucose and venous blood gas analysis:

  ◦ arterial blood gas may be obtained, but adds little additional diagnostic information when compared with venous blood gas, unless there are concerns about oxygenation

Acute Medicine: Clinical Cases Uncovered. By C. Roseveare.
Published 2009 by Blackwell Publishing, ISBN: 978-1-4051-6883-0

Table 69 Common precipitants of diabetic ketoacidosis (DKA)

Infection, e.g. urinary tract, respiratory, viral illness, gastroenteritis, soft tissue infection, etc.	Fever and focal symptoms may not be present in patients with diabetes; look closely for more unusual sites of infection – examine external genitalia in men for evidence of balanitis; look in skin folds for evidence of candida or cellulitis; inspect teeth for evidence of dental sepsis A raised white cell count is a common finding in DKA and not always suggestive of infection C-reactive protein is often not elevated in patients with diabetes and infection
Acute pancreatitis	Measure amylase level for all patients presenting with DKA; abdominal pain may be a presenting symptom of DKA – does not always reflect intra-abdominal pathology
Myocardial infarction	Patients with diabetes are more prone to ischaemic heart disease; look closely at admission ECG and measure cardiac enzymes; mild elevation of troponin is not uncommon in DKA and does not necessarily imply myocardial infarction
Omission of insulin dose (for patients with pre-existing Type 1 diabetes)	May be inadvertent or deliberate – sometimes relates to poor understanding of their condition. Careful history is required and early involvement of diabetes specialist team to ensure appropriate re-education

- Measure the capillary ketone level using a ketonemeter (if available)
- Test urine for the presence of glucose and ketones
- Attach to a cardiac monitor
- Perform an ECG
- Commence an intravenous infusion of normal saline – 1 L to be infused over 30 min:
  - tachycardia, hypotension and increased capillary refill time suggest dehydration, which is common in DKA, as a result of osmotic diuresis and vomiting
- Commence an intravenous insulin sliding scale (see Table 70) – Actrapid 50 units diluted to 50 mL with 0.9% saline, starting at 6 units/h via a syringe pump
- Consider insertion of a nasogastric tube if the patient is vomiting or drowsy

Miss Kappel's airway is confirmed as patent and protected with a total GCS of 12/15. The cardiac monitor reveals a sinus tachycardia, which is confirmed on a 12-lead ECG.

Venous blood gas reading is as follows:
- *pH 7.01, pCO_2 2.8, pO_2 6.8, HCO_3 10.2, base excess −18.6, lactate 2.3*
- *Na 131, K 6.1*
- *glucose 25.9 mmol/L*

Table 70 Suggested insulin sliding scale for patients with diabetic ketoacidosis (DKA)*

Blood glucose (mmol/L)	Insulin infusion rate (u/h)
<4.0	See hypoglycaemia guidance below
4.0–7.0	1
7.1–10.0	2
10.1–14.9	3
>14.9	6

Hypoglycaemia guidance

Blood glucose <2.5 or symptomatic with blood glucose <4:

Treat with 25 mL of 50% glucose i.v.

Stop insulin for 15 min then restart at 0.5 u/h, checking blood glucose every 15 min for 1 h

Asymptomatic with blood glucose 2.5–4:

Stop insulin for 15 min then restart at 0.5 u/h, checking blood glucose every 15 min for 1 h

*Use human Actrapid 50 units diluted to 50 mL with normal saline via syringe pump.

- capillary beta-hydroxybutyrate level 4.5 mmol/L (normal range 0–1 mmol/L)

What do the blood gases suggest and what management should be instituted?

- **There is severe metabolic acidosis** (low bicarbonate and negative base excess) with attempted respiratory compensation (low pCO_2), which accounts for the Kussmaul respiration. The pH is low (acidaemia), indicating that respiratory compensation is inadequate for the degree of metabolic acidosis
- **Although the lactate reading is high**, this is not enough to account for the degree of metabolic acidosis; another acid is likely to be responsible – in this case the ketone β-hydroxybutyrate
- **The glucose reading is high**, confirming the diagnosis of diabetes mellitus: this, in combination with the metabolic acidosis and ketonaemia, confirms the diagnosis of DKA (see Table 71)
- **The potassium level is high** – this will almost certainly fall rapidly following initiation of insulin therapy; close monitoring will be required
- **Fluid resuscitation and intravenous insulin** will be the mainstay of the initial management

The first litre of fluid has now finished. Miss Kappel continues to exhibit Kussmaul breathing, but her pulse has fallen to 100 beats/min with blood pressure 100/50. Miss Kappel has passed 600 mL of dilute urine. She appears less confused and drowsy (GCS 13/15). .

Further venous blood gas analysis is as follows:
- *pH 7.13, pCO_2 2.9, pO_2 5.9, HCO_3 12.5, base excess –16, lactate 1.9*
- *Na 133, K 5.1*
- *glucose 21.6*

Table 71 Criteria for the diagnosis of diabetic ketoacidosis

Glucose >11 mmol/L

pH <7.30

HCO_3 <15 mmol/L

Ketonaemia >3 mmol/L (if available)

Presence of ketonuria

What further fluid is now required and how quickly should it be infused?

- Normal (0.9%) saline is the usual fluid of choice for initial resuscitation; some clinicians (particularly intensivists) prefer to use Hartman's or Ringer's lactate solution to prevent excessive accumulation of chloride, which can exacerbate acidosis. However, there is no evidence to suggest that this makes a clinically significant difference in most cases
- Adults with DKA usually require an average of 6 L of fluid over the first 16 h – a suggested infusion regimen is given in Table 72
- Excessively rapid fluid replacement can result in cerebral oedema – this is more common in children and adolescents, in whom calculation of fluid requirement based on body weight is recommended (see Fig. 44)
- As the potassium level falls, potassium chloride (KCl) will need to be added to the fluid infused; it is usually recommended to add 40 mmol KCl to each litre of fluid once the serum potassium falls below 5.5; if the potassium falls below 3.5, 60–80 mmol KCl should be added to each litre of fluid
- The maximum recommended infusion rate for potassium is 20 mmol/h; if the fluid is being infused more rapidly than is permitted by the potassium concentration, two separate infusions may be required
- Bicarbonate solution is rarely indicated; attempts to correct acidosis in this way paradoxically increase cerebral acidosis and increase the risk of cerebral oedema. Bicarbonate be considered in cases of severe acidosis (pH < 6.8) but only in consultation with a senior physician or intensivist

Table 72 Suggested fluid resuscitation regimen for adults with diabetic ketoacidosis

Fluid	Rate
0.9% saline	500 mL/h for 1 h
0.9% saline with 40 mmol/L KCL	500 mL/h for 5 h
0.9% saline with 40 mmol/L KCL	300 mL/h for 10 h

The fluid infusion regimen should be adjusted according to response; when the blood glucose falls <15 mmol/L the fluid should be changed to dextrose/saline or 5% dextrose. If this occurs within the first 16 h, saline should be continued as above and 5% dextrose should be infused via a second cannula at a rate of 125 mL/h (or 10% glucose if blood glucose <7 mmol/L).

Step 1: assess degree of dehydration

- <3% – dehydration not clinically detectable; normal skin turgor
- 5% (mild) – dry mucous membranes, sunken eyes
- 7.5% (moderate) – as above with reduced skin turgor
- 10% (or more) – as above and severely unwell with poor perfusion (capillary refill >2 s), skin turgor reduced (skin recoil >2 s), thready rapid pulse; hypotension

Step 2: calculate fluid deficit

- Deficit (litres) = % dehydration × body weight

(using 10% as maximum figure for % dehydration)

Step 3: calculate maintenance requirement for 48 h

- 200 mL/kg/48 h for first 10 kg body weight
- 100 mL/kg/48 h for second 10 kg body weight
- 40 mL/kg/48 h for anything over 20 kg

$$\text{Hourly rate} = \frac{\text{48-h maintenance} + \text{deficit} - \text{resuscitation fluid already given}}{48}$$

Figure 44 Calculation of fluid requirement by body weight (recommended for children, adolescents and young adults).

Miss Kappel is prescribed a further litre of normal saline to run over the next 2 h, followed by a litre over 2 h containing 40 mmol KCl. The current infusion rate of insulin is 6 units/h, with a blood glucose recording of 21.3 mmol/L. Her pulse is 90 beats/min and blood pressure 110/70. Miss Kappel has passed a further 200 mL of urine in the past hour.

Miss Kappel is now much more alert and no longer confused (GCS 15/15). She is now able to give a reliable history.

Miss Kappel tells you that she has not felt well for at least four weeks. Her appetite has been reduced and she has felt tired most of the time. Miss Kappel initially attributed this to a flu-like illness, but the symptoms persisted. She first noted the need to pass more urine three weeks ago, and has been excessively thirsty throughout this time. In the past few days Miss Kappel has also noted a burning sensation on micturition. Miss Kappel started vomiting two days ago and has not kept much food or fluid down since then. Yesterday she noted pain in her left flank area and she felt feverish before going to bed, but she remembers little else until her arrival in hospital. The pain is still present, and described as a constant ache, worsened by moving and lying on her left side.

Miss Kappel has no significant past history and she takes no regular medication. There is no family history of diabetes, but her mother suffers from an overactive thyroid. Miss Kappel is a non-smoker and drinks only occasional alcohol. She drives a car and works as a trainee hairdresser.

Her periods have been regular. She agrees to undergo a pregnancy test.

An examination reveals a mild pyrexia (37.7°C) with cardiovascular signs as above. There is a soft ejection systolic murmur in the aortic area, which does not radiate to the carotids. Respiratory examination is normal apart from the Kussmaul breathing pattern which appears less obvious. There is marked tenderness in the left renal angle and suprapubic area but no abdominal masses or organomegaly.

Laboratory blood results are now available as follows:

- *haemoglobin 145 mg/L, white cell count 16.7, platelets 265*
- *Na 131, K 6.2, urea 13.6, creatinine 90*
- *albumin 31, alanine transaminase 40, alkaline phosphatase 135, bilirubin 15*
- *C-reactive protein 219*
- *amylase 45*
- *glucose 28*
- *pregnancy test: negative*
- *the sample was taken before the patient was started on intravenous fluid or insulin*
- *chest radiograph: normal*

Is there a precipitating cause of the diabetic ketoacidosis?

- DKA may be the presenting symptom of Type 1 diabetes, as in this case
- In some cases the deterioration in the patient's condition leading to the development of DKA results from

another medical condition – this is particularly important in patients with pre-existing diabetes that has been well controlled in the past, but should also be considered for patients presenting for the first time

• Some of the common precipitating causes are listed in Table 68

• In this case Miss Kappel is exhibiting symptoms and signs of acute pyelonephritis, which is likely to have complicated her new diagnosis of Type 1 diabetes, resulting in the development of diabetic ketoacidosis

• The raised C-reactive protein (CRP) and white cell count support the suspicion of infection as the precipitating cause

• The absence of nitrites and leucocytes from the urine does not exclude urinary tract infection in this context: extreme dilution of the urine in the context of the osmotic diuresis in DKA can lead to false-negative urinalysis

• Urine should be sent to the laboratory for culture in all cases

A urine specimen is sent for culture and Miss Kappel is started on intravenous cefuroxime 750 mg 8 hourly.

Six hours have now passed since Miss Kappel's arrival in hospital. Her breathing pattern now appears normal and her latest blood glucose reading is 14.4 mmol/L. She has not vomited since admission to hospital although she still feels nauseous and is reluctant to eat.

Miss Kappel has received 3 L of normal saline.

Repeat venous blood gas is as follows:
• *pH 7.30, pCO$_2$ 3.6, HCO$_3$ 18, base excess −3.5*
• *Na 137, K 4.4*
• *glucose 14.9*

What further management should be undertaken?

• Miss Kappel remains acidotic but the pH is now near normal

• The potassium level has fallen and will need to be monitored with further supplementation

• The glucose level has fallen significantly: ideally this should be maintained between 11 and 15 in the first 16 h (see Table 69)

A second cannula is sited and an infusion of 5% dextrose is commenced at a rate of 125 mL/h in addition to the saline/KCl infusion, which is now running at 300 mL/h; you plan to repeat the venous blood gas and potassium in 2 h, and to adjust the potassium supplementation dose if required.

For how long should Miss Kappel remain on intravenous insulin?

• Before stopping the intravenous insulin the following criteria should be met:
  ○ the acidaemia should have resolved (pH >7.3)
  ○ Miss Kappel should be able to eat

• If a ketonemeter is available, this can be used as a guide to cessation of intravenous insulin:
  ○ continue intravenous insulin until ketones are no longer present in the blood (<0.3 mmol/L)
  ○ urinary ketones may remain present for many hours after the disappearance of ketones from the blood and are therefore a less useful guide to resolution of ketosis

• Subcutaneous insulin should be administered 1 h before discontinuation of the intravenous infusion, since acidosis can rapidly recur as the intravenous insulin clears from the blood

What further considerations are required prior to discharge?

• Miss Kappel should be referred to the inpatient specialist diabetes team while on the ward; they will be able to provide advice regarding the most appropriate form of insulin for this patient

• Miss Kappel will require careful education about the nature and significance of the diagnosis of Type 1 diabetes; most hospitals have a diabetes nurse specialist, who will be able to start this process and arrange appropriate follow-up

• Miss Kappel should be warned about the symptoms of hypoglycaemia and what action to take should this occur

• If Miss Kappel drives a car or motorbike she is required to inform the DVLA and her vehicle insurance company; she will still be able to continue to drive (although she may have to change her car insurance company as some will refuse to provide insurance in this situation). The DVLA will issue a licence that has to be renewed every three years. Discontinuation of driving is only required if Miss Kappel experiences frequent hypoglycaemic attacks or other complications (e.g. visual impairment, neuropathy) that may affect her ability to drive

Miss Kappel remains on intravenous insulin for 24 h at the end of which the acidosis has fully resolved and her appetite has returned. Miss Kappel is visited by the diabetes specialist nurse, who provides her with some background information about diabetes and suggests a subcutaneous insulin regimen, which is commenced before lunch on the day after admission. Miss Kappel is given instruction on self-administration of insulin and is observed giving herself two doses without difficulties.

After 24 h of intravenous cefuroxime the loin pain has resolved and there is no longer any renal angle tenderness or dysuria. Miss Kappel's temperature is normal. Urine culture reveals a fully sensitive Escherichia coli infection.

Miss Kappel is switched to an oral cephalosporin and advised to complete a one-week course.

Follow-up is arranged in the diabetes clinic in one week and the diabetes specialist nurse arranges to contact Miss Kappel by phone within the next two days.

Miss Kappel is advised of the requirement to contact the DVLA and vehicle insurance company to inform them of the diagnosis of diabetes.

CASE REVIEW

This case describes a 25-year-old woman who is brought to hospital exhibiting symptoms and signs consistent with diabetic ketoacidosis. Miss Maria Kappel is not known to have diabetes, but gives a recent history of polydipsia, polyuria and weight loss. Miss Kappel has started vomiting in the past 48 h and has become drowsy and confused on the day of admission.

Initial results demonstrate a severe metabolic acidosis with hyperglycaemia and hyperkalaemia. Urinalysis confirms ketonuria. Miss Kappel is started on intravenous normal saline and intravenous insulin with close monitoring of cardiac rhythm and conscious level. Over the next few hours there is gradual improvement in her conscious level and metabolic status with a reduction in the hyperglycaemia. Potassium falls, requiring supplementation.

When Miss Kappel's confusion resolves she gives a recent history of left loin pain and dysuria; she has a mild pyrexia and tenderness in the renal angle consistent with pyelonephritis. Laboratory results show elevation of white cell count and CRP, which is consistent with infection as the precipitating cause. She is started on intravenous cefuroxime, which is switched to an oral equivalent after 24 h.

After 24 h of intravenous insulin Miss Kappel's acidosis has resolved and she is able to eat; she is reviewed by the diabetes specialist team on the ward and starts a subcutaneous insulin regimen, which she is taught to self-administer before discharge from hospital.

Because Miss Kappel responded rapidly to treatment she was managed safely on the acute medical unit; however, very close observation is required in the early stages, and transfer to a high dependency unit or intensive care should always be considered for patients with severe acidosis (pH <7.1) or a reduced level of consciousness. Gradual improvement in the conscious level should be the aim, with normalisation of acidosis over 12 h and a fall in blood glucose of around 3–5 mmol/L each hour. Deterioration in the conscious level after initiation of therapy should raise concerns about the possibility of cerebral oedema. Although this is more common in children, it has also been described in adults, and is usually caused by excessively rapid fluid infusion over the first few hours. Older patients and patients with co-existent cardiac or renal disease (both common in patients with established diabetes) can run into problems with fluid overload, resulting in pulmonary oedema. In such cases, central venous monitoring may be necessary to avoid overhydration.

It should always be remembered that a new diagnosis of insulin-dependent diabetes is a major life event for a young patient. As in Miss Kappel's case, the patient has often been healthy until the diagnosis is made, and this can have major implications for their lifestyle. It is important not to bombard the patient and their family with large amounts of information too quickly, and to involve the diabetes specialist team at the earliest opportunity. Some patients will have significant concerns about self-injection and this issue may need to be introduced in a sensitive way.

KEY POINTS

- DKA is a serious complication of Type 1 diabetes, and can be the presenting symptom of this condition.
- An underlying precipitant for DKA should always be sought – urinary and respiratory infections are common triggers; for patients with pre-existing diabetes, omission of insulin is an important cause of DKA.
- Fluid replacement and intravenous insulin is the mainstay of treatment for DKA – most adults require around 6 L of fluid in the first 12–24 h.
- Close monitoring of conscious level, heart rhythm and fluid balance are essential – in some cases this will require transfer to a high dependency or intensive care unit.
- The acid–base balance should be monitored regularly using venous or arterial sampling, which will also enable measurement of potassium level.

- Potassium will need to be supplemented as the level falls after initiation of insulin therapy.
- Bicarbonate should only be used in cases of extreme acidosis (pH <6.8) and only following discussion with a senior physician or intensivist.
- Prior to discontinuation of intravenous insulin the patient should be able to eat normally and there should be resolution of the acidosis.
- The diabetes specialist team should be involved in the patient's care as soon as possible after admission, to start education of the patient and discuss future management.

Further reading

British Society for Paediatric Endocrinology and Diabetes. BSPED consensus statement for the management of DKA. www.bsped.org.uk/professional/guidelines/docs/BSPDD-KAApr04.pdf

Dunger DB, Sperling MA, Acerini CL *et al.* ESPE/LWPES consensus statement on diabetic ketoacidosis in children and adolescents. *Arch Dis Child* 2004; **89**: 188–94

Hammersley MS, Edge JA. The management of diabetic keto-acidosis. *Acute Med* 2007; **6**(1): 3–8

Savage MW, Kilvert A. ABCD guidelines for the management of hyperglycaemic emergencies in adults. *Pract Diabetes Int* 2006; **23**: 227–31

Sprigings D, Chambers JB. Diabetic ketoacidosis. In: *Acute medicine: a practical guide to the management of medical emergencies,* 4th edition. Blackwell Publishing, Oxford, 2008

A 73-year-old man with abnormal renal function

PART 2: CASES

You are called by a GP who has just received some blood results of one of her patients. Mr Da Costa is a 73-year-old man who had been to see his GP as he had been feeling tired and unwell for the past week with nausea and vomiting. The GP sent some blood for tests, including renal function (urea and electrolytes, U&E), and has just been called by the laboratory as the results are abnormal. She tells you that Mr Da Costa has creatinine of 540 and urea of 42, with potassium of 6.4. She would like Mr Da Costa admitted for investigation and further treatment.

What challenges will this patient present?

• Mr Da Costa's blood tests suggest acute renal failure (ARF)

• Although ARF may be suspected clinically (see Table 73), many of the symptoms are non-specific

• The diagnosis is often not considered until the results of blood tests are available. The organization of local laboratory services often means that results of abnormal tests are telephoned to GPs at the end of the day; this will often result in admission to hospital outside normal working hours

• Although patients with ARF often appear relatively well, the consequences can be significant, particularly if there is hyperkalaemia, which can result in life-threatening arrhythmias

• Early-warning scoring systems used in hospital (see p. 6) will often not trigger the need for urgent assessment of patients with ARF

• There are many causes of ARF, which is often a reflection of a serious underlying condition; it is crucial to consider the possible causes in the patient's initial work-up

Acute Medicine: Clinical Cases Uncovered. By C. Roseveare.
Published 2009 by Blackwell Publishing, ISBN: 978-1-4051-6883-0

Mr Da Costa walks into the admissions ward, accompanied by his wife. He looks slightly pale but otherwise appears well. Mr Da Costa's initial observations reveal a pulse rate of 80 beats/min, blood pressure 130/70, respiratory rate 14 breaths/min and oxygen saturation of 98% while breathing room air. Mr Da Costa is complaining of nausea but has no other specific symptoms. The nurse who undertook his initial assessment has triaged him as non-urgent. Mr Da Costa is placed in a bed towards the end of the ward and is not connected to a cardiac monitor.

While Mr Da Costa is awaiting medical review, his wife suddenly notes that he has become unresponsive, pale and clammy. She alerts the nurse caring for him, who is unable to find a pulse. Mrs Da Costa is connected to a cardiac monitor, which reveals a broad complex tachycardia (see Fig. 45).

The cardiac arrest team is called and Mr Da Costa receives a single 200 J DC shock, following which he reverts to sinus rhythm with a rate of 100 beats/min. His cardiac output returns with a blood pressure of 130/70. Mr Da Costa regains consciousness and is breathing spontaneously.

What immediate management is required?

Mr Da Costa has almost certainly experienced an episode of pulseless ventricular tachycardia. The likely cause of this, given the information supplied by the GP, is the hyperkalaemia identified on the blood tests taken earlier in the day.

The following actions are required.

• Confirm that Mr Da Costa's airway is secure and that oxygenation is adequate

• Obtain intravenous access

• Send further blood to the laboratory for confirmation of U&E (along with full blood count (FBC), liver function tests (LFT), calcium, C-reactive protein (CRP))

• Obtain an arterial blood gas sample for immediate analysis (this should give immediate confirmation of the potassium level)

• Obtain an ECG

Table 73 Symptoms and signs of acute renal failure

Symptoms

Fatigue

Loss of appetite

Nausea and vomiting

Confusion, agitation and coma

Thirst and dry mouth (if dehydrated)

Postural symptoms (if dehydrated)

Pruritus

Signs

Reduced or absent urine output

Jugular venous pressure raised (if fluid overloaded) or lowered (if dry)

Peripheral oedema (if fluid overloaded)

Signs of pulmonary oedema (if fluid overloaded)

Hypertension (if fluid overloaded)

Hypotension/postural BP drop (if dehydrated)

Tachycardia

Metabolic flap

Myoclonus

Pericardial/pleural rub

Table 74 ECG changes in hyperkalaemia

Small or absent P-waves

Prolongation of the PR interval

Widening of the QRS complex

Tall, triangular 'tented' T waves

Sine wave morphology

Complete heart block

• Move Mr Da Costa to an observable bed within the acute admissions ward and ensure that he is connected to a cardiac monitor

• Request an urgent portable chest radiograph – to look for evidence of fluid overload

Arterial blood gas analysis reveals the following results:
• *PaO_2 14.8 kPa, $PaCO_2$ 3.9 kPa, pH 7.31, HCO_3^- 19 mmol/L*
• *Na 130, K 7.1*
An ECG is performed and shows sinus rhythm with broad QRS complexes and prominent triangular T-waves in the anterior chest leads – see Fig. 46.
  Mr Da Costa is connected to a cardiac monitor, which reveals frequent ventricular ectopic beats.

How should these results be interpreted?

• The predominant abnormality is severe hyperkalaem-

ia. Mr Da Costa also has a mild, compensated metabolic acidosis and hyponatraemia

• The ECG changes are consistent with hyperkalaemia (see Table 74)

• Severe hyperkalaemia (>6.5 mmol/L or any elevation in the context of ECG abnormalities or recent arrhythmia) should be considered a life-threatening medical emergency

• In some cases hyperkalaemia should be interpreted with caution: haemolysis caused by trauma to red blood cells during phlebotomy, transit or due to delay in sample analysis, can result in a falsely high reading

• In this case Mr Da Costa has already experienced a severe arrhythmia and is continuing to experience frequent ectopic beats, with ECG evidence of hyperkalaemia; immediate action is therefore required to lower this level

How should the hyperkalaemia be treated?

A summary of the treatment of hyperkalaemia is given in Box 31; in this case the following immediate management should be instituted.

• Give 10 mL of 10% calcium gluconate by slow intravenous injection

• Administer 10 units of fast-acting insulin (e.g. Actrapid) along with 50 mL of 50% glucose by infusion over 20 min

• Prescribe 15 mL of calcium resonium orally four times daily

• Repeat the ECG and serum potassium after 30 min

• Continue to monitor Mr Da Costa closely and undertake hourly blood glucose readings for 4 h following administration of the insulin

• A continuous insulin/dextrose infusion may be necessary

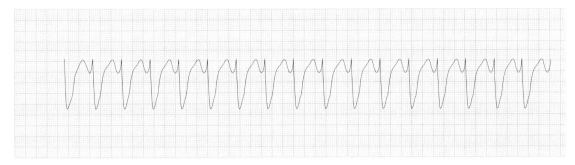

Figure 45 Rhythm strip showing regular broad complex tachycardia.

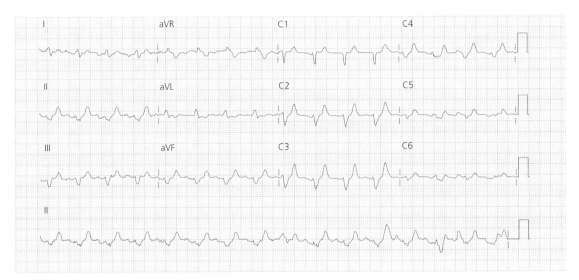

Figure 46 ECG following DC cardioversion. The patient is in sinus rhythm; P-waves are difficult to identify (most easily seen in lead II and on the rhythm strip), where the P–R interval is at the upper limit of normal (200 ms). The QRS complexes are broad (120 ms) with prominent, tall T-waves in leads V2–V4. These features are typical of hyperkalaemia.

Mr Da Costa is given the treatment listed above and reassessed 30 min later. He remains alert and orientated with a pulse of 100 beats/min and blood pressure 90/50. There are now only occasional ectopics on the monitor. No further serious arrhythmias have been observed. Mr Da Costa has vomited once since arrival on the ward.

Mr Da Costa feels cool peripherally and his mucous membranes appear dry. Capillary refill time is noted to be prolonged. He has not passed any urine since arrival in hospital. Jugular venous pressure is not elevated.

Mr Da Costa appears slightly breathless (respiratory rate 18 breaths/min) but his chest is clear on examination.

The repeat ECG shows normalisation of the QRS duration with less prominent T-waves (see Fig. 47).

A chest radiograph shows slight cardiomegaly but no evidence of pulmonary oedema.

Repeat arterial blood gas measurement is as follows:
- *pH 7.32, pCO$_2$ 3.56, pO$_2$ 14.3, HCO$_3$ 18.5*
- *Na 131, K 6.2*

What further emergency management is indicated?

- Mr Da Costa's potassium is falling and the improvement in his ECG appearance is reassuring, although he will require further treatment for the hyperkalaemia and continued cardiac monitoring
- The initial observations suggest that Mr Da Costa may be hypovolaemic, perhaps due to dehydration resulting from vomiting
- Fluid resuscitation is required, although this will need to be given with caution to prevent fluid overload. A

Box 31 Treatment of hyperkalaemias

The principles of treatment for hyperkalaemia can be summarised as follows.

1 Stop potassium accumulation
Any drips containing potassium or drugs which can elevate the serum K$^+$ should be stopped immediately
- ACE inhibitors, angiotensin II receptor blockers, direct renin inhibitors
- spironolactone, amiloride
- Heparin
- NSAIDs
- Beta-blockers, digoxin

This reduces further K$^+$ build-up and aids the effectiveness of K$^+$-displacing therapies

2 Protect the heart
If ECG changes are present, give 10 mL of 10% calcium gluconate by slow intravenous injection

This is cardioprotective, providing calcium ions, which prolong the plateau phase of the cardiac action potential and so prevent tachyarrhythmias. However, it only lasts for 20–30 min. If ECG changes continue or recur, multiple doses may be necessary (up to 50 mL).

Calcium in high concentrations is potentially toxic and this drug should always be given slowly via a central line, or large-bore peripheral cannula that flushes easily with no evidence of extravasation, to reduce the incidence of chemical tissue injury.

If the patient is on digoxin, rapid administration of calcium can precipitate toxicity.

3 Use insulin and beta-agonists to shift potassium into cells

Insulin promotes K$^+$ transport into cells, which can lower the serum K$^+$ by about 1 mmol/L for a few hours. Dextrose is given to prevent hypoglycaemia, and also stimulates the pancreas to produce its own insulin. Blood sugar level needs to be tested hourly for 4–6 h after the infusion.

Sympathetic stimulation also drives K$^+$ from the serum to the intracellular space. High-dose nebulisers are as effective as i.v. salbutamol and easier to administer. The effect lasts up to 2 h and may be super-additive with that of insulin.

4 Remove K$^+$ from the body

Calcium resonium is an exchange resin that leaches K$^+$ ions from the gut in exchange for Ca^{2+}. It can cause constipation and so needs to be given with laxatives such as lactulose 10 mL bd to ensure good gut transit. It takes several hours to show an effect, so repeat courses of the measures in step 3 may be necessary.

If the patient is unable to take oral calcium resonium it can be given as a 30 g enema. This needs to be retained in the rectum for 6–9 h then washed out, i.e. with a phosphate enema, and the process repeated.

Measures to reverse the acute renal failure (where this is the cause of hyperkalaemia) may result in a rapid return of urine output and enable the kidneys to excrete the excess potassium in the urine.

If, despite treatment, potassium continues to rise or there are persisting ECG changes then acute haemodialysis or haemofiltration may be required. Contact your local specialist renal or intensive care service.

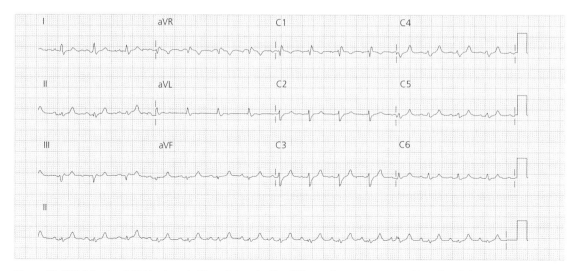

Figure 47 ECG following initial treatment of hyperkalaemia. The QRS complexes are narrower (80 ms) and the T-waves are less prominent.

250–500 mL bolus of normal saline should be administered initially, over 30–60 min
• Insertion of a central venous cannula should be considered to enable accurate titration of fluid infusion volumes; if there is evidence of fluid overload or pulmonary oedema, urgent referral to the critical care team will be required
• Administration of an antiemetic should be considered if Mr Da Costa continues to vomit
• Insertion of a urinary catheter should be undertaken to enable monitoring of urine output and exclusion of urinary retention as a cause of renal failure (see later)
• Mr Da Costa's acidosis does not require specific action at present (see Box 32)

Mr Da Costa is commenced on an intravenous glucose/insulin sliding scale and given 500 mL of normal saline over 30 min. Following this Mr Da Costa's blood pressure improves to 110/70 with no evidence of fluid overload. A urinary catheter is inserted and drains 100 mL of concentrated urine. Your specialist registrar reviews the patient and decides not to insert a central venous cannula at present, as Mr Da Costa is apparently responding to initial treatment.

Mr Da Costa is prescribed cyclizine 50 mg tds i.v.

What further management is required?
• Mr Da Costa's condition has now been stabilized with improvement in his potassium level and circulatory status
• It is now important to consider the underlying cause of Mr Da Costa's renal dysfunction, which will require a detailed history and examination
• While taking the history the clinician should consider the many causes of renal impairment (see Table 75), bearing in mind that there may be more than one contributory factor

• In considering the possible cause, it is also important to determine whether Mr Da Costa has any underlying/previous chronic renal impairment
• It will also be necessary to review the results of the recent laboratory blood tests and compare these to any old results that may be available

Mr Da Costa gives a past history of tablet-controlled diabetes and hypertension, but was relatively well until four days earlier when he developed diarrhoea and vomiting. Mr Da Costa's wife had been unwell with a similar illness the previous day. He had profuse watery diarrhoea for 48 h associated with vomiting, during which time he had only been able to take small quantities of fluid orally; following this Mr Da Costa had felt persistently nauseated with intermittent vomiting. He had been passing small quantities of urine until yesterday, but had not passed any urine for 24 h.

Over the past year Mr Da Costa has noticed that he has been requiring to pass urine more frequently, and that the stream had been narrower; there has also been difficulty initiating the urine flow and some dribbling after micturition. Mr Da Costa needs to get up at least twice each night to pass urine. His GP has referred him to a urologist but he is awaiting an appointment.

Current medication comprises aspirin 75 mg daily, simvastatin 40 mg daily, ramipril 5 mg daily, gliclazide 80 mg daily, bisoprolol 2.5 mg daily. None of these drugs has been started recently. Mr Da Costa has not taken any over-the-counter medications.

A full clinical examination reveals no other cardiovascular or respiratory abnormality. His jugular venous pressure is not elevated following 1 L of fluid and there are no basal crackles on respiratory examination. A rectal examination reveals an enlarged, smooth prostate.

Box 32 Management of acidosis in acute renal failure

Metabolic acidosis is common in patients with acute renal failure
Acidosis impairs myocardial contractility, affects tissue oxygen delivery, and can affect the central nervous system function in addition to a range of deleterious metabolic effects.

However, rapid correction of acidosis with intravenous sodium bicarbonate can cause a worsening of intracellular acidosis and tissue oxygenation; unless the acidosis is severe, it is best to allow the acidosis to correct by:

• compensation by the respiratory system, with hyperventilation blowing off CO_2
• restoration of renal function as quickly as possible by identifying and treating the cause of renal failure
If there is severe or intractable acidosis, haemodialysis or filtration on a specialist renal or intensive care unit will be required.

Location	Process	Examples
Pre-renal	Low blood pressure 　　Hypovolaemia	Shock, sepsis, dehydration
	Low renal blood flow 　　Renovascular disease 　　Renal vasoconstriction	Renal artery stenosis, renal infarction Hepatorenal syndrome
	Low renal oxygenation 　　Hypoxaemia	Respiratory disease, anaemia
Renal	Impaired autoregulation Nephrotoxicity	ACE-is, A2RBs, DRIs, NSAIDs
	Drugs	Aminoglycosides, contrast media
	Myoglobin	Rhabdomyolysis
	Urate	Tumour lysis syndrome
	Allergic inflammation	
	Acute interstitial nephritis	Drugs, particularly penicillins
	Glomerulopathy	IgA disease, nephrotic syndromes
	Primary	
	With systemic vasculitis	Wegener's, microscopic polyangiitis
	With systemic illness	Endocarditis, hepatitis C
	Anti-GBM disease	Goodpasture's syndrome
	Infection	
	Local/systemic sepsis	Urinary tract infection, pneumonia
	Renal infections	Legionella, tuberculosis, hantavirus
	Infiltration	Sarcoid, amyloid, lymphoma
Post-renal	Urethral obstruction	
	Intraurethral	Urethral stricture, blocked catheter
	At bladder outflow	Prostatic hypertrophy, bladder stone
	Ureteric obstruction	
	Bilateral intraureteric	Stones, tumours, papillary necrosis
	Unilateral intraureteric	As above if single functioning kidney
	Retroperitoneal	Retroperitoneal fibrosis, tumours
	Tubular obstruction	
	Cast nephropathy	Myeloma, rhabdomyolysis

Table 75 Causes of acute renal failure: these are often classified as 'pre-renal', 'renal' and 'post-renal'

ACE-is, angiotensin-converting enzyme inhibitors; A2RBs, angiotensin 2 receptor blockers, DRIs, direct renin inhibitors; NSAIDs, non-steroidal anti-inflammatory drugs; GBM, glomerular basement membrane.

How should the clinical features be interpreted?

• Mr Da Costa's recent diarrhoeal illness and poor fluid intake may suggest dehydration as a contributory factor

• Mr Da Costa's underlying diabetes and hypertension may have resulted in a degree of underlying renal vascular disease

• The history of poor urine flow, frequency of micturition, hesitancy and terminal dribble are suggestive of chronic urinary obstruction; however, the small residual urine volume does not suggest acute urinary retention as the cause for his renal failure

This patient's blood test results are given below:

	On arrival*	At GP this morning	6 months ago
Sodium	141 mmol/L	139 mmol/L	144 mmol/L
Potassium	7.1 mmol/L	6.4 mmol/L	4.4 mmol/L
Urea	47.3 mmol/L	41.9 mmol/L	7.2 mmol/L
Creatinine	593 μmol/L	540 μmol/L	114 μmol/L
eGFR	9 mL/min	10 mL/min	58 mL/min

*Blood was sent to the laboratory prior to treatment of hyperkalaemia.

How should the renal function tests be interpreted?

A guide to interpretation of renal function test results is given in Box 33.

Box 33 Interpretation of renal function tests

Creatinine is used as a surrogate marker for glomerular filtration rate (GFR). As creatinine is produced by muscle cells a 'normal' level varies with body composition: a tall, muscular male will have a higher creatinine than a small, frail, old woman. The normal GFR declines with age. In young adults, GFR would be expected to be around 120 mL/min, and a fall to as little as 60 mL/min in old age is still considered within the normal range.

Creatinine has a reciprocal relationship with GFR, such that small changes in creatinine occur with large changes in GFR at near-normal levels, whereas in near-endstage kidney disease large changes in creatinine may only represent small changes in GFR. This means that a creatinine only just outside the normal range (e.g. 100 µmol/L) may represent a significant drop in GFR (e.g. by >30%).

eGFR is an estimation of the glomerular filtration rate calculated using the serum creatinine and demographic data such as the patient's age, sex, and race. The formula to perform this calculation is based on patients with chronic kidney disease, and assumes that the serum creatinine is in a steady state. In acute renal failure the serum creatinine may be rapidly changing, and this invalidates the eGFR calculation. eGFR alone is therefore a poor guide as to actual renal function in the acute setting; however, rate of change of creatinine can give a guide as to whether renal function is improving or worsening.

Urea is a waste product produced by nitrogen metabolism, e.g. of protein digestion and turnover. Absolute urea levels correlate poorly with clinical state. However, urea can be a helpful guide as to the *cause* of renal impairment. Usually, the serum urea level in mmol/L is less than one-tenth of the serum creatinine level in µmol/L. If the kidney is underperfused, however, there will be excess urea reabsorption as the tubule tries to conserve salt and water. Creatinine is not reabsorbed, however, and will still be lost in the urine. The serum urea will therefore rise disproportionately. A urea–creatinine ratio of greater than 1:10 may therefore indicate a pre-renal element to the renal failure.

Comparison between current and old blood tests can help decide whether this entire episode is acute, or if there is a background of some renal impairment with an additional process causing a recent change (acute-on-chronic renal failure).

- The blood tests from six months ago show a degree of mild chronic kidney disease with an estimated glomerular filtration rate (eGFR) just below the acceptable range. The current results therefore reflect *acute-on-chronic* renal failure
- The aim of treatment should be to return renal function to as near to the patient's baseline as possible, in this case to get back to a creatinine of around 114 µmol/L
- Although the urea is undoubtedly high, the urea–creatinine ratio is still below 1:10, suggesting that this is not *solely* a pre-renal problem resulting from dehydration and hypovolaemia

Does Mr Da Costa require dialysis or other renal supportive therapy?

Indications for haemodialysis or haemofiltration are given in Box 34.

Mr Da Costa appears to be responding to therapy and further renal support is therefore not required at this time.

What other investigations/management may be helpful?

- **Urine dipstick analysis**: failure of the glomerular filter to retain plasma proteins and blood cells causes leakage of protein and blood in the urine, which may be detected on dipstick testing. The absence of haematuria or proteinuria makes intrinsic renal disease very unlikely (<3%)
- **Laboratory urine analysis**: dipstick testing is only *semi-quantitative* and sensitive but not specific for renal disease. There can be other sources of blood or protein loss from the lower urinary tract, such as with infection or catheterisation. Laboratory testing to quantify the protein output more accurately, with a urinary protein–creatine ratio, and microscopy to look at red cell morphology or the presence of casts, can give additional guidance
- **Renal tract ultrasound**: this will enable exclusion of hydronephrosis resulting from post-renal obstruction; this may require the insertion of a nephrostomy tube. Ultrasound should always be undertaken where obstruction is considered as a possible cause or if the urine flow does not start following catheterisation. Assessment of the size of the kidneys will also give useful information: if the kidneys appear small, this implies an element of *chronic* renal failure
- **Discontinuation of any nephrotoxic drugs** or drugs that may exacerbate dehydration or reduce renal perfusion (e.g. diuretics, angiotensin-converting enzyme (ACE) inhibitors, antihypertensives, non-steroidal anti-inflammatory drugs, etc.); many drugs are excreted by the kidneys and can therefore accumulate in the blood in

---

> **Box 34 Indications for haemodialysis/ haemfltration**
>
> In cases where failure of excretion results in accumulation of fluid, electrolytes, drugs or acid which does not respond to medical therapy, additional renal support may be required. There are no absolute indications for haemodialysis or haemofiltration, but the following may be used as a guide.
> - Severe fluid overload refractory to treatment (e.g. pulmonary oedema causing cardiorespiratory compromise)
> - Hyperkalaemia not settling with medical therapy
> - Refractory acidosis (e.g. pH <7.1 and not improving)
> - Symptomatic uraemia (usually when urea >50)
> - Pericardial rub or effusion
> - Change in mental status or coma
> - Severe renal failure which is likely to progress to any of the above

the presence of renal failure. Refer to the British National Formulary to determine if the dose of any drugs taken by the patient should be reduced or the drug level checked
- **Involvement of a specialist nephrologist**: if your hospital has one, their advice should be sought at the earliest opportunity; ongoing management can be complex and it may be necessary to consider formal renal support if the patient's condition does not improve. A nephrologist may also be able to advise on further blood tests and the need for renal biopsy in some cases

Mr Da Costa's medication is all withheld apart from aspirin 75 mg daily. Mr Da Costa is given a further 1000 mL of fluid over 4 h and continues with the insulin sliding scale. Mr Da Costa's urine output over the next 4 h is 30 mL/h and his blood pressure rises to 130/70.

Repeat arterial blood gas testing is as follows:
- *pH 7.39, pCO_2 4.1, pO_2 13.7, HCO_3 20.4*
- *Na 133, K 5.9*
- *dipstick testing of the catheter specimen shows blood ++, protein +++. the sample is sent for culture and protein–creatinine ratio*

Further blood results are as follows:
- *Hb 101, white cell count 14.5 (neutrophils 10.5), platelets 195*
- *C-reactive protein 65*

The suggested diagnosis is acute renal failure secondary to dehydration on a background of pre-existing chronic renal impairment related to hypertension, diabetes and obstructive uropathy.

Over the next 24 h Mr Da Costa's urine output increases from 30 mL/h to 140 mL/h. He is referred to the nephrology consultant, who agrees to take over his care during his hospital stay. Mr Da Costa spends a further week on the ward, during which his urea and creatinine gradually fall and his serum potassium level normalises. His antihypertensive medication is restarted and he is converted back from insulin to his oral gliclazide. While on the ward Mr Da Costa is reviewed by the urology team, who arrange for outpatient assessment and treatment of his prostatic enlargement.

CASE REVIEW

This case describes a 73-year-old man, referred to hospital after blood results indicate acute renal failure with hyperkalaemia. The GP had checked Mr Da Costa's renal function after he presented with malaise, nausea and vomiting after a recent diarrhoeal illness. Although Mr Da Costa appears well on arrival, his condition suddenly deteriorates shortly after admission with an episode of pulseless ventricular tachycardia, which is treated promptly with DC cardioversion. Mr Da Costa's severe hyperkalaemia is confirmed on blood analysis and he is also noted to have ECG features consistent with this. Mr Da Costa is treated with calcium gluconate, intravenous insulin and glucose infusion, which results in an improvement in his potassium level and stabilisation of his cardiac rhythm.

Further blood testing confirms the acute renal failure,

and comparison with previous results is suggestive of some pre-existing chronic renal impairment. A careful history reveals that Mr Da Costa has tablet-controlled diabetes and hypertension along with symptoms suggestive of chronic urinary outflow obstruction prior to the onset of the diarrhoea and sickness earlier that week. During the acute illness, Mr Da Costa's fluid intake had been very poor and he had felt persistently nauseous since. He had been anuric for the past 24 h.

Mr Da Costa appears clinically dehydrated and is therefore treated with intravenous fluid; antihypertensive therapy is withheld and his insulin is continued to provide diabetic control as well as maintenance of the potassium level. His urine output gradually improves over the next 24 h.

KEY POINTS

- Renal failure may be asymptomatic and present as an isolated finding on blood testing.
- Symptoms and signs are often non-specific but can give clues as to whether the patient is intravascularly over- or underfilled.
- Hyperkalaemia with ECG changes is a medical emergency requiring immediate treatment.
- Severe hyperkalaemia, acidosis, uraemia or fluid overload

that is unresponsive to treatment is an indication for dialysis/filtration.
- Hypoperfusion and nephrotoxic drugs often complicate renal failure of any cause.
- Initial management should be directed at resuscitative care (ABCs), renal ultrasound scan and urine dip, and treatment for any co-existent medical problem such as sepsis.

Further reading

Firth JD. The clinical approach to the patient with acute renal failure. In: Winnearls C, Cameron JS *et al* (eds). *Oxford textbook of clinical nephrology*, 3rd edition. Oxford University Press, Oxford, 2005

Hilton R. Acute renal failure. *BMJ* 2006; **333**: 786–90

Sprigings D, Chambers JB. Potassium disorders. In: *Acute medicine: a practical guide to the management of medical emergencies*, 4th edition. Blackwell Publishing, Oxford, 2008

Case 20 A 55-year-old man with pyrexia of unknown origin

You are contacted by a GP who is concerned about a 55-year-old man whom he has seen several times over the past few weeks complaining of fever and malaise. Last week he arranged for Mr Paul Biggins to have a chest radiograph and some blood tests. The radiograph was reported as normal, but the blood tests revealed a raised erythrocyte sedimentation rate (ESR) of 115 and C-reactive protein (CRP) of 198, along with a mild normocytic anaemia. The GP had initially planned to refer Mr Biggins to the outpatient clinic for further investigation. However, today Mr Biggins requested a home visit because he felt worse. The GP found Mr Biggins to have a pyrexia of 38°C but no obvious focus of infection. Given Mr Biggins' apparent deterioration he feels that the patient now justifies hospital admission for further investigation and treatment.

What challenges will this patient present?

• The patient with a persisting fever with no cause identified despite initial investigations is often described as having a pyrexia of unknown origin or PUO
• The differential diagnosis of PUO is broad, and extensive investigation fails to identify a cause in a significant proportion of patients (see Table 76)
• Most diagnostic information will come from the history – it will be necessary to take this in meticulous detail, including many direct questions that clinicians would not normally ask
• Try to formulate a differential diagnosis while taking the history, and target clinical examination and investigation specifically to test out your suspicions
• Many of the investigations required can be difficult to obtain quickly on an outpatient basis; a prolonged inpatient stay may be required, particularly if the patient's condition is deteriorating

Acute Medicine: Clinical Cases Uncovered. By C. Roseveare.
Published 2009 by Blackwell Publishing, ISBN: 978-1-4051-6883-0

Mr Biggins is brought to hospital by his partner and manages to walk into the admissions ward with her assistance, although Mr Biggins is clearly uncomfortable and weak. Initial observations reveal a regular pulse of 100 beats/min, with blood pressure 130/70. Mr Biggins appears slightly breathless with a respiratory rate of 14 breaths/min, although oxygen saturation reads 99% on room air. His temperature is 37.5°C.

What immediate management is required?

• Mr Biggins' airway is not threatened and breathing and circulation are stable at present
• Although there will probably be other patients who are being admitted who require more urgent attention, it is important not to leave Mr Biggins' assessment until too late in the day, as some of the required investigations may be easier to obtain during normal working hours
• Further assessment will require a detailed history and thorough examination to determine the likely cause of his symptoms
• When taking the history it is important to consider the broad differential diagnosis in this situation (see Table 75)

Mr Biggins says he has been unwell for approximately four weeks. Initially he noticed generalised aching and tiredness and thought he was suffering from a viral infection. Mr Biggins had mild shortness of breath and a slight cough, but this was non-productive and seemed to settle. Subsequently he felt hot and recorded his own temperature at 38.3°C.

Over the past four weeks the symptoms of muscle aching and lethargy have fluctuated but Mr Biggins has never felt 'right'. His temperature has risen most evenings, usually to around 38°C. Mr Biggins' shoulders and hips have been particularly painful and stiff, but he had not noticed any specific joint swelling or redness. Mr Biggins' appetite has been reduced and he thinks he has lost around 1 stone (approximately 6 kg) in weight.

Table 76 Classification of causes of pyrexia of unknown origin (PUO)

Cause	Symptoms	Signs	Comments
Infective	See Table 77	See Table 77	
Rheumatological conditions/ connective tissue diseases (systemic lupus erythematosus, Sjögrens syndrome, rheumatoid arthritis, adult Still's disease)	Joint pains/swelling Raynaud's phenomenon Dry mouth/eyes ('sicca' syndrome) Skin rashes	Skin rash Joint swelling/effusion/deformity Muscle tenderness in polymyositis	Adult Still's disease is a diagnosis of exclusion in patients with PUO
Vasculitis e.g. polymyalgia rheumatica (PMR), temporal arteritis (TA), polyarteritis nodosa (PAN)	Shoulder girdle/hip girdle pain in PMR Headache/jaw claudication in TA Skin rashes in other vasculitides	Temporal artery tenderness in TA Purpuric rash Microscopic haematuria in PAN	May be difficult to diagnose without biopsy of inflamed vessel (e.g. temporal artery or renal biopsy)
Haematological malignancy	Often non-specific Drenching night sweats in lymphoma Bone pain/fractures in myeloma	Pallor Lymph node/splenic enlargement	Patients with haematological malignancy also more prone to infection resulting in fever
Solid organ malignancy	Usually age >40 Prolonged weight/appetite loss Symptoms related to site of malignancy (e.g. change of bowel habit, cough, haematuria, pain, etc.)	Cachexia Mass, organomegaly or lymph node enlargement Remember breast examination for women and testicular/ prostate examination for men	Any solid organ malignancy may result in PUO

Mr Biggins saw his GP after one week, who confirmed his self-diagnosis of a viral infection and advised him to return if his symptoms failed to settle. Last week he re-presented to the GP, who arranged some investigations.

Over the past three days the symptoms have become much more noticeable; Mr Biggins' fever has persisted and has risen to 39°C at times with drenching sweats at night; the muscular aching now makes it difficult for him to get out of bed. Mr Biggins also feels more short of breath. He has eaten very little for the last two days but has continued to take fluid. Mr Biggins is passing urine but his bowels have not been open for the past 48 h.

What other specific information should be sought in the history?

• Because infection is one of the most common causes of PUO, Mr Biggins should be asked specifically if there

have been any symptoms to suggest infection pertaining to any body area (see Table 77)

• Possibility of exposure to, or symptoms of, sexually transmitted disease should be considered

• A careful dental history should be taken – dental sepsis is a possibility and dental treatment may precipitate infective endocarditis

• Ask specifically about prior history of or exposure to tuberculosis in the past. Enquire about previous surgery involving the insertion of a prosthesis (e.g. heart valves or metal plates in bones) – these are potential sources of occult infection

• A history of intravenous recreational drug abuse should be sought: infection may occur at injection sites and i.v. drug use may predispose to HIV and infective endocarditis

• A recent travel history should be sought, including the possibility of travel to any malaria-endemic area

Table 77 Symptoms/signs suggestive of infection related to body systems

System	Symptoms	Signs
Upper respiratory tract	Sore throat, dry cough	Enlarged, inflamed tonsils Inflamed tympanic membranes
Lower respiratory tract	Productive cough Breathlessness Pleuritic chest pain	Signs of pulmonary consolidation (crepitations, bronchial breathing) Signs of pleural effusion (dullness, reduced breath sounds)
Alimentary system	Diarrhoea, abdominal pain, vomiting	Abdominal tenderness
Cardiovascular system	Pericarditic pain (sharp pain worsened by inspiration, lying flat and leaning forward) Breathlessness/orthopnoea	Pericardial rub in pericarditis Murmur in endocarditis Stigmata of infective endocarditis (see below) Bibasal crackles of pulmonary oedema
Central nervous system	Headache Neck stiffness Photophobia Confusion/drowsiness	Altered conscious level Neck stiffness Positive Kernig's sign
Musculoskeletal system	Pain over area of bony prosthesis Painful, swollen joint (usually single joint)	Hot, swollen, tender joint Evidence of joint effusion Tenderness, erythema or swelling over prosthesis
Urogenital system	Penile/vaginal discharge Pain/irritation around testicular/vaginal area Dysuria Urinary frequency Renal angle pain	Renal angle/groin/suprapubic tenderness Erythema/tenderness over penis/scrotal area Prostatic tenderness on rectal examination Cervical tenderness on vaginal examination
Dental system	Recent trips to dentist Toothache	Tenderness over jaw or gums Inflamed/swollen gums

- Risk factors for immunosuppression should be considered, including recent immune suppressant drugs (e.g. cancer chemotherapy) or possible HIV infection
- Given the possibility of underlying malignancy, a history of prior weight loss, change of bowel habit, prostatic symptoms (for men) or breast lumps (for women) should be sought
- Ask about symptoms of Raynaud's phenomenon (white or blue discolouration of hands in cold weather), dry mouth/eyes (sicca syndrome) or skin rashes that may suggest a connective tissue disease such as systemic lupus erythematosus or scleroderma

Detailed systematic review reveals no other symptoms pertaining to the urinary or gastrointestinal systems. Mr Biggins has not had a prior sexually transmitted disease and no history of penile discharge. He broke his right femur as a teenager and a metal plate was inserted; this area has been aching recently, but no more so than other areas of the body.

One month prior to the onset of symptoms Mr Biggins underwent a dental extraction and root canal work; he has seen his dentist since then, who was happy with his progress with no cause for concern. Mr Biggins has not had any dental pain since this time.

He travelled to Africa two months prior to the onset of symptoms, during which he took malaria prophylaxis. Mr Biggins has also made two trips to Thailand during the past year; he had an unprotected sexual encounter during one of his trips to Thailand, but tested negative for HIV on his return. Mr Biggins is heterosexual, and in a stable relationship for the past six months. There is no history of intravenous drug abuse and no previous tuberculosis.

There are no symptoms of prostatism, and prior to the onset of symptoms Mr Biggins' weight was stable with no change of bowel habit or rectal bleeding. His father died from colonic carcinoma at the age of 60.

There is no history of Raynaud's phenomenon and no skin rashes or arthritis.

Mr Biggins smokes 20 cigarettes per day. He works as a freelance journalist and consumes around 30 units alcohol per week. Hobbies include coarse fishing and gardening. Mr Biggins is not taking any medication and has no known allergies.

What is the differential diagnosis following the history?

• Respiratory infection (possibly with an unusual organism) given the initial cough and recent shortness of breath
• Malaria: despite taking prophylaxis the onset of symptoms in relation to his travel to Africa requires this to be excluded
• Infective endocarditis: given the dental treatment prior to onset of symptoms
• Dental infection (despite the reassurances of his dentist)
• Weil's disease (leptospirosis) – Mr Biggins' fishing has probably exposed him to rats, which are the main vectors of this infection
• HIV-related illness: a single HIV test undertaken after his unprotected sexual encounter does not exclude HIV as seroconversion may not have occurred
• Prosthetic infection of the bone plate in Mr Biggins' right femur
• Vasculitis – e.g. polymyalgia rheumatica, given the history of shoulder and hip girdle pain
• Lung or bowel malignancy (given the smoking and family history)
• Haematological malignancy, given the drenching night sweats

What specific areas should be considered during physical examination?

Careful consideration should be given to each of the possible differentials during examination, including:
• A search for peripheral stigmata of infective endocarditis (see Table 78)
• Thorough examination of all lymph node areas and spleen
• Evidence of bony tenderness over his prosthesis
In addition do not forget:

Table 78 Peripheral stigmata of endocarditis

Petechial haemorrhages: found on limbs, trunk and mucous membranes

Splinter haemorrhages: may be seen in fingers and toes; also caused by trauma/excessive manicure, etc.

Roth spots: haemorrhages on fundi, often with central pale area

Osler's nodes: hard, tender erythematous nodules in pulps of fingers and toes and over thenar/hypothenar eminences of hands

Janeway lesions: transient, non-tender erythematous areas on palms and soles of feet – rarely seen in practice

Finger clubbing: although often described as a feature of endocarditis, in reality this is only a feature of chronic, untreated disease so rarely seen in the acute setting

Splenomegaly: common but may be quite subtle; often more prominent in patients with chronic endocarditis, but variable

Haematuria/proteinuria: a common finding; usually due to renal infarction or mild glomerulonephritis

• Examination of the tympanic membranes and throat, and palpation for sinus tenderness
• Examination of the external genitalia
• A rectal examination, with palpation of prostate for tenderness (prostatitis) or irregularity (malignancy) and rectal masses
• Breast examination for lumps (more relevant in women)
• Examination of all joints for evidence of erythema, swelling, effusion or tenderness

On examination Mr Biggins remains pyrexial (37.5°C). His ears and throat are normal. There is mild tenderness over the frontal sinus.

There are several splinter haemorrhages in his finger nails but no other peripheral stigmata of infective endocarditis.

There is no finger clubbing or lymphadenopathy.

Cardiovascular examination reveals a regular tachycardia of 100 beats/min and blood pressure 130/70. Heart sounds are normal with a soft pansystolic murmur audible over the apex and radiating to the axilla. His jugular venous pressure is not visible.

There are inspiratory crackles at the bases of both lungs, which fail to clear with coughing.

An abdominal examination is unremarkable, including a rectal examination and examination of external genitalia. The liver and spleen are not enlarged and there are no renal masses.

There is mild tenderness of the major muscle groups and Mr Biggins' shoulders and knees are painful on movement, but there is no joint swelling, erythema or effusion.

No skin rashes are noted.

Bedside urinalysis reveals 2+ blood and 1+ protein but no leucocytes or nitrites.

How has the differential been refined by examination?

• The combination of splinter haemorrhages and a systolic murmur increase the likelihood of infective endocarditis; remember that splinter haemorrhages can also follow nail trauma (Mr Biggins is a keen gardener) and asymptomatic mitral regurgitation is not uncommon in healthy individuals
• The bibasal crackles on the chest examination may reflect respiratory infection; alternatively, this appearance could reflect a fibrotic process (e.g. associated with connective tissues disease) or pulmonary oedema
• The absence of lymph node enlargement does not exclude haematological malignancy
• The lack of leucocytes and nitrites on urinalysis makes urine infection less likely; microscopic haematuria is a non-specific finding, but can be a sign of renal tract malignancy and is also commonly found in patients with infective endocarditis

What further investigations are required?

Suggested blood tests for the initial investigation of patients presenting with PUO are listed in Table 79.

Remember to review all the tests sent off by the GP before repeating these; although it will usually be helpful to repeat inflammatory markers, full blood count renal and liver function, some of the more complex immunological tests (e.g. immunoglobulins, autoimmune markers) are expensive and unlikely to change over a short space of time. If the GP has already checked these and found them to be normal, repeating them may be unnecessary.

In addition the following tests should be undertaken.
• **Chest radiograph**: although this has been undertaken recently by the GP and was reported as normal, Mr Biggins has become more unwell since and now has symptoms and signs in the chest

• **Dental radiograph**: to look for evidence of bony infection from a dental abscess (may require review by maxillofacial surgeon or hospital-based dentist)
• **Transthoracic echocardiogram (TTE)**: the systolic murmur has raised the possibility of infective endocarditis as a cause; although TTE is not a sensitive test for the diagnosis of infective endocarditis, the finding of 'vegetations' on the mitral valve would support this and indicate the need for further tests
• **Abdominal ultrasound**: although Mr Biggins does not have specific symptoms related to the abdomen, ultrasound is non-invasive and does not require X-ray exposure. The finding of a solid organ mass (e.g. renal cell carcinoma, liver metastasis, etc.) would help to direct further investigations. Collections of pus in the subphrenic or pelvic areas may also be identified by ultrasound
• **ECG**: may show signs of pericarditis in association with infection, or co-existent myocardial ischaemia; conduction abnormalities may be associated with infective endocarditis

Investigation results are as follows:
• *haemoglobin 98, white cell count 19.5 (neutrophils 14.8), platelets 197*
• *ESR 110, CRP 277*
• *Na 137, K 4.6, urea 2.9, creatinine 80*
• *albumin 30, total protein 96, bilirubin 22, alanine transaminase 35, alkaline phosphatase (ALP) 490*
• *prostate-specific antigen normal*
• *malarial film negative (no parasites seen)*
• *immunoglobulins: raised IgG with polyclonal alpha-2 region consistent with acute phase response; no monoclonal bands*
• *autoimmune profile: all negative*
• *HIV test: negative*
• *viral serology: Epstein Barr virus IgG positive (consistent with previous infection); all others negative.*
• *Chest radiograph: upper lobe venous diversion consistent with mild pulmonary oedema; no evidence of infection*
• *ECG: sinus tachycardia; no other abnormality*
• *abdominal ultrasound: mild splenomegaly (12 cm); no other abnormalities; normal liver and biliary tree*
• *transthoracic echocardiogram: mild left ventricular dilatation with mild systolic dysfunction. Moderate mitral regurgitation; possible vegetation on anterior leaflet of mitral valve*
• *Three sets of blood cultures have been sent and results are awaited (usually take approx 48 h)*

Table 79 Initial blood tests for patients with pyrexia of unknown origin

Test	Justification	Comments
Full blood count	Raised white cell count (WCC) in infection Low WCC may suggest haematological malignancy or risk of unusual infection Microcytic anaemia in gastrointestinal malignancy Raised platelets in haematological malignancy or acute inflammatory disease	Remember that raised neutrophil count is not a specific feature of infection and can be found in many inflammatory conditions
Urea and electrolytes	Renal impairment in vasculitis, connective tissue disease	Patients with chronic renal failure may be more prone to infection
Liver function tests (LFT)	Raised transaminases/alkaline phosphatase (ALP) bilirubin in biliary sepsis Abnormal LFT in malignant infiltration Low albumin suggestive of severe/chronic sepsis/inflammation	ALP is often raised in context of inflammation of any cause – does not necessarily imply liver disease
C-reactive protein	Elevated in acute inflammatory/infective conditions	Often higher in context of bacterial than viral infection; very non-specific – raised level will not identify cause of inflammation
Erythrocyte sedimentation rate	Elevated in infective/inflammatory conditions	Non-specific, but values >100 are suggestive of haematological malignancy, vasculitis or chronic suppurative infection
Autoimmune profile	Positive anti-nuclear antibody (ANA) in most connective tissue diseases (including systemic lupus erythematosus) Positive rheumatoid factor in rheumatoid arthritis Anti-neutrophil cytoplasmic antibody (ANCA) in patients with polyarteritis nodosa and Wegener's granulomatosis	Ensure not recently measured before requesting – these are expensive tests
Immunoglobulins	Monoclonal bands in patients with myeloma Polyclonal raised IgG in patients with any inflammatory condition	Also send urine for Bence Jones protein in patients with suspected myeloma
Prostate-specific antigen (in men)	Usually elevated in prostate cancer especially metastatic disease	Normal level does not exclude prostate cancer; may also be elevated in patients with prostatitis
Blood culture	May reveal bacteraemia as the cause for fever	At least three sets of cultures for patients with suspected endocarditis

PART 2: CASES

What do the investigation results suggest?

• The raised white cell (neutrophil) count, high ESR and CRP and polyclonal IgG rise all support a diagnosis of significant bacterial infection; ALP can be an 'acute phase' protein (similar to CRP) and albumin frequently falls in association with severe infection

• The chest radiograph finding of pulmonary oedema

rather than pulmonary consolidation or fibrosis as a cause for the crackles suggests a cardiac rather than a respiratory cause for Mr Biggins' breathlessness
• The finding of a possible vegetation on the mitral valve supports the clinical suspicion of infective endocarditis; this may also account for the mild splenomegaly

Table 80 Duke criteria for diagnosis of infective endocarditis (IE)

Pathological criteria

Micro-organisms demonstrated by culture or histology

Pathological lesions – histological confirmation of vegetations or abscesses

Clinical criteria (see below)

Two major criteria, or

One major and three minor criteria, or

Five minor criteria

Major criteria

Positive blood culture – at least two separate blood cultures drawn 12 h apart, or all of three blood cultures, or a majority of four blood cultures with first and last drawn 12 h apart.

Evidence of endocardial involvement on echocardiogram

Clinical evidence of new valvular regurgitation

Positive serology for Q-fever or other causes of culture-negative IE, e.g. *Bartonella*

Identification of a micro-organism from blood culture or excised tissue using molecular biology methods

Minor criteria

Predisposition – predisposing heart condition or i.v. drug use

Fever >38.0°C

Vascular phenomena – major arterial emboli, septic pulmonary infarcts, mycotic aneurysm, intracranial haemorrhage, conjunctival haemorrhage, Janeway lesions, new finger clubbing, splinter haemorrhages, splenomegaly

Immunological phenomena – glomerulonephritis, Osler's nodes, Roth spots, positive rheumatoid factor, elevated erythrocyte sedimentation rate (>1.5× upper limit of normal), elevated C-reactive protein (>100 mg/L)

Microbiological evidence – positive cultures, but not meeting above criteria

A working diagnosis of infective endocarditis is made and Mr Biggins is referred to the cardiology team for review. The cardiology consultant suggests that Mr Biggins undergoes a transoesophageal echocardiogram for further evaluation of the valve and confirmation of the diagnosis. The cardiologist agrees with the provisional diagnosis on the basis of the Duke criteria (see Table 80). Microbiological confirmation would be preferable.

A further two sets of blood cultures are taken.

Mr Biggins is transferred to a monitored bed within the acute medical unit and connected to a cardiac monitor in case of the development of cardiac conduction defects. Observation frequency is increased to hourly (blood pressure, pulse and respiratory rate) in case of sudden decompensation caused by acute failure of the valve. Mr Biggins is placed on the list for transfer to a cardiac bed as soon as one is available.

What is the likely causative organism and what treatment should be started?
• The majority of native valve infective endocarditis is caused by viridans *streptococci* (50–70%), *Staphylococcus*

Table 81 Antibiotics and their use in infective endocarditis

Antibiotic	Dose/route	Duration
Treatment of IE due to penicillin-sensitive organisms		
Benzylpenicillin	7.2–12 g i.v./24 h	4–6 weeks
+gentamicin	3–5 mg/kg i.v./24 h	2 weeks
For patients with penicillin allergy		
Vancomycin	30 mg/kg in 24 h	4 weeks
+gentamicin	3–5 mg/kg i.v./24	2 weeks
Treatment of IE due to staphylococci on native valve		
Penicillin-sensitive staphylococci		
Benzylpenicillin	12–14 g i.v./24 h	6 weeks
+gentamicin	3–5 mg/kg i.v./24 h	3–5 days
Methicillin-sensitive staphylococci		
Flucloxacillin	8–12 g i.v./24 h	6 weeks
+gentamicin	3–5 mg/kg i.v./24 h	3–5 days
Methicillin-resistant staphylococci		
Vancomycin	30 mg/kg i.v./24 h	6 weeks
+gentamicin	3–5 mg/kg i.v./24 h	3–5 days

aureus (25%), and *enterococcus* (10%). In prosthetic valve endocarditis *S. epidermidis* and *S. aureus* are the most common organisms

• Antibiotic treatment should be directed against these organisms empirically while awaiting blood culture results and then revised when sensitivities are known (see Table 81)

• Ensure that a large number of blood culture specimens have been taken before starting antibiotics – ideally take two sets from each arm on several different occasions

• Blood cultures are negative in approximately 14% of cases, often delaying diagnosis and treatment with a profound impact on clinical outcome. Negative cultures are most commonly related to the previous administration of antibiotics, but may be associated with pathogens including *Legionella*, *Coxiella*, the HACEK group (*Haemophilus* species, *Actinobacillus actinomycetemcomitans*, *Cardiobacterium hominis*, *Eikenella*

corrodens, and *Kingella kingae*), and fungi such as *Candida*, *Histoplasma* and *Aspergillus* species. Serological testing can be particularly useful for investigating the possibility of *Coxiella burnetti* (Q fever) and *Bartonella* infection and should be carried out in all patients who are initially culture negative. Other techniques for pathogen isolation include histological samples and polymerase chain reaction

Mr Biggins starts intravenous benzylpenicillin and gentamicin pending culture results. The following day these reveal fully sensitive Streptococcus viridans bacteraemia.
Mr Biggins undergoes a transoesophageal echocardiogram, which confirms the presence of vegetations on the mitral valve and deteriorating valvular regurgitation. Mr Biggins is transferred to the cardiology ward and undergoes urgent mitral valve replacement the following day, from which he makes a full recovery.

CASE REVIEW

A 55-year-old man is admitted with a four-week history of intermittent fever, associated with myalgia, anorexia and weight loss. Apart from a slight cough at the outset, there are no symptoms pertaining to a specific body system; in the days before admission Mr Paul Biggins became more unwell with the development of breathlessness, more persistent fever and drenching night sweats. The symptoms started two weeks after undergoing a dental extraction; other complicating factors in the history include recent travel to Africa, risk factors for HIV and a previous bone plate in his femur.

An examination reveals splinter haemorrhages and a soft systolic murmur along with bibasal crackles and microscopic haematuria. Inflammatory markers and the white cell count are significantly elevated, and a chest radiograph shows evidence of pulmonary oedema; transthoracic echo is suggestive of a vegetation on the mitral valve.

Mr Biggins starts intravenous antibiotics on the basis of a working diagnosis of infective endocarditis. This diagnosis is subsequently confirmed by the finding of

Streptococcus viridans bacteraemia; a transoesophageal echo supports the diagnosis and suggests the need for urgent valve surgery, which is undertaken successfully 24 h later.

The case highlights the complexity of differential diagnosis for patients with PUO, and the need for a careful history, examination and targeted investigation. Although in this case the diagnosis was reached relatively quickly, in many cases of PUO detailed investigations over a prolonged period fail to identify a cause. Sometimes detailed imaging scans of the chest, abdomen and pelvis are required to look for evidence of lymph node enlargement, occult malignancy or collections of pus. A radioisotope bone scan should be considered if osteomyelitis is possible. Radioisotope-labelled white cell scanning may also be helpful to identify a possible source of sepsis, although this will not be available in many hospitals. Patients with immunodeficiency (e.g. HIV infection) present specific challenges because of the wide variety of infections of which they may be at risk; early involvement of specialists in infectious diseases or microbiology is advised in such cases.

KEY POINTS

- PUO can be a complex problem requiring a thorough history/examination and the ability to think laterally.
- The differential diagnosis is wide, but may be narrowed down by careful probing during the initial assessment.
- Investigations should be targeted at any area of suspicion aroused by the history/examination.
- Always consider endocarditis in any patient with a PUO and prior dental work, previous valvular abnormality or prosthesis.

- If endocarditis is suspected, ensure that a large number of sets of blood cultures are taken before commencing antibiotic therapy.
- Early involvement of the cardiology team is necessary to ensure that those patients at risk of valvular failure undergo early surgical valve replacement.

Further reading

Arnow PM, Flaherty JP. Fever of unknown origin. *Lancet* 1997; **350**: 575–80

Baddour LM, Wilson WR, Bayer AS *et al.* Infective endocarditis: diagnosis, antimicrobial therapy, and management of complications: a statement for healthcare professionals from the Committee on Rheumatic Fever, Endocarditis, and Kawasaki Disease, Council on Cardiovascular Disease in the Young, and the Councils on Clinical Cardiology, Stroke, and Cardiovascular Surgery and Anesthesia, American Heart Association: endorsed by the Infectious Diseases Society of America. *Circulation* 2005; **Jun 14**: 111(23)

Horstkotte D, Follath F, Gutschik E *et al.* Guidelines on prevention, diagnosis and treatment of infective endocarditis executive summary: the Task Force on Infective Endocarditis of the European Society of Cardiology. *Eur Heart J* 2004; **25**(3): 267–76

Mourad O, Palda V, Detsky AS. A comprehensive, evidence-based approach to fever of unknown origin. *Arch Int Med* 2003; **163**: 545–51

A 25-year-old woman admitted
following an overdose

A 25-year-old woman is brought to hospital, accompanied by her boyfriend. Earlier that evening Miss Felicity Jones and her boyfriend had argued and he had walked out of the house. On his return two hours later he found Miss Jones lying on the sofa. There was evidence of her having consumed alcohol and there were a number of empty packets of pills lying on the floor next to her. Miss Jones admitted to having taken these approximately one hour earlier; he called 999 and the ambulance brought Miss Jones to hospital.

What challenges will this patient present?
• The history may be difficult to obtain because of the effects of drugs, alcohol or co-existent psychiatric illness
• Miss Jones may be uncooperative because of her emotional state
• Miss Jones may attempt to self-discharge or abscond from hospital prior to full assessment being undertaken
• There may be a risk of further self-harm while Miss Jones is a medical inpatient
• The damaging effects of some drugs may require a prolonged period of observation in a medical ward, which may struggle to manage Miss Jones's psychiatric needs

Overdose is a common cause for hospital admission, particularly among younger adults. In some cases the consequences are severe, and around 4000 people die from deliberate self-poisoning in the UK every year. However, it should be noted that >80% of these never reach hospital. Since overdose accounts for over 300 000 hospital admissions per year it can be deduced that the vast majority of these are discharged back to the community. It is important to remember that a significant proportion of those discharged from hospital following

overdose will make a further attempt at suicide during the following 12 months. Most hospitals therefore require that all patients undergo some form of psychiatric risk assessment prior to discharge.

On arrival Miss Jones is conscious and smells strongly of alcohol; her speech is slurred and incoherent, but she is breathing spontaneously with oxygen saturation of 99% on room air. Her pulse is 100 beats/min with blood pressure 90/60. The Glasgow Coma Score (GCS) is calculated at 14/15 (see p. 127). Blood glucose is 4.7.

What immediate management is required?
• Re-assessment of airway/breathing/circulation:
  ○ in this case Miss Jones' airway is patent and she is adequately oxygenated with a normal respiratory rate
  ○ she is slightly tachycardic and hypotensive
  ○ i.v. access should be established and intravenous fluid administered
• Take blood for full blood count (FBC), urea and electrolytes (U&E), liver function tests (LFT), clotting profile
• Take an extra serum sample for possible later use to check drug levels
• Measure capillary blood glucose
• Consider venous or arterial blood gas analysis
• Attach to a cardiac monitor
• Obtain an ECG

Miss Jones is uncooperative but reluctantly agrees to the insertion of a cannula, and 500 mL of normal saline is administered over 30 min, after which her blood pressure is 110/70 with pulse 96 beats/min. Blood is sent to the laboratory as above. Miss Jones refuses an arterial blood gas. Miss Jones is connected to a cardiac monitor, which shows a sinus tachycardia, confirmed on ECG. Having stabilised Miss Jones you now wish to proceed to take a history. Miss Jones' partner, who has accompanied the

Acute Medicine: Clinical Cases Uncovered. By C. Roseveare.
Published 2009 by Blackwell Publishing, ISBN: 978-1-4051-6883-0

patient into hospital, is standing by the bedside clutching her hand. He appears reluctant to leave the room at the moment.

Should Miss Jones' partner be sent out of the room?

This can be a difficult question to answer, and the decision needs to be taken in the context of the situation at the time. The following issues should be considered.

• Sometimes it is helpful to allow a family member/partner to stay with the patient during the initial assessment process: a familiar face may help to reassure and calm the patient

• On other occasions the presence of a family member/partner may exacerbate the patient's behaviour, particularly if an argument was the precipitant

• Issues of confidentiality will arise as soon as discussions start regarding the reasons for the overdose

• If the patient is coherent enough to give a history it is advisable to send any relatives outside before such discussions occur, and to ask the patient's permission before speaking to any family member or friend

• **Remember to keep a chaperone with you at all times**: this should apply even if the patient is the same sex as the doctor.

Miss Jones is reluctant to talk to the admitting doctor, saying she 'just wants to go to sleep'. Miss Jones admits that she took some tablets but does not know what they were, and cannot be precise about when she took them.

How can you establish what Miss Jones has taken, and when she took it?

• It is not uncommon for patients to be vague about what they took and when

• Alternatively the patient may be unconscious or confused and unable to respond to questions

• However, the importance of this information cannot be overstated

• Seventy percent of all overdoses involve consumption of a medication prescribed to the patient or a member of their household

• Most of the remainder have taken over-the-counter drugs

• Paracetamol is more commonly taken in overdose than aspirin

• Most laboratories can easily measure paracetamol and aspirin (salicylate) levels, although interpretation of

the level usually requires knowledge of the timing of consumption

Useful sources of information regarding which drugs may have been taken will include:

• **The ambulance crew**: they may have documented the number/nature of the empty packets; they will also have information on the timing of the call for help and may have obtained further information from those present at the scene

• **The patient's GP** should be able to provide a list of medication prescribed to the patient and household, along with the dates of the last prescriptions to give an idea of quantities available to the patient

• **The accompanying family member/partner** should be able to provide information regarding the patient's prior medical history, prescribed medication and which drugs were kept in the house (remembering to be wary of issues of confidentiality)

• **Previous hospital/accident and emergency records**: frequently patients will have a previous history of self-harm, psychiatric or medical problems that have required hospital assessment or treatment

For patients with reduced conscious level the clues described in Table 82 will often help in identifying which sedative drug has been consumed.

Miss Jones' partner indicates that the empty bottles/packets of medication were labelled as paracetamol 500 mg; it would appear that Miss Jones took around 16 g of paracetamol. From his earlier discussion with Miss Jones he believes that she took all the medication together approximately two hours ago.

Is there a specific antidote/treatment that can limit the effects of the drug?

• Specific treatments are available to reverse or ameliorate the effects of many drugs taken in overdose. Some of these are noted in Table 82. On-line resources such as TOXBASE are now easy to access for clinicians and will provide information about the appropriate treatment and recommended monitoring following overdose of most drugs

• Most hospital departments involved in the management of patients following overdose will be registered to use TOXBASE. Further information can be obtained from: www.hpa.org.uk/chemicals/toxbase.htm

• Gastric lavage (stomach pump) is now rarely used as a means of reducing absorption of a drug. Unless the drug

Table 82 Clues that may be helpful in identifying the drug causing unconsciousness

Clinical features	Likely drug precipitant	Comments	Antidote
Small/pinpoint pupils Respiratory depression	Opiate (e.g. morphine)	May have been taken as recreational overdose rather than deliberate self-poisoning	Naloxone (see Case 13)
Dilated pupils with sluggish reaction Tachycardia/short PR interval on ECG Urinary retention Bilateral upgoing plantar response	Tricyclic antidepressant (e.g. amitriptylline)	Pupillary, urinary and cardiac effects are due to anticholinergic properties; may occur with other anticholinergic drugs Upgoing plantar response is quite common, but further investigation may be required (e.g. cranial CT)	None
Bradycardia Hypothermia Hyporeflexia Blistering at points of skin trauma	Barbiturate (e.g. phenobarbitone)	Now rarely prescribed so not common – sometimes seen in elderly patients who may have secreted supplies prescribed in the past	None
Deeply unconscious Respiratory depression Normal pulse/blood pressure/pupils	Benzodiazepine (e.g. diazepam)	Often appear deeply asleep, but haemodynamically stable with normal pupils; effects may be prolonged (especially with diazepam)	Flumazenil (best avoided unless profound respiratory depression – risk of seizure: see p. 130)

has been consumed very recently, it is *unlikely* that the tablets will remain in the stomach for long enough for this to be effective. There is also a considerable risk of the patient aspirating their stomach contents during the procedure without formal airway protection, particularly if they have taken a sedating drug or alcohol

• In some cases the oral administration of activated charcoal liquid may reduce absorption of the drug. TOXBASE will usually provide guidance about the benefit; in most cases benefit will only accrue from administration within one hour of the overdose. Activated charcoal is unpleasant to take, and many patients may refuse. Administration via a nasogastric tube may be considered, particularly if the patient is sedated or intubated

> *Miss Jones has taken paracetamol; TOXBASE recommends that the patient be started on intravenous N-acetyl cysteine while awaiting a paracetamol level to be taken at 4 h (see below).*

What further management is required?

A full medical history and careful examination is required for a number of reasons.

• There may be a co-existent medical complaint that has precipitated the overdose: Miss Jones may have taken the paracetamol to relieve a severe headache (see Case 11) or a chronic illness may have resulted in depression

• Co-existent renal failure, liver disease or other chronic illness may influence the metabolism/excretion of the drug

• Unexpected clinical findings might suggest that Miss Jones has taken something in addition to that which has been reported (e.g. anticholinergic symptoms/signs, pupillary abnormalities – see Table 82)

• A careful drug history can help to identify other agents that the patient may have consumed – the laboratory may be able to check blood levels to determine whether a toxic dose has been consumed (e.g. phenytoin, carbamazepine, digoxin, etc.); many laboratories will routinely measure the salicylate level to enable exclusion of aspirin toxicity

In addition, it is important to consider formal assessment of the patient's mental state at the time of initial clerking. This will help the clinician to establish the risk of further self-harm while on the ward or after leaving; if the patient subsequently requests to self-discharge it will have been helpful to have documented the likely risk in the medical notes.

Miss Jones is carefully examined, with a chaperone present. Her pulse is 100 beats/min but cardiovascular and respiratory examination is otherwise unremarkable. Pupils are 3 mm, equal and reactive; neurological examination is normal, apart from slurred speech consistent with alcohol excess. There are no stigmata of chronic liver disease and the liver is not palpable or tender.

Investigations have revealed normal electrolytes, renal and liver function. The paracetamol level is measured at 1.35 mmol/L, 4 h after consumption of the drug. The salicylate level is normal.

What is the relevance of the raised blood paracetamol level and what treatment is required?

• Paracetamol overdosage can result in irreversible liver damage, occasionally resulting in fulminant hepatic failure; the mechanism of liver damage is described in Box 35

• In some cases liver transplantation is the only available treatment option to prevent death

• The likelihood of paracetamol-induced liver injury can be predicted by measuring the paracetamol level; interpretation of this figure will depend on the time since consumption of the drug

• The earliest that this figure can be interpreted with accuracy is at 4 h; after 16 h, interpretation of the level becomes more difficult

• The value of the paracetamol level can be plotted on the graph (see Fig. 48) – a value above the treatment line indicates that 60% of patients would develop significant liver damage if untreated; the patient should be started on treatment with *N*-acetyl cysteine (see Box 35, Table 84)

• Patients on hepatic enzyme-inducing drugs (e.g. phenytoin, carbamazepine), those with a history of chronic alcohol abuse and malnourished patients are at higher risk of liver injury – a lower treatment line (high-risk line) should be used for these patients (see Fig. 48)

• For patients who have taken a 'staggered' overdose (i.e. several overdoses spread out over a period of hours or

> **Box 35 Mechanism of paracetamol-induced liver damage and treatment**
>
> Liver damage is dose dependent – the more paracetamol has been consumed, the more likely it is to occur. Under normal circumstances around 5–10% of paracetamol is metabolised by mixed-function oxidase enzymes in the liver to a highly toxic metabolite. This is normally deactivated by conjugation with glutathione. Following overdose, glutathione stores become depleted and the toxic metabolite causes hepatocyte necrosis. Anything that induces the action of these enzymes will tend to increase the likelihood of paracetamol-induced liver damage (see Table 83). Glutathione depletion due to malnutrition or anorexia may also exacerbate the toxic effects of the drug.
>
> In the UK, the mainstay of treatment following paracetamol overdose is intravenous *N*-acetyl cysteine (NAC). This drug is a glutathione precursor, replenishing hepatic stores of glutathione to enable more effective conjugation of the active metabolite. Methionine is an oral agent that has similar properties as a glutathione precursor and can be administered as an alternative to NAC. Oral methionine is more commonly used than intravenous NAC in the USA.

Table 83 Factors which increase likelihood of paracetamol-induced liver injury (requiring treatment at the high-risk line on Fig. 48)

Factor	Example
Hepatic enzyme-inducing drugs	Carbamazepine, phenytoin Chronic alcohol use
Chronic malnutrition	Anorexia nervosa; HIV/AIDS
Chronic liver disease	Alcoholic liver disease

days), interpretation of the level can be impossible, and treatment should be started empirically

• Empirical treatment should also be started while awaiting results of paracetamol level for patients who report taking >16 g paracetamol; the treatment can be stopped if the level proves to be below the treatment line and the time of ingestion is clear

Miss Jones starts intravenous N-acetyl cysteine using the regimen shown in Table 84. Miss Jones has been transferred to an observable bed on the acute medical unit. The effects

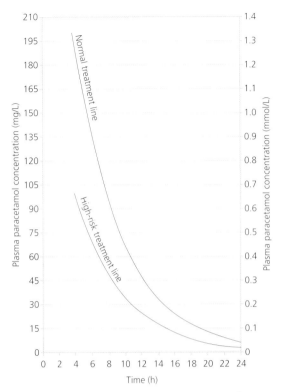

Figure 48 Paracetamol treatment lines: treatment with *N*-acetyl cysteine is recommended if the paracetamol level is above the appropriate line; this graph assumes that the drug has all been consumed at the same time and that the time of ingestion is known. For staggered overdose or when the time of ingestion is unclear, empirical treatment is recommended until the likelihood of liver damage can be excluded (usually after a minimum of 24 h).

Table 84 Dosing regimens for drugs used in paracetamol overdose

Drug	Route of administration	Dosing regimen
N-acetyl cysteine	Intravenous	150 mg/kg in 200 mL of 5% dextrose over 15 min then: 50 mg/kg in 500 mL 5% dextrose over 4 h then: 100 mg/kg in 1000 mL 5% dextrose over 16 h
Methionine	Oral	2.5 g stat then 2.5 g 4 hourly for 12 h

of the patient's presentation. In some cases, mental health teams may be reluctant to conduct a formal assessment of the patient until they have been declared medically fit.

How can the possibility of liver failure be identified/excluded following paracetamol overdose?

• The effects of liver injury following paracetamol overdose may not become apparent for a number of hours. Hepatic enzymes (e.g. alanine transaminase, ALT, aspartate transaminase, AST) will rise first, implying *hepatocyte damage*. However, it is the tests of liver *function* that give the best guide to prognosis

• The liver produces a number of proteins, including those involved in the coagulation cascade (clotting factors). Of these, factor VII has the shortest half-life; if production of proteins by the liver stops, due to hepatocellular damage, the level of factor VII in the blood will drop rapidly

• This can be measured by looking at the international normalised ratio (INR) or prothrombin time (PT). Rising INR or PT suggests impaired liver function, but is usually not apparent for at least 24 h

• Treatment with *N*-acetyl cysteine should be continued until this result is available

• If the liver function tests, renal function and INR are entirely normal 24 h after the time of overdose, *N*-acetyl cysteine treatment can usually be discontinued

---

of the alcohol are wearing off, and at present she remains cooperative with her treatment. Miss Jones asks how long she will have to stay on the drip and when she will be able to leave hospital.

What further observation/investigation is required prior to discharge?

Two further issues need to be considered.

• Identification or exclusion of the medical complications of the drug overdose (in Miss Jones' case liver damage as a result of paracetamol)

• Assessment of risk of further self-harm (see Box 36)

Although the first of these may appear to be the most crucial in terms of the patient's immediate management, it is very important not to ignore the psychiatric aspects

Box 36 Risk assessment following overdose

Psychiatric risk assessment using the SAD PERSONS scale; score 1 point for each line

Criterion	Comment
Sex (male = 1 point)	Although women self-harm more commonly than men, suicide is more common in men than women
Age >45 or <19	Older and younger people are at higher risk of suicide
Depression	10–20% of patients hospitalised for treatment of depression will subsequently commit suicide
Previous attempts	Previous suicide attempts dramatically increase risk of subsequent attempts
Ethanol abuse	Approximately 15% of patients with history of ethanol abuse commit suicide
Rational thinking lost	Psychosis increases risk of suicide
Social supports lacking	Social isolation increases risk of suicide
Organised plan	If patients have made an organised plan (e.g. storing tablets, suicide note, etc.) the risk is higher
No spouse/partner	Particularly for older patients if widowed
Sickness/chronic illness	Presence of chronic illness increases the risk of suicide

Score 7–10 = high risk
Score 5–6 = moderate risk
Score 3–4 = mild risk
Score 1–2 = low risk

These figures should be used as a general guide only; a patient who scores only 1 or 2 on this scale may be at higher risk; if in doubt, early discussion with a specialist in mental health should be undertaken.

- If the liver function is abnormal or INR is >1.2, further monitoring is required with repeat blood testing after a further 12 h
- Detailed discussion of the management of paracetamol-induced liver failure is beyond the scope of this chapter. If a patient is deemed to be developing this condition, early discussion with a specialist liver unit is required. Some of the principles of ongoing management in this situation are outlined in Table 85

> The infusion of N-acetyl cysteine is continued using the regimen shown in Table 84. It is felt that formal psychological assessment should be deferred until the following morning, at which time Miss Jones' INR will also be measured to establish whether the N-acetyl cysteine can be discontinued.
>
> Two hours later you are called back to the ward to speak to Miss Jones, who has announced that she wants to self-discharge. Miss Jones has disconnected her N-acetyl cysteine infusion, and has removed her cannula.

Should Miss Jones be detained in hospital against her will?

Two issues need to be considered.

1 Does Miss Jones have the mental capacity to understand the consequences of leaving hospital against medical advice? (see Table 86)

2 Does Miss Jones have a psychiatric condition that may require further assessment or treatment?

Patients who lack mental capacity may be detained in hospital if it is deemed to be in their best interests to stay; the justification for this should be documented in the medical notes. This situation commonly applies for patients who are acutely confused because of the effects of a medical condition, drug or alcohol consumption.

Patients who have mental capacity but who are deemed to have a psychiatric condition requiring ongoing assessment may be detained under the Mental Health Act (MHA). Various Sections of the Act exist for use in different situations. In practice, Section 5(2) is most commonly used on a medical ward. The following points should be noted.

- Section 5(2) requires the signature of the resident medical officer (RMO – usually the on-call medical SpR or SHO) and the duty hospital manager
- Patients can only be 'sectioned' if they are deemed to be at risk to themselves or to others as a result of a psychiatric illness

Table 85 Principles of management for patients with rising international normalized ratio (INR) following paracetamol overdose (should be followed in combination with advice from a regional liver specialist unit)

Management	Comments
Continuous pulse oximetry/cardiac monitoring and hourly temperature, blood pressure and conscious level assessment	Arrhythmias may occur. Reduced conscious level >72 h after onset may suggest hepatic encephalopathy
Monitor blood glucose hourly	Hypoglycaemia may occur due to impaired gluconeogenesis; if conscious level drops within first 72 h following overdose, hypoglycaemia is more likely than hepatic encephalopathy
Continue N-acetyl cysteine at 16 hourly rate	Although paracetamol metabolism is likely to be complete, continued treatment has been shown to reduce need for transplantation: mechanism unclear but may relate to altered intrahepatic blood flow improving hepatocellular recovery
Monitor INR twice daily	Rapid rise in INR is a poor prognostic sign and should trigger further discussion with the specialist unit. Never attempt to correct a rising INR unless the patient is actively bleeding since this will remove the utility of this measurement as a prognostic marker
Regular arterial blood gas measurement (1 or 2 times per day)	Acidaemia (pH < 7.3) without other explanation is an independent indication for transplantation
Monitor urine output and renal function	Deteriorating renal function is a poor prognostic sign. Keep well hydrated with i.v. fluids and insert a catheter for hourly monitoring of urine output
Prophylactic antibiotic/antifungal treatments	Patients are at high risk of sepsis due to impaired liver function; choice of antimicrobial agent will vary depending on guidance by the local liver unit

• Detention is permitted for up to 72 hours, although a formal psychiatric review will normally be undertaken before this

• Detention in hospital on a Section 5(2) does not allow you to *treat* the patient against their will; continuation of the N-acetyl cysteine infusion will require the patient's agreement

• Once sectioned, the patient cannot be released from hospital until they have been seen by a consultant psychiatrist, who will determine whether their period of detention should be extended to enable further treatment. It may be that the patient will agree to this voluntarily

Consider the following in dealing with this scenario.

• **Talk to the patient**: find out why they wish to leave. Sometimes it is something simple like wanting a cigarette or a wash or to talk to their partner; if you can convince them to stay voluntarily, this will save considerable time later

Table 86 Assessment of mental capacity

A competent patient must be able to:

Comprehend and retain information

Believe the information given

Weigh up the information to make an informed choice

• **Establish if the patient has the mental capacity to make their own decisions** (see Table 86)

• **Reassess suicide risk** (see Box 36): if doubt persists discussion with a trained mental health practitioner is advisable

• **Ensure that the patient understands the seriousness of the medical condition,** if self-discharging despite the need for ongoing medical treatment. This is particularly true of a paracetamol overdose, where symptoms may not arise for several days; prevention of liver damage is only possible if treatment is given early. This should be made very clear

• **Document your discussions carefully** in the medical notes

• **Contact the patient's GP** to ensure that appropriate community follow-up is undertaken

• **Always remember a chaperone;** security staff should be alerted if a patient is to be detained against their will in hospital; physical restraint is occasionally necessary. If a patient on a 'Section' manages to abscond from the ward the police should be informed immediately.

Miss Jones agrees to stay overnight following a long discussion. Miss Jones' cannula is resited and she completes the full 20-h infusion of N-acetyl cysteine. Her INR is 1.1 (prothrombin time 15 s), 30 h after the overdose and repeat liver and renal function is also normal. After formal risk assessment by the psychological medicine team the next morning, Miss Jones is deemed to be at low risk of repeating the overdose, and has no evidence of a mental illness. Miss Jones is given the number of an organisation providing relationship counselling, but appears to have made up with her boyfriend. It appears that Miss Jones is consuming more alcohol than is normally recommended and she is advised to cut this down prior to discharge from hospital.

CASE REVIEW

A 25-year-old woman is brought to hospital by her boyfriend after having taken an overdose of tablets combined with alcohol. Miss Felicity Jones is initially uncooperative and vague about what medication she has taken; however, Miss Jones' boyfriend is able to inform the medical admitting team that she has taken around 16 g of paracetamol approximately two hours before arrival in hospital. Miss Jones is moved to a medical ward and the paracetamol level, taken four hours after the time of ingestion, is measured at 1.35 mol/dL, which requires treatment with N-acetyl cysteine. Shortly after admission Miss Jones asks for the infusion to be discontinued and informs the staff that she wishes to discharge herself from the ward. Because no formal risk assessment has been undertaken, the medical SHO is called urgently to the ward so that Miss Jones' mental competence and psychiatric risk can be assessed, along with her understanding of the potential severity of the medical consequences of the overdose. Miss Jones agrees to stay and to continue the treatment, following discussion with the SHO; formal detention under the Mental Health Act is not required. Measurement of her liver enzymes and clotting profile >24 h after ingestion of the paracetamol indicate that there has been no liver damage. The N-acetyl cysteine infusion is discontinued.

The following day Miss Jones undergoes a formal interview with the mental health team, who establish that the risk of further self-harm is low. Miss Jones is discharged with advice to seek relationship counselling and reduce her alcohol intake.

This case highlights some of the issues relating to initial management of patients following overdose. Although the medical consequences of the overdose are usually the main priority in the early stages following admission, the psychiatric issues should not be ignored. Medical teams involved with such cases should be prepared to undertake a psychiatric risk assessment as soon as possible after admission; this will help to clarify whether detention under the Mental Health Act is likely to be necessary if the patient attempts to leave the hospital.

KEY POINTS

- Initial assessment of a patient following overdose should include attempts to identify what drug(s) have been consumed and the timing of ingestion.
- Having identified which drugs have been consumed, access to a database such as TOXBASE will assist the clinician in the specific management options which are required.
- Following suspected paracetamol overdose, measurement of the level should be deferred until at least 4 h after ingestion.

- N-acetyl cysteine should be commenced if the patient's level lies above the treatment line, or empirically if they have taken a staggered overdose, consumed more than 16 g of paracetamol, or if presentation is delayed >16 h after consumption.
- Mental health risk assessment should be carried out at the earliest opportunity; this will identify whether detention under the Mental Health Act is likely to be required should the patient wish to leave the hospital.

Further reading

Butler J, Longhitano C. Self harm. *Medicine* 2008; **36**(9): 455–8

Sprigings D, Chambers JB. Poisoning: general approach. In: *Acute medicine: a practical guide to the management of medical emergencies*, 4th edition. Blackwell Publishing, Oxford, 2008

Sprigings D, Chambers JB. Poisoning with aspirin, paracetamol and carbon monoxide. In: *Acute medicine: a practical guide to the management of medical emergencies*, 4th edition. Blackwell Publishing, Oxford, 2008

Wallace CL *et al*. Paracetamol overdose: an evidence based flow-chart to guide management. *Emerg Med J* 2002; **19**: 202–5

A 35-year-old woman with an acutely swollen leg

You are called to the acute medical unit to review a 35-year-old woman who has presented to hospital complaining of pain and swelling in her right leg. This came on gradually over the past week but is now restricting her mobility. Joanna Polydorou was initially assessed on the ward by a specialist nurse in the acute medical unit's deep vein thrombosis (DVT) clinic. The nurse arranged for Ms Polydorou to undergo a duplex scan of her leg veins. This has apparently shown no evidence of a DVT. You have been asked to review Ms Polydorou prior to discharge.

What challenges will this patient present?

DVT is a potentially serious diagnosis, although most hospitals now have protocols in place which enable treatment to be initiated in the community without the need for an inpatient stay. Clinics set up to manage DVT are often nurse led, and the degree of involvement of medical staff will vary depending on local protocols. Some hospitals will require that all patients are seen by a doctor irrespective of the test results, whereas others may have protocols that only require medical involvement if the nurse has specific concerns. In this situation the nurse is often considerably more experienced than the doctor; the junior doctor would therefore be well advised to listen carefully to his/her concerns, which may include:
• The possibility of an alternative serious diagnosis requiring hospital treatment
• Concern about the presence of a DVT despite the negative duplex scan
• The possibility of a co-existent pulmonary embolism, complicating an undiagnosed DVT
• Other co-existent illness that needs to be addressed before discharge
• The need for symptom control prior to discharge

The nurse explains that she is concerned that Ms Polydorou has significant pain and swelling despite the negative duplex scan.

Ms Polydorou appears flushed and is unable to walk without significant discomfort. The nurse has completed a set of observations that reveal a pulse of 96 beats/min, blood pressure 130/70, temperature 37.8°C, oxygen saturation 99% while breathing room air.

What immediate management is required?

Apart from some oral analgesia (e.g. paracetamol) Ms Polydorou does not appear to require any specific treatment at present. In general, a patient with a swollen leg does not require immediate intervention, and may be given quite a low priority by the busy on-call junior doctor. However, the following should always be remembered.
• DVT may precede the development of pulmonary embolism (PE): the patient should be in an area where they can be observed
• A significant proportion of patients with DVT have asymptomatic PE: a patient who is tachycardic and/or hypoxic may need more urgent assessment
• Don't leave your assessment until too late in the day: if further investigation is required this may not be possible outside normal working hours
• A long delay for the patient may add to your workload: you will have to waste time apologising for the delay, and the patient is less likely to go away feeling satisfied

Has the assessment to date satisfactorily excluded DVT?

No test for DVT is 100% sensitive – in other words you can never rely entirely on a single investigation to exclude DVT. Following a negative initial investigation it is important to consider:
• The clinical probability of DVT
• The sensitivity of the investigation already undertaken

Acute Medicine: Clinical Cases Uncovered. By C. Roseveare. Published 2009 by Blackwell Publishing, ISBN: 978-1-4051-6883-0

• What other investigations could be used to corroborate the findings

Ms Polydorou describes a two-day history of right leg swelling. This started gradually, initially affecting her right calf but spreading gradually up to the knee level. Ms Polydorou gives a past history of a DVT affecting the same leg during a pregnancy and comments that this leg has swelled up periodically since then; however, this feels different. Ms Polydorou smokes 20 cigarettes per day, and takes no medication. Ms Polydorou has not undergone any recent surgery, although she undertook a 4-h coach trip two weeks ago. Ms Polydorou has felt generally unwell for the past two days and felt feverish and shivery the previous evening.

On examination Ms Polydorou has a mild pyrexia (37.8°c); the right calf is slightly warmer than the left and mildly swollen compared with the left side (4 cm difference in calf circumference) with pitting oedema at the ankle level; there is marked erythema, extending to just above the knee level with clear demarcation of the proximal limit (see Plate 6). Ms Polydorou has mild tinea pedis (athlete's foot) between the toes of both feet.

What is the clinical probability of DVT?

Clinical assessment is a notoriously unreliable tool in the assessment of suspected DVT. When taking a history and examining a patient with a swollen leg it is worth considering the following.
• Are the appearances compatible with the diagnosis of DVT? (see Table 87)
• Are there risk factors for venous thrombosis? (see p. 40)
• Is an alternative diagnosis more likely? (see Table 88)

In addition it may be appropriate to calculate a formal risk score as part of your objective assessment. The most commonly used score is the Wells score (see Table 89); however, it should be remembered that this cannot be used in isolation, and does not excuse proper clinical assessment.

Although there are risk factors for DVT (immobility on coach trip, previous DVT, cigarette smoking), the clinical appearances, fever, systemic upset and potential entry site for infection (athlete's foot) are more suggestive of cellulitis as the cause for her symptoms. The Wells score would be 1 (+1 for previous DVT, +1 for swelling. +1 for oedema; –2 for alternative diagnosis being at least as likely as DVT).

Table 87 Clinical features of deep vein thrombosis (DVT)

Clinical feature	Comments
Swelling of affected limb	Almost invariable unless the clot is non-occlusive. Extent of swelling may give a guide to the extent of DVT (i.e. total leg swelling to groin level suggestive of iliofemoral DVT), although this cannot be relied upon
Erythema	May be quite subtle. Marked discolouration is more suggestive of cellulitis. Erythema is usually diffuse without clear demarcation
Warmth	Feel the temperature with the back of your hand and compare to the other side – remember to expose both legs for the same period of time. Again often only subtle differences in temperature in DVT; marked warmth is more suggestive of cellulitis
Tenderness	Particularly over deep veins – calf, medial aspect of thigh and/or groin; marked, superficial tenderness is more suggestive of thrombophlebitis. Demonstration of Homan's sign (pain elicited by flexion of ankle) is unreliable and painful for the patient
Prominence of superficial veins	With deep venous occlusion superficial veins produce 'collateral' drainage. Marked asymmetry of superficial veins is suggestive of this

What is the sensitivity of the investigations already undertaken?

A variety of diagnostic tests are available for the investigation of suspected DVT. These vary in their complexity, availability, sensitivity and specificity (see Table 90).
• Ms Polydorou has undergone lower limb duplex scan, which has limited sensitivity for below-knee DVT
• The fact that the scan shows no evidence of a DVT makes it extremely unlikely that there is a DVT between the popliteal vein and the pelvis

Table 88 Differential diagnosis of unilateral leg swelling

Diagnosis	Features	Comments
Deep vein thrombosis (DVT)	See Table 87	
Cellulitis	Systemic upset – fever, etc. Marked erythema/warmth with clear demarcation of proximal extent of erythema May be entry site for infection (bite, cut, athlete's foot, etc.)	DVT and cellulitis occasionally co-exist Infection with streptococci or staphylococcus is the usual cause
Trauma/muscle tear	May be apparent from history Abrupt onset of pain with subsequent swelling around the site Localised tenderness	DVT may develop in leg that is immobilised following trauma, or due to vascular damage at the time of injury
Venous insufficiency	Long history of recurrent/persistent leg swelling, ulceration, varicose veins, etc. Often bilateral May follow previous DVT	Venous incompetence may be demonstrated on duplex scan
Ruptured Baker's cyst	Calf pain and swelling often indistinguishable from DVT May be history of knee pain/swelling/arthritis	May be apparent at the time of lower limb ultrasound as hypoechoic lesion
Extrinsic compression of veins	Usually occurs in pelvis – swelling extends to groin level Clinically indistinguishable from DVT History may suggest underlying malignancy (weight loss, malaise, etc.)	Pelvic malignancy is the commonest cause in women; prostatic cancer for men Examine carefully for groin lymph nodes; perform rectal examination and consider pelvic examination for women
Rheumatological causes (gout, inflammatory or septic arthritis)	Swelling/pain/erythema usually centred around knee/ankle joints – calf and thigh relatively spared May be effusion in knee joint	
Soft tissue tumours	May be localised mass lesion	Muscle sarcomas are rare; may be shown as hypoechoic lesions on ultrasound; MRI scanning required for diagnosis

Table 89 Wells score for DVT assessment

Wells score or criteria: (possible score –2 to 9)
1 Active cancer (treatment within last 6 months or palliative) – 1 point
2 Calf swelling >3 cm compared with other calf (measured 10 cm below tibial tuberosity) – 1 point
3 Collateral superficial veins (non-varicose) – 1 point
4 Pitting oedema (confined to symptomatic leg) – 1 point
5 Swelling of entire leg – 1 point
6 Localised pain along distribution of deep venous system – 1 point
7 Paralysis, paresis, or recent cast immobilisation of lower extremities – 1 point
8 Recently bedridden >3 days, or major surgery requiring regional or general anaesthetic in past 12 weeks – 1 point
9 Previously documented DVT – 1 point
10 Alternative diagnosis at least as likely – subtract 2 points

Interpretation:
Score of 2 or higher – deep vein thrombosis is likely.
Score of less than 2 – deep vein thrombosis is unlikely.

Table 90 Diagnostic tests for suspected deep vein thrombosis (DVT)

Test	Sensitivity	Specificity	Comments
D-dimer	High	Low	Simple to take; near-patient testing kits available Elevated in the context of inflammation of any cause, malignancy, following surgery, pregnancy May be useful in distinguishing new clot (raised D-dimer) from old 'chronic' thrombosis (D-dimer often normal)
Duplex scan	Intermediate	High	Non-invasive, ultrasound-based test: usually easily available Generally less sensitive for below-knee thrombosis (operator dependent) Will miss isolated pelvic thrombosis (approximately 1% of DVT) Unable to distinguish 'new' from 'old' clot
Impedance plethysmography	Intermediate	Intermediate	Equipment not universally available, but is portable and may be used at the bedside by ward staff after limited training May identify patients who require further assessment with duplex
Ascending venography	High	High	Requires cannulation of foot vein Painful for patient; time consuming for radiology department Intravenous contrast injection required More sensitive than duplex scanning for identification of below-knee thrombosis
CT/MR venography	High	High	Particularly useful for imaging pelvic veins May identify causes of extrinsic compression where veins are clear Limited availability requires selective use

What other investigation could be used to corroborate the findings?

A small calf vein thrombus remains possible; however, given that the clinical likelihood of DVT is considered to be low, and an alternative diagnosis (cellulitis) is more likely, further imaging of this area is not required in this case. In cases where suspicion of calf vein thrombosis persists, repeat duplex scan or venography may be warranted.

D-dimer is unlikely to be helpful in distinguishing DVT from cellulitis, since both conditions will usually produce elevated levels.

Further investigations in this case should include:
• Full blood count (raised white cell count will support the diagnosis of cellulitis)
• Urea and electrolytes (U&E) (to exclude electrolyte abnormalities and underlying renal dysfunction)
• C-reactive protein (CRP) (almost invariably raised in the presence of cellulitis)

• Blood glucose (cellulitis may complicate undiagnosed diabetes)

Blood cultures may be warranted if the patient is pyrexial; swabs of any open wounds or discharging abscesses should be sent.

Investigations reveal a white cell count of 14.7 (neutrophils 10.4) and CRP 37. Electrolytes, renal function and blood glucose are normal.

Ms Polydorou starts oral amoxicillin 500 mg tds and flucloxacillin 500 mg qds to ensure adequate treatment of staphylococci and streptococci, the most likely causative organisms. Ms Polydorou is also given topical clotrimazole cream for treatment of her tinea pedis. She is advised to take regular paracetamol and allowed home with a recommendation to visit her GP if the symptoms fail to settle within the next few days. Ms Polydorou is also advised not to drive until the pain and swelling in her leg have settled. She makes an uneventful recovery.

CASE REVIEW

A 35-year-old woman has been referred to hospital for investigation of a swollen right leg. The GP has asked for DVT to be excluded. Initial investigation revealed a normal duplex scan of the deep veins of that leg. Ms Joanna Polydorou has a number of risk factors for DVT, including cigarette smoking, recent prolonged coach travel and a previous DVT in the same leg. Examination confirms that the leg is swollen, warm and erythematous,; however, the clear demarcation of the erythema, co-existent fever and malaise are more suggestive of cellulitis as the cause for the symptoms. Formal risk scoring using the Wells score reveals a low probability of DVT; when combined with the clinical impression of cellulitis and negative duplex scan it is considered that DVT has been satisfactorily excluded.

Ms Polydorou is treated for cellulitis with oral flucloxacillin and amoxicillin and makes an uneventful recovery.

Given the low sensitivity and specificity of many of the diagnostic tests for DVT, careful clinical assessment is essential. Establishing an alternative diagnosis is a key element of the process; as well as helping in the exclusion of DVT it will also enable appropriate treatment to be given. DVT can occasionally co-exist with cellulitis, because of immobility and increased coagulability of the blood during active inflammation. Further imaging may be required if the swelling fails to settle. In addition, lower limb cellulitis frequently fails to respond adequately to oral antibiotic therapy, in which case intravenous treatment is required. Once-daily treatment regimens using intravenous ceftriaxone may enable patients to be treated with intravenous antibiotics without hospital admission, provided they are systemically well.

KEY POINTS

- Although most patients referred to hospital with an acutely swollen leg require exclusion of DVT, alternative diagnoses should always be considered.
- Initial assessment of a patient with a swollen leg should enable the clinician to establish the clinical likelihood of DVT.
- Use of a formal risk score may assist the clinician in their initial assessment but should not be used in isolation.

- No single investigation is 100% specific or sensitive for the diagnosis of DVT.
- Identification of an alternative cause for the swelling will enable appropriate treatment to be initiated and will help in the exclusion of DVT when investigations are non-diagnostic.

Further reading

Goodacre S *et al.* Meta-analysis: the value of clinical assessment in the diagnosis of deep venous thrombosis. *Ann Intern Med* 2005; **143**: 129–39

Jones GR. Principles and practice of antibiotic therapy for cellulitis. *CPD J Acute Med* 2002; **1**(2): 44–9

MCQs

For each situation choose the single option you feel is most correct.

1 *Pleuritic chest pain . . .*

a. is a characteristic presenting symptom of myocardial infarction
b. is typically described as a dull ache, exacerbated by exertion
c. is the main presenting symptom in most cases of pulmonary embolism
d. may be the presenting symptom in pneumothorax
e. usually starts abruptly if caused by pulmonary embolism

2 *A 25-year-old woman with no previous medical history presents to hospital with a 24-hour history of breathlessness on exertion. She is a non-smoker. Chest examination and chest radiograph are normal; she has a sinus tachycardia of 110 beats/min, tachypnoea (respiratory rate 22 breaths/min) and is mildly hypoxic, and hypocapnoeic (pO$_2$ 9.8, pCO$_2$ 3.1, pH 7.51). What is the most likely diagnosis?*

a. hyperventilation related to anxiety
b. acute asthma
c. pneumothorax
d. pulmonary embolism
e. diabetic ketoacidosis

3 *Which of the following is **not** a criterion for measurement of the Wells score for pulmonary embolism?*

a. previous malignancy
b. symptoms and/or signs of deep vein thrombosis
c. current use of oral contraceptive pill
d. tachycardia >100 beats/min
e. haemoptysis

4 *A 45-year-old man presents to hospital describing 2 days of black, tarry stools and a single episode of fresh haemetemesis. He has no significant prior history but drinks approximately 40 units of alcohol per week. He has been experiencing mild 'indigestion' symptoms for many years. On examination he is tachycardic (110 beats/min) with blood pressure 90/60. There are no stigmata of chronic liver disease and no ascites. Rectal examination confirms the typical appearance and smell of melaena stool. What is the most likely cause for his gastrointestinal bleed?*

a. oesophagitis
b. oesophageal varices
c. Mallory–Weiss tear
d. peptic ulcer
e. colonic diverticular disease

Acute Medicine: Clinical Cases Uncovered. By C. Roseveare.
Published 2009 by Blackwell Publishing, ISBN: 978-1-4051-6883-0

PART 3: SELF-ASSESSMENT

5 *An 80-year-old woman presents to hospital with a 3-day history of fresh rectal bleeding. She gives a long history of 'indigestion', for which she uses antacids and takes regular aspirin after a previous myocardial infarct. The blood is bright red and mixed with formed stool. On examination she appears well and is haemodynamically stable with a blood pressure of 140/70 and pulse 70 beats/min. There is mild epigastric and left iliac fossa tenderness, but no masses. Rectal examination reveals hard stool with some fresh blood on the glove on inspection. What is the most likely cause for her gastrointestinal bleeding?*

a. colonic diverticular disease
b. peptic ulcer
c. oesophageal varices
d. ulcerative colitis
e. oesophagitis

6 *A 50-year-old man has just returned to the ward after upper gastrointestinal endoscopy. He was admitted earlier in the day with melaena and endoscopy has revealed a large duodenal ulcer with a visible vessel that has been injected with adrenaline. Which of the following treatments is most likely to be effective in reducing his risk of ongoing bleeding?*

a. intravenous ranitidine 200 mg bd
b. *Helicobacter* eradication therapy
c. intravenous terlipressin 2 mg 6 hourly
d. intravenous omeprazole: 80 mg bolus followed by infusion of 8 mg/hour over 72 hours
e. oral omeprazole 40 mg daily

7 *A 27-year-old woman presents to hospital with a 6-week history of diarrhoea with rectal bleeding; over the past week the diarrhoea has been occurring more than 10 times per day and waking her several times during the night. She has lost ½ stone in weight. There has been some blood with each stool. Today she has a mild fever and appears dehydrated with a pulse of 100 beats/min and blood pressure 90/40. What is the most likely diagnosis?*

a. irritable bowel syndrome
b. ulcerative colitis
c. rectal carcinoma
d. thyrotoxicosis
e. salmonella enteritis

8 *Which of the following is **not** an appropriate immediate investigation for a patient presenting to hospital with suspected acute colitis?*

a. stool culture
b. electrolytes and liver function tests
c. urgent colonoscopy
d. abdominal radiograph
e. rigid sigmoidoscopy and biopsy

9 *Which of the following statements is correct in relation to a patient presenting to hospital with acute-onset diarrhoea?*

a. hyperkalaemia is a common finding at presentation
b. ischaemic colitis rarely results in bloodstaining of the stool
c. irritable bowel syndrome is more likely if the patient is woken at night by the need to open their bowels
d. hypoalbuminaemia usually indicates associated renal protein loss
e. isolation in a side room is recommended even if initial stool culture is negative

10 *A 50-year-old man presents to hospital after developing a sudden, severe headache 2 hours earlier. He has no prior history of note. Which of the following statements is correct?*

a. thunderclap migraine is the most likely diagnosis
b. a normal CT brain scan will exclude subarachnoid haemorrhage in >95% of cases
c. lumbar puncture should be undertaken as soon as possible after the patient's arrival in hospital if CT scan is normal
d. subarachnoid haemorrhage is unlikely if there are no focal neurological signs
e. reduced conscious level is an adverse prognostic sign

11 *Following the diagnosis of subarachnoid haemorrhage, which of the following statements is **incorrect**?*

a. urgent referral to a neurosurgical unit is usually required
b. intravenous nimodipine is recommended to reduce blood pressure
c. regular neurological observations should be undertaken
d. fall in conscious level should lead to urgent repeat CT brain scanning
e. surgical or radiological treatment of an aneurysm may prevent recurrence

12 *When a patient presents to hospital following an episode of unexplained syncope, which of the following clinical features is **not** indicative of a high risk of a cardiac cause for their collapse?*

a. age <50 years
b. sinus bradycardia of 45 beats/min
c. family history of sudden death
d. previous myocardial ischaemia
e. co-existent ejection systolic murmur

13 *Which of these statements is correct in relation to a patient presenting to hospital with unexplained transient loss of consciousness?*

a. the patient can continue to drive after discharge, provided that the admitting clinician is confident that the episode was not caused by a seizure
b. transient ischaemic attack is a common cause in older people
c. prolonged drowsiness suggests syncope is the likely cause
d. hyperglycaemia is a common cause
e. the patient may shake violently following an episode of syncope

14 *Which of the following clinical signs is **not** a common feature of deep venous **thrombosis**?*

a. pallor of limb with absence of foot pulses
b. warmth of limb in comparison to unaffected side
c. unilateral swelling of lower limb
d. tenderness over medial aspect of thigh
e. dilatation of superficial veins over the shin

15 *A 50-year-old woman is referred to hospital by her general practitioner because of a painful, swollen left calf. Which of the following statements is **incorrect**?*

a. lower limb venous duplex scan is a sensitive test for exclusion of above-knee deep vein thrombosis
b. raised D-dimer is usually considered diagnostic of deep vein thrombosis in this context
c. cellulitis is a possible diagnosis
d. recent surgery increases the likelihood that deep vein thrombosis is the cause
e. ruptured Baker's cyst is a possible explanation

16 *A 27-year-old woman presents to hospital complaining of palpitations and light-headedness. Examination reveals a regular pulse of 180 beats/min with a blood pressure of 100/60. ECG reveals a narrow complex tachycardia. Which of the following diagnoses is most likely?*

a. atrial fibrillation
b. atrial flutter
c. supraventricular tachycardia
d. sinus tachycardia
e. ventricular tachycardia

17 *Which of the following statements is correct in relation to a patient presenting to hospital with a broad complex tachycardia following a recent myocardial infarction?*

a. the most likely diagnosis is supraventricular tachycardia
b. thyrotoxicosis is a common cause
c. DC cardioversion is the treatment of choice if the patient is haemodynamically compromised
d. adenosine is likely to be an effective treatment
e. amiodarone is contraindicated

18 *A 50-year-old man presents to hospital with a 2-week history of mild chest discomfort, palpitations and shortness of breath on exertion; ECG reveals an irregularly irregular tachycardia with a heart rate of 130 beats/min. Blood pressure is 160/70; heart sounds are normal and chest is clear. Which of the following statements is **incorrect**?*

a. atrial fibrillation is the most likely diagnosis
b. digoxin is an appropriate treatment to provide rate control
c. alcohol is a possible underlying cause
d. urgent DC cardioversion is the treatment of choice
e. amiodarone may result in chemical cardioversion

19 *A 19-year-old woman with known asthma is brought to hospital by ambulance. She has become increasingly wheezy over the past 24 hours and has not responded to her normal inhalers. Which of the following statements is correct?*

a. normal pCO_2 is usually suggestive of a relatively mild asthma attack
b. she should be given 28% oxygen initially, pending the results of arterial blood gases
c. the main reason for undertaking a chest radiograph is to exclude underlying infection as the cause for her wheeze
d. absence of wheeze is an indicator of life-threatening asthma
e. tachycardia suggests anxiety is the cause of her symptoms

20 *Which of the following statements is **incorrect** in relation to an acute asthma exacerbation?*

a. bacterial pneumonia is a common cause
b. allergy to house dust mite is a possible trigger
c. intravenous magnesium sulphate may be effective for the treatment of severe exacerbations of asthma
d. salbutamol may be administered intravenously
e. oxygen should be used as the driving gas for the administration of nebulised bronchodilators

21 *Which of the following is **not** a strong indication for urgent CT brain scanning following the admission of a confused patient with a history of alcohol dependency to hospital?*

a. evidence of focal neurological deficit
b. evidence of recent head injury
c. deterioration in conscious level following admission
d. a history of previous seizure
e. clinical evidence of raised intracranial pressure

22 *A 49-year-old man with a long history of chronic alcohol abuse is brought to hospital after he was noted to be confused and unsteady on his feet for the past 48 hours. Which of the following statements is correct?*

a. hypoglycaemia is unlikely unless the patient suffers from diabetes
b. administration of oral thiamine is likely to be effective in preventing Wernicke's encephalopathy
c. Korsakoff's psychosis is usually reversible
d. administration of intravenous glucose may precipitate Wernicke's encephalopathy
e. Wernicke's encephalopathy is unlikely in the absence of ophthalmoplegia

23 *A 19-year-old woman is brought to hospital by her boyfriend, after consuming approximately 16 g of paracetamol 2 hours previously. Which of the following statements is correct?*

a. measurement of plasma paracetamol level should be undertaken as soon as she arrives in hospital
b. drowsiness and pinpoint pupils on admission are suggestive of acute liver failure
c. treatment with *N*-acetyl cysteine is likely to be necessary if the patient consumed the drug over a prolonged period
d. the finding of normal liver function and INR at the time of admission indicates that liver damage is unlikely to occur
e. if the paracetamol level is below the treatment line at 4 hours, treatment with N-acetyl cysteine is likely to be necessary

24 *Which of the following is not likely to increase the likelihood of liver damage following paracetamol overdose?*

a. a history of anorexia nervosa
b. long-standing chronic alcohol abuse
c. alcohol ingestion at the time of paracetamol overdose
d. use of carbamazepine as treatment for epilepsy
e. previous chronic liver disease

25 *Following a patient's admission with paracetamol overdose, the paracetamol level is found to be above the treatment line and she is treated with N-acetyl cysteine. Which of the following statements is correct in relation to her further treatment and investigation?*

a. the finding of an isolated rise in alanine transaminase suggests acute liver failure and is an indication for referral to a specialist liver unit
b. Section 5(2) of the Mental Health Act will allow detention in hospital for up to 28 days of psychiatric treatment
c. repeat measurement of paracetamol level will often provide valuable prognostic information
d. if the INR is found to be elevated, correction with fresh frozen plasma is recommended
e. treatment with *N*-acetyl cysteine should be continued if the INR is elevated after 24 hours

26 *A 75-year-old man is brought to hospital in the early hours of the morning having been woken by acute shortness of breath. He has a past history of mild chronic obstructive pulmonary disease and has had a previous myocardial infarct, although he was well in the days prior to this admission. On arrival he appears sweaty and pale with a regular pulse of 100 beats/min and blood pressure 140/70. Respiratory examination reveals bilateral coarse crepitations to both midzones. What is the most likely diagnosis?*

a. pulmonary embolism
b. pulmonary fibrosis
c. exacerbation of COPD
d. acute left ventricular failure
e. bilateral pneumonia

27 *A 25-year-old woman is being treated for acute asthma. After initially stabilising with nebulised salbutamol, the nurses are concerned that her condition is deteriorating. She has been receiving regular salbutamol nebules and was treated with 40 mg of prednisolone orally on arrival in hospital. You find her to be slightly drowsy but easily rousable with a pulse of 110 beats/min. Oxygen saturation is 99% on high-flow oxygen. Her breathing is more laboured than when you assessed her earlier in the day, and the breath sounds are now quiet with only scanty audible wheeze. She is currently receiving salbutamol 5 mg via a nebuliser. Blood gases are as follows: pH 7.27, pCO_2 7.4, pO_2 16.9, HCO_3 22.4. What is the most appropriate immediate management plan?*

a. reduce the inhaled oxygen concentration to 28% and repeat the arterial blood gas in 30 minutes
b. administer 100 mg hydrocortisone intravenously
c. arrange an urgent chest radiograph
d. fast-bleep the on-call intensive care specialist to the ward and consider urgent transfer to the intensive care unit
e. administer 2 g of magnesium sulphate intravenously

28 *A 60-year-old man is brought to hospital complaining of central crushing chest pain over the past 2 hours. He has a past history of hypertension and has a family history of ischaemic heart disease. His admission ECG shows 2 mm ST segment elevation in leads II, III and AVF (see figure below). Which of the following statements is correct?*

a. the likely diagnosis is anterior ST elevation myocardial infarction (STEMI)
b. normal troponin I on blood taken shortly after admission makes myocardial infarction unlikely
c. thrombolysis is unlikely to be beneficial
d. complete heart block is a recognised early complication
e. the patient should be given 75 mg of aspirin on arrival in hospital

29 *Which of the following is not a contraindication to thrombolytic therapy for suspected STEMI?*

a. recent evidence of gastrointestinal bleeding
b. recent haemorrhagic stroke
c. major surgery within past 4 weeks
d. onset of symptoms >12 hours prior to admission to hospital
e. left bundle branch block on admission ECG

30 *Which of the following is **not** a recognised cause of hypercalcaemia?*

a. primary hyperparathyroidism
b. bronchial carcinoma
c. myeloma
d. secondary hyperparathyroidism
e. sarcoidosis

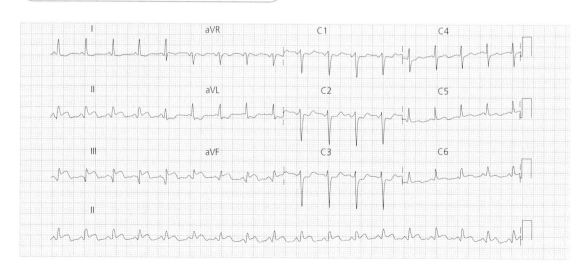

EMQs

1 Arterial blood gases

a. Uncompensated metabolic acidosis
b. Partially compensated metabolic acidosis
c. Compensated metabolic acidosis
d. Compensated metabolic alkalosis
e. Uncompensated respiratory acidosis
f. Compensated respiratory acidosis
g. Partially compensated respiratory acidosis
h. Uncompensated respiratory alkalosis
i. Compensated respiratory alkalosis

Which of the above terms best describes the acid–base disturbance demonstrated in the examples below?

1. A 25-year-old woman with insulin-dependent diabetes who is brought to hospital with drowsiness and hyperglycaemia. Blood gases are as follows: pH 7.09, pCO_2 2.15, pO_2 18.5, HCO_3 9, base excess −15

2. A 30-year-old man who has been brought to hospital with tachypnoea and tachycardia; blood gases are as follows: pH 7.66, pCO_2 2.4, pO_2 18.7, HCO_3 21, base excess 1.2

3. A 60-year-old woman with long-standing COPD who is incidentally noted to be cyanosed while being assessed in the accident and emergency department following admission after a fall: pH 7.37, pCO_2 8.6, pO_2 8.1, HCO_3 37.4, base excess +13

4. A 25-year-old woman with asthma who has become drowsy after initial stabilisation with nebulised salbutamol: pH 7.28, pCO_2 7.9, pO_2 15.6, HCO_3 21, base excess 1.5

2 ECG abnormalities

a. ST segment elevation in leads II, III and AVF
b. ST segment depression in leads V2–V4
c. ST segment elevation in Leads II, III, AVF, V5 and V6
d. ST segment elevation in V2–V4
e. ST segment elevation in leads V2–V6, I and AVL
f. ST segment elevation in leads V5, V6, I and AVL
g. ST segment elevation in all leads except V1 and AVR

Which of the above ECG abnormalities is most likely to be represented by the diagnoses listed below?

1. Anterior ST elevation myocardial infarction
2. Inferior ST elevation myocardial infarction
3. Inferolateral ST elevation myocardial infarction
4. Lateral myocardial infarction
5. Acute pericarditis
6. Anterior ischaemia

3 The unconscious patient

a. Opiate overdose
b. Benzodiazepine overdose
c. Amitriptylline overdose
d. Hypoglycaemia
e. Intracranial bleed
f. Meningococcal septicaemia
g. Post-ictal state following seizure
h. Hepatic encephalopathy

Which of the above diagnoses is likely to be suggested by the following clues, when assessing a patient who is brought into hospital with reduced conscious level?

1. Young man with pyrexia and evidence of petechial rash over his trunk
2. Middle-aged man with jaundice and ascites
3. Young woman with pinpoint pupils and reduced respiratory rate
4. Middle-aged man with pallor and profuse sweating
5. Elderly woman with unilateral fixed, dilated pupil

Acute Medicine: Clinical Cases Uncovered. By C. Roseveare.
Published 2009 by Blackwell Publishing, ISBN: 978-1-4051-6883-0

6. Young male with extensive upper torso bruising and evidence of urinary incontinence
7. Middle-aged man with dilated, sluggishly reactive pupils and bilateral upgoing plantars

---

4 Acute shortness of breath
a. Acute asthma
b. Pneumothorax
c. Pulmonary embolism
d. Bronchopneumonia
e. Left ventricular failure
f. Hyperventilation
g. Pleural effusion

Which of the above diagnoses would be suggested by the following clinical scenarios?

1. A 25-year-old woman who takes the oral contraceptive pill who was referred to hospital complaining of breathlessness of sudden onset; on examination she is tachycardic (100 beats/min) and tachypnoeic with oxygen saturation of 90% when breathing room air. Chest examination reveals good air entry throughout with no added sounds or wheeze.
2. A 20-year-old man with no prior significant history who has been referred to hospital after developing breathlessness of sudden onset, accompanied by severe right-sided pleuritic chest pain. On examination he is noted to be tall and slim and there is reduced expansion and reduced breath sounds over the right lung field.
3. A 79-year-old woman with a past history of ischaemic heart disease who is brought to hospital complaining of an abrupt onset of shortness of breath which woke her from sleep. Examination reveals bilateral basal crackles and elevation of the jugular venous pressure.
4. A 30-year-old man with a short history of fever and malaise followed by the development of breathlessness, and cough productive of discoloured sputum. Examination reveals bronchial breathing at the right base.
5. A 70-year-old man who has become increasingly breathless over the past week, after recovering from a respiratory infection. Examination reveals reduced breath sounds at the left base, which is also stony-dull to percussion.

---

5 Gastrointestinal bleeding
a. Peptic ulcer
b. Mallory-Weiss tear
c. Colonic carcinoma
d. Oesophageal variceal bleed
e. Oesophagitis
f. Gastric carcinoma

Which of the above diagnoses is suggested by the clinical scenarios described below?

1. A 60-year-old man with a 5-month history of weight loss, poor appetite and early satiety. In the past week he has started vomiting after meals and today has noted a small quantity of blood with the vomit.
2. A 55-year-old woman who has been taking regular ibuprofen for her rheumatoid arthritis. Recently she has developed heartburn and epigastric pain, which has been worse after meals. Over the past 48 h she has noted a change in the colour of her stool, which is now black and tarry in consistency with a pungent odour.
3. A 27-year-old man with a history of heavy alcohol consumption, but no prior admissions to hospital. Today he consumed approximately 10 pints of beer after which he vomited repeatedly. He noticed blood in the second vomit and subsequently vomited a further 250 mL of fresh blood.
4. A 48-year-old man who has been admitted to hospital for investigation of jaundice and abdominal distension. Shortly after admission he vomits approximately 500 mL of fresh blood. He is tachycardic and hypotensive.

---

6 Diarrhoea
a. Acute ulcerative colitis
b. Salmonella enterocolitis
c. Ischaemic colitis
d. Pseudomembranous colitis
e. Viral gastroenteritis
f. Diarrhoea-predominant irritable bowel syndrome
g. Thyrotoxicosis
h. Carcinoma of the colon

Which of the above diagnoses is suggested by the following clinical presentations?

1. A 60-year-old woman with a past history of atrial fibrillation presenting with a 3-day history of fresh

rectal bleeding associated with approximately six loose, watery stools per day. On examination she has an irregular pulse but appears relatively well with mild left iliac fossa tenderness only.

2. A 25-year-old man with a 6-week history of gradually worsening diarrhoea, becoming very loose and frequent in the past week with up to 15 watery stools per day. In the past 24 h there has been associated bleeding with each stool. He has lost around 1 stone in weight over the past month. On examination he is tachycardic and mildly pyrexial with generalised mild abdominal tenderness and quiet bowel sounds.

3. A 30-year-old woman with a 2-year history of frequent loose stools, up to 10 times per day, usually occurring in the morning and never waking her from sleep. Her weight has increased over the past year and there has been no rectal bleeding. On examination she is not tachycardic and appears well with a soft abdomen and active bowel sounds.

4. A 49-year-old man who developed diarrhoea abruptly 3 days before admission to hospital. He has felt very unwell, with associated fever, anorexia and cramping abdominal pain. The stool has a green, watery appearance and contained a small quantity of blood on one occasion only. On examination he appears unwell with a pyrexia of 38.5°C, pulse 100 beats/min and generalised mild abdominal tenderness; bowel sounds are active.

5. A 75-year-old woman who developed diarrhoea 1 week ago, the day after discharge from hospital following treatment for pneumonia. The stool is watery in consistency and contains some blood. On examination she is apyrexial and appears dehydrated.

---

7 Arrhythmias

a. Ventricular tachycardia

b. Supraventricular tachycardia

c. Fast atrial fibrillation

d. Complete heart block with ventricular 'escape' rhythm

e. Mobitz type 1, second-degree heart block

f. Sinus tachycardia

g. Sinus bradycardia

h. Atrial flutter with 2 : 1 block

i. First-degree heart block

Which of the following ECG appearances best describes the abnormalities listed above?

1. A broad complex tachycardia, with QRS complexes >140 ms in diameter; there is concordance of polarity across the chest leads and dissociation of P-waves from the QRS complex.

2. A rate of 50 beats/min with P waves before every QRS complex and PR interval of 120 ms.

3. An irregularly irregular tachyarrhythmia with no clearly defined P-waves; all QRS complexes have similar morphology.

4. A regular tachycardia with a rate of exactly 150 beats/min.

5. A slightly irregular rhythm where the PR interval is noted to lengthen with each beat; every fourth P-wave is not followed by a QRS complex.

6. A very slow bradyarrhythmia of 30 beats/min; the P-waves appear to be dissociated from the QRS complexes which are broad (>120 ms).

7. A regular rhythm with rate of 70 beats/min but prolongation of the PR interval (220 ms).

---

8 Stroke

a. Total anterior circulation infarction

b. Partial anterior circulation infarction

c. Lacunar infarction

d. Posterior circulation infarction

Which of the above descriptions describes each of the following presentations?

1. A 70-year-old man who is brought into hospital with a sudden onset of dense left-sided weakness; examination reveals loss of power and sensation on the left, but normal visual fields. Reflexes are brisk on the left with upgoing plantar response.

2. A 64-year-old woman who is brought to hospital complaining of right arm and leg weakness. Examination reveals normal sensation and visual fields; however, there is weakness (grade 3/5) affecting all muscle groups of her right arm and right leg. Reflexes are brisk on the right with an upgoing right plantar response. Speech is normal.

3. An 82-year-old man who was found collapsed on the floor in his nursing home. He is not moving his right arm or leg and his eyes are deviated to the left. He appears to be unaware of his right-hand side and has not spoken at all since being found. He is unable to follow simple commands. Examination reveals a dense right hemiparesis with apparent sensory neglect of the right and receptive/expressive aphasia.

Reflexes are brisk on the right with upgoing right plantar response.

4. A 55-year-old woman who has noted right-sided facial weakness associated with left arm and leg weakness on waking this morning. Examination reveals a right-sided Horner syndrome and right upper motor neurone facial nerve weakness, with pyramidal distribution weakness (grade 4/5) affecting the left arm and leg. There is also mild ataxia noted on assessment of her gait.

---

9 The acutely confused older person

a. Urinary tract infection
b. Alcohol withdrawal
c. Drug-induced confusion
d. Chronic cognitive impairment
e. Hypoxia
f. Respiratory tract infection
g. Myocardial infarction
h. Cerebrovascular event
i. Electrolyte disturbance
j. Subdural haematoma

What is the most likely cause of the following patients' confusion?

1. A 94-year-old woman with a past history of hypertension and congestive cardiac failure. She takes a combination of ramipril, furosemide, bendrofluazide and aspirin. She has recently recovered from a diarrhoeal illness, during which her diuretics were continued. Over the past 24 h the staff in her nursing home have noticed that she is becoming increasingly confused; today she is refusing all food and drink.

2. A 73-year-old woman who lives alone. She was brought into hospital 2 days earlier following a mechanical fall during which she fractured her pubic ramus. There was no evidence of head injury at a CT brain scan was normal. You have been called to see her because she has become severely agitated. She is tremulous, sweaty and shouting abuse at the nursing staff and other patients and will not allow you to examine her.

3. A 81-year-old woman who lives alone, with a long-standing history of mild dementia; her daughter normally visits daily but was away last week and arranged for a neighbour to check on her. On the daughter's return she found her mother to be much more confused than normal. She takes an array of medication for a combination of ischaemic heart disease, atrial fibrillation, hypertension and congestive cardiac failure.

4. An 87-year-old man who has had fluctuating confusion over the past week. He has had a number of falls over the past year. Approximately 2 weeks ago he was brought to the emergency department following a fall and required three stitches to his scalp; a skull radiograph at that time showed no fracture. He has not described headache and there is no focal neurological disturbance on examination.

5. A 77-year-old man with a long history of pulmonary fibrosis related to previous asbestos exposure. He has become increasingly breathless over the past 6 months. His wife reports that in the past week he has become intermittently confused. On examination he has a respiratory rate of 35 breaths/min and bilateral coarse crackles to the midzones.

---

10 The patient with a swollen leg

a. Below-knee deep vein thrombosis
b. Iliac vein thrombosis
c. Cellulitis
d. Ruptured Baker's cyst
e. Chronic venous insufficiency
f. Dependent oedema
g. Calf muscle tear

Which of the above diagnoses is suggested by the following clinical presentations?

1. A 35-year-old woman with a history of a recent insect bite to her right foot. Twenty-four hours later she felt unwell and developed a localised erythematous area at the site of the bite, which subsequently spread to affect her right shin and calf. On examination she is pyrexial and has a clearly defined area of erythema over the right shin, which is warm and tender to touch.

2. A 70-year-old man with a past history of arthritis affecting his knees that limits his mobility. One week ago he developed sudden pain behind his left knee; since then his left calf has been swollen and painful. On examination the calf is swollen on the left with tenderness over the calf muscles and popliteal fossa. The calf feels warm to touch but there is no erythema.

3. A 35-year-old man who developed a sudden pain in his right calf 3 days ago while playing football; since then he has been unable to walk without pain. On examination there is localised tenderness in the calf muscle; there is slight swelling of the right foot, but no warmth or erythema.

4. A 35-year-old woman who takes the oral contraceptive pill and whose left leg has been immobilised in a splint after injuring her ankle 4 weeks ago. On removal of the splint her calf is noted to be swollen, warm and erythematous. The calf muscle is tender on examination. Duplex scan shows no evidence of a DVT.

5. A 75-year-old man with a past history of prostatic carcinoma who has developed extensive swelling of his right leg over the past week. Examination reveals swelling of the leg that extends to the groin level.

SAQs

1 *A 52-year-old man presents to hospital complaining of central chest pain which started 4 hours earlier. On examination he is sweaty and remains in some discomfort with a blood pressure of 140/60 and pulse 70 beats/min. ECG shows ST segment elevation in leads V2–V4 (see figure below).*

a. What is the likely diagnosis?

b. What immediate treatment should be prescribed and what further history should be obtained?

c. What complications may arise during this patient's hospital stay, and how should he be monitored?

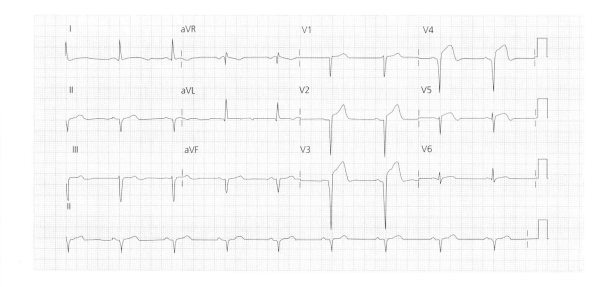

2 *A 60-year-old woman is admitted to hospital describing 2 days of black, tarry stool with an offensive odour. She feels light-headed on standing, and fainted shortly before hospital admission. On examination she appears pale with a slight tachycardia (100 beats/min); blood pressure is 140/70 while supine, falling to 90/50 on standing.*

a. What is the likely diagnosis and cause for these symptoms?

b. What is the significance of the episode of fainting and pulse/blood pressure readings?

c. What immediate treatment should be provided?

d. What further information should be sought in the history and what investigations are required?

Acute Medicine: Clinical Cases Uncovered. By C. Roseveare.
Published 2009 by Blackwell Publishing, ISBN: 978-1-4051-6883-0

3 *A 25-year-old woman with a past history of asthma is brought to hospital complaining of acute wheeze, which is not relieved by her usual inhalers. On examination she is tachycardic (110 beats/min) and unable to speak in full sentences. Respiratory rate is 30 breaths/min and peak flow is 150 L/min (previous best peak flow 400 L/min). Chest examination reveals widespread expiratory wheeze.*

a. How would you classify the severity of this attack?
b. What immediate treatment is required?
c. What further treatment options should be considered if the patient's condition fails to settle?

4 *An 88-year-old man is brought to hospital after neighbours found him wandering in the street outside his house in his pyjamas. According to the neighbours he has a history of mild dementia but normally cares for himself. They had seen him 24 hours earlier and noted him to be a bit 'chesty', but was not apparently more confused than normal at that time. Currently, he is unable to give any further history and scores 0/10 on a mini-mental test score. Examination reveals him to be pyrexial (38.4°C) with bibasal crackles on respiratory examination. He has an irregular tachycardia (110 beats/min) with blood pressure 170/100. Neurological and abdominal examinations are unremarkable.*

a. What further information should be sought and what sources can be used to acquire this further history?
b. What is the differential diagnosis based on the information given?
c. What further investigations may be helpful?

5 *A 25-year-old man is brought to hospital by his father. His father had visited his son's flat where he was noted to be very drowsy; there was an empty bottle of vodka next to him along with empty packets of 16 × 500 mg paracetamol tablets. His father also found a hand-written suicide note beside him. He has been very withdrawn recently after breaking up with his partner and has seen his GP who arranged for some counselling; he has no history of prior overdose or documented psychiatric illness. On arrival in hospital he appears drowsy (Glasgow Coma Score 11/15) and smells strongly of alcohol. He has pinpoint pupils and his respiratory rate is 8 breaths/min.*

a. What is the significance of the pinpoint pupils and reduced respiratory rate?
b. What investigation and treatment are likely to be required?
c. Once medically stable, what psychiatric management may be required?

6 *A 50-year-old woman is brought to hospital after collapsing at home with a sudden severe headache. She does not normally experience headaches and has never experienced a headache of this intensity. She has vomited twice. She has been seen by the accident and emergency team who have arranged for a CT brain scan which is normal. The headache has now improved after she was given analgesia.*

a. What possible diagnoses should be considered?
b. What further investigations are required, and how should the results be interpreted?

7 *A 28-year-old man is referred to hospital by his GP. He is known to suffer with ulcerative colitis which has been well controlled over the past year. However, for the past week he has noticed a progressive increase in his stool frequency which is now up to 10 times per day and waking him twice each night. He has lost 6 kg in weight. The stool is watery in consistency and there is blood mixed in. On examination he is apyrexial with a pulse of 100 beats/min. There is mild left iliac fossa tenderness with active bowel sounds but no distension or peritonism. An abdominal radiograph shows an empty colon that is not distended.*

a. What is the most likely diagnosis?
b. How can the severity of the problem be assessed?
c. What treatment should be prescribed?

8 *A 19-year-old man is brought to hospital. He was diagnosed with Type 1 diabetes at the age of 14 and has been treated with insulin since then. Over the past 24 hours he has felt increasingly unwell. Initially he noticed cramp-like abdominal pain which was followed by diarrhoea and vomiting. His mother noticed that he appeared breathless and checked his blood glucose which read 'high' on his glucometer. She has brought him to hospital. He appears slightly drowsy and mucous membranes are dry. Pulse is 120 beats/min with blood pressure 90/40. Urinalysis reveals 4+ ketones and 3+ glucose.*

a. What is the likely diagnosis, and how should this be confirmed?
b. What are the possible causes?
c. How should he be treated?

9 *A 60-year-old woman is brought to hospital by her husband. She has been unwell for the past 2 days with generalised malaise, weakness and fever. In the past 24 hours she has taken to her bed where she has become increasingly confused and drowsy. Her fluid intake has been minimal during this time. She has a past history of ischaemic heart disease and congestive cardiac failure, and takes furosemide, ramipril, aspirin and simvastatin. On arrival in hospital she looks extremely unwell. She has a pyrexia of 39°C and is drowsy with Glasgow Coma Score of 12/15 (disorientated speech, eyes open to command and localises painful stimuli). Pulse is 130 beats/min and appears of good volume, with blood pressure 80/30. There are a few bibasal crackles in her chest and a soft ejection systolic murmur. There also appears to be some tenderness in the right renal angle and suprapubic area.*

a. Give a differential diagnosis and some of the possible underlying causes.
b. What initial treatment is required?
c. How should she be investigated further?

10 *A 50-year-old man with a long history of chronic obstructive airways disease is referred to hospital by his GP. He has been experiencing increasing breathlessness over the past week associated with a cough productive of green sputum. The general practitioner has started him on oral amoxicillin and prednisolone 2 days ago but there has been no improvement. On arrival in A&E he appears breathless and cyanosed, and is using accessory muscles of respiration. There is poor air entry throughout both lung fields with a few expiratory wheezes, but no other added sounds. Arterial blood gases while breathing room air are as follows: pH 7.37, pCO_2 7.94, pO_2 6.45, HCO_3 35, base excess +8, saturation 83%.*

a. What abnormalities are demonstrated on the arterial blood gases and what is their significance?
b. What initial treatment is required and what further monitoring should be undertaken?
c. What further treatment options are indicated if the CO_2 level rises after initiation of treatment?

MCQs answers

1. d. Pleuritic chest pain is typically described as a sharp, stabbing pain, exacerbated by inspiration and coughing. Causes include pneumothorax and pleural infection (bacterial or viral). Although pleuritic chest pain may occur in the context of pulmonary infarction following pulmonary embolism, this is usually of gradual onset. Breathlessness is a more common presenting symptom in most cases of pulmonary embolism and can be of abrupt onset. Ischaemic cardiac pain is not usually pleuritic in nature.

2. d. The combination of tachycardia, tachypnoea, hypoxia with normal chest examination and a normal radiograph is suggestive of pulmonary embolism. Although there are no clear risk factors for pulmonary embolism she may have an underlying thrombotic tendency. Anxiety-induced hyperventilation may produce tachycardia and respiratory alkalosis (low pCO_2 and elevated pH), but would not account for the hypoxia, which is significant in a patient of this age without previous lung disease. Pneumothorax would normally be apparent on a chest radiograph, whereas diabetic ketoacidosis would normally result in a low pH.

3. c. Although use of an oral contraceptive pill containing oestrogen increases the likelihood of pulmonary embolism its use does not constitute a criterion for calculation of the Wells score (see p. 40).

4. d. In the absence of evidence of portal hypertension or chronic liver disease, peptic ulcer is more likely than oesophageal varices as the cause of significant upper gastrointestinal bleeding, even in patients who drink large quantities of alcohol. Mallory–Weiss tear and oesophagitis are recognised causes of haematemesis, but do not commonly result in melaena. Colonic diverticular disease is a recognised cause of fresh rectal bleeding, but would not account for haematemesis.

5. a. Although brisk upper gastrointestinal bleeding can result in fresh rectal bleeding, the patient would normally be haemodynamically compromised in this context. Lower gastrointestinal bleeding is more likely and diverticular disease would be the most common cause in a patient of this age. Bleeding due to ulcerative colitis is usually accompanied by diarrhoea.

6. d. Although terlipressin reduces portal pressure and may be useful to reduce the risk of rebleeding in the context of variceal bleeding there is no evidence for its use in peptic ulcer bleeding. Acid suppression with intravenous omeprazole has been shown to reduce the risk of rebleeding following endoscopic treatment of a bleeding peptic ulcer. Clot stability is improved when the gastric pH is raised above 4, which cannot be achieved with oral omeprazole or intravenous ranitidine. *Helicobacter pylori* eradication will reduce the likelihood of ulcer recurrence after healing, but does not affect risk of rebleeding.

7. b. The history of nocturnal diarrhoea, rectal bleeding and weight loss makes irritable bowel syndrome unlikely. Thyrotoxicosis may present with diarrhoea, weight loss and tachycardia, but this is uncommon and would not explain the rectal bleeding. Infective causes should always be considered in this situation, although the long history makes ulcerative colitis more likely. Rectal carcinoma may result in a change of bowel habit (including the onset of diarrhoea) and rectal bleeding but would be very uncommon in this age group.

8. c. Colonoscopy is generally contraindicated in patients with acute colitis as air insufflation may

Acute Medicine: Clinical Cases Uncovered. By C. Roseveare.
Published 2009 by Blackwell Publishing, ISBN: 978-1-4051-6883-0

precipitate toxic dilatation and the friable mucosa may risk colonic perforation. Rigid sigmoidoscopy and biopsy may enable confirmation of the presence of colitis, and is still undertaken in some circumstances, although flexible sigmoidoscopy may give more useful diagnostic information about the nature and extent of inflammation. An abdominal radiograph will provide useful information about the distribution of colitis and will enable identification of toxic megacolon. Hypokalaemia and hypoalbuminaemia are relatively common in severe colitis; stool culture has low sensitivity, but may enable appropriate targeting of antibiotic therapy if positive.

9. e. Hypokalaemia is common as a result of potassium loss; hyperkalaemia is unusual except in the context of associated acute renal failure or excessive potassium replacement. Ischaemic colitis usually results in heavy blood loss, often disproportionate to the extent and severity of inflammation. Nocturnal diarrhoea usually implies an inflammatory or secretory problem – motility-related diarrhoea rarely wakes the patient from sleep. Hypoalbuminaemia is a common accompaniment of severe colitis and may reflect chronic inflammation or gastrointestinal protein loss; renal protein loss is not common in this situation. Infection control precautions including isolation are advisable for any patient presenting with diarrhoea; the low sensitivity of stool culture should lead to caution in the interpretation of negative results, unless an alternative diagnosis is clear-cut.

10. e. Migraine can present suddenly, but would be unusual as a first presentation in a man of this age. Normal CT brain is generally considered to exclude only around 90% of subarachnoid haemorrhages. Lumbar puncture should generally be delayed until >12 h from the onset of symptoms to enable the appearance of bilirubin in the cerebrospinal fluid; this will help to distinguish the appearance of contamination from a traumatic lumbar puncture. Subarachnoid rarely results in focal neurological signs, although reduced conscious level is associated with a larger bleed and therefore worse overall prognosis.

11. b. Nimodipine is generally given orally or via a nasogastric tube to prevent cerebral vasospasm following subarachnoid haemorrhage; intravenous use requires delivery via a central venous cannula, so is not normally recommended.

12. a. The risk of a cardiac cause of syncope is increased in patients **over** the age of 50; coexistent ischaemic heart disease, tachy- or bradyarrhythmias, family history of sudden death and valvular heart disease also suggest the need for further cardiac investigations.

13. e. Violent shaking following a syncopal episode can mimic the features of a seizure, causing diagnostic difficulties; this is particularly relevant in relation to the patient's future driving status. Unless the clinician is confident that the loss of consciousness was caused by a simple faint, the patient should be advised not to drive and to contact the DVLA for further advice. A transient ischaemic attack rarely results in loss of consciousness. Prolonged drowsiness is more in keeping with a seizure, rather than syncope; hypoglycaemia (rather than hyperglycaemia) is commonly associated with loss of consciousness.

14. a. Pallor and absence of pulses are suggestive of arterial rather than venous obstruction. Occasionally very extensive, proximal venous thrombosis can result in arterial occlusion due to the degree of swelling; however, this is not a common feature. The other features are recognised signs of DVT.

15. b. D-dimer is a very non-specific test and raised level cannot be considered diagnostic of DVT. Elevations can also be seen in the presence of inflammatory diseases and infection as well as in the presence of co-existent malignancy, following surgery and during pregnancy. Lower limb venous duplex scan is highly sensitive for the diagnosis of above-knee thrombosis, although it is less sensitive for below-knee thrombosis.

16. c. A regular narrow complex tachycardia at this rate is likely to be supraventricular tachycardia. Atrial flutter will usually produce a heart rate very close to 150 beats/min, whereas atrial fibrillation is irregular. Sinus tachycardia is unlikely to produce a tachycardia at this rate, while ventricular tachycardia almost always produces broad complexes.

17. c. Although supraventricular tachycardia can result in broad complexes when combined with a bundle branch block, ventricular tachycardia is much more likely after myocardial infarction. For this reason

adenosine is unlikely to be effective and amiodarone is a more appropriate initial treatment if the patient is haemodynamically stable; emergency DC cardioversion is required if the patient is hypotensive or developing cardiac failure. Thyrotoxicosis should be considered, but is not common in this context.

18. d. DC cardioversion may be required, but should normally be delayed until the patient has been anticoagulated for at least 4 weeks, unless haemodynamically compromised or the onset is clearly within 48 h of presentation. Rate control with digoxin or beta-blockers may improve symptom control for such patients. Alcoholic cardiomyopathy is a relatively common cause of atrial fibrillation in this situation.

19. d. Absence of wheeze in the context of acute asthma may result from extreme bronchospasm with inadequate air entry; this is therefore usually considered a life-threatening feature. Tachycardia is also a feature of severe asthma, and may also result from regular use of beta-stimulant bronchodilators (e.g. salbutamol). During a mild asthma attack patients breathe rapidly, resulting in depression of pCO_2; normal or raised pCO_2 may suggest that the patient is tiring and is normally considered a sign of more severe asthma. High-flow oxygen should be administered on admission for all patients with acute asthma – unlike in the patient with chronic obstructive pulmonary disease where controlled oxygen therapy may be required. The main reason for undertaking a chest radiograph is to exclude pneumothorax.

20. a. Viral infections are common precipitants of acute asthma, but bacterial infection is a relatively unusual precipitant. Intravenous salbutamol is as effective as nebulised salbutamol and may be particularly useful if the patient's bronchospasm is so severe that inhaled agents are not likely to reach the small airways. Air is often used as the driving gas for nebulisers where the patient has chronic obstructive pulmonary disease and there is a concern about a rising pCO_2; however, this is not likely in acute asthma where oxygen should always be used as the driving gas. Magnesium sulphate may be of benefit in severe asthma, although there is limited evidence for its use in mild or moderate attacks.

21. d. Focal neurological deficit or clinical evidence of raised intracranial pressure may suggest significant intracranial pathology as the cause for the confusion; a recent head injury or deterioration in condition after admission raises the suspicion of intracranial bleeding which may be amenable to surgical intervention. Seizure is common in patients with a history of alcohol dependence, and is often a result of lowered seizure threshold due to chronic alcohol misuse, or alcohol withdrawal. Although CT scanning may be required if seizures continue, this will often not be required if the patient's condition stabilises.

22. d. Hypoglycaemia is a relatively common finding in patients with alcohol dependency; this may result from impaired hepatic gluconeogenesis, as a reactive hypoglycaemia following acute alcohol ingestion. Administration of intravenous glucose in this situation may result in an increased cerebral requirement for thiamine; if the patient is thiamine deficient this may precipitate acute Wernicke's encephalopathy. Oral thiamine is poorly absorbed and will not generally increase the plasma thiamine adequately to cross the blood–brain barrier and prevent Wernicke's encephalopathy following an acute presentation to hospital. Failure to treat acute Wernicke's encephalopathy may result in Korsakoff's psychosis, which is usually considered irreversible. Only around 10% of patients with Wernicke's encephalopathy have the classic triad of ataxia, confusion and ophthalmoplegia; the commonest finding at presentation is acute confusion.

23. c. Accurate interpretation of the paracetamol level and the likelihood of liver damage requires the level to be compared with the 'treatment line'. Patients whose paracetamol level is above the line are more likely to sustain liver damage and their prognosis is improved by treatment with *N*-acetyl cysteine. Given that the paracetamol level can continue to rise for up to 4 h, accurate interpretation requires that measurement is delayed for 4 h from the time of consumption. Interpretation of the level is much more difficult if the patient has taken a staggered overdose, and empirical treatment with *N*-acetyl cysteine is therefore usually required, pending measurement of liver function and INR after at least 24 h. It

usually takes at least 24 h before abnormalities of liver function become apparent; the finding of abnormal INR or other liver function tests at the time of admission usually reflects pre-existing liver disease, warfarin consumption or an earlier overdose.

24. c. Hepatic enzyme-inducing drugs (e.g. carbamazepine, phenytoin) increase the production of the toxic metabolites following paracetamol overdose and therefore make liver damage more likely. Liver enzymes are also induced by chronic liver disease, chronic alcohol ingestion and malnutrition. Anorexia also depletes hepatic glutathione stores that are usually required to deactivate toxic metabolites of paracetamol. Acute alcohol ingestion results in inhibition of the enzymes, and therefore may paradoxically reduce the risk of liver damage.

25. e. Elevation of the INR following paracetamol overdose suggests synthetic liver dysfunction and may progress to fulminant hepatic failure. Continued treatment with *N*-acetyl cysteine may reduce the likelihood of progression to liver failure. An isolated rise in liver transaminases is relatively common – although this usually reflects some degree of liver damage it is of no prognostic significance in the absence of elevation of the INR. Serial measurement of the INR gives useful prognostic information; however, repeat measurement of the paracetamol level is rarely helpful, unless there are reasons to believe that the patient has taken more of the drug following admission to hospital. Given the importance of the INR in determining prognosis and the need for liver transplantation, correction of this with fresh frozen plasma should be avoided unless the patient is acutely bleeding. Section 5(2) of the Mental Health Act will allow detention of a patient who is deemed to be at risk to themselves or to others, due to a psychiatric illness, for up to 72 h; if more prolonged detention is required the section will need to be converted into a Section 2 or Section 3 by a registered psychiatrist.

26. d. The clinical findings are typical of pulmonary oedema. The acute onset of symptoms is not typical for pneumonia or an exacerbation of chronic obstructive pulmonary disease, which would usually be pre-dated by symptoms of infection. Pulmonary embolism cannot be excluded; bilateral pleural rub associated with extensive pulmonary infarction can occasionally mimic the signs of pulmonary oedema, but this is much less likely. The crackles of pulmonary fibrosis can also mimic the features of pulmonary oedema, but this is normally a chronic condition that would not normally present acutely.

27. d. The elevated pCO_2 in the context of acute asthma is a sign that the patient is tiring; the normal bicarbonate and low pH suggest that this has come on acutely and respiratory arrest may be imminent. Urgent transfer to intensive care is likely to be necessary and it may be necessary for the patient to be intubated and ventilated prior to transfer. Intravenous bronchodilators such as salbutamol or aminophylline may be helpful, pending arrival of the anaesthetist, but intravenous hydrocortisone has a slow onset of action and the benefit of magnesium in this situation is limited. Reducing the FiO_2 in this situation would be disastrous; this is in contrast to the situation in relation to a patient with COPD and rising CO_2 where controlled flow oxygen may result in a fall in the CO_2 level.

28. d. ST segment elevation in II, III and AVF is suggestive of inferior STEMI, which usually indicates occlusion of the right coronary artery. Since the right coronary artery also supplies the sinus node and atrioventricular node, bradyarrhythmias including complete heart block are relatively common. Thrombolysis or primary percutaneous coronary intervention therapy is indicated for any patient presenting within 12 h of the onset of their symptoms. Patients should all receive 300 mg of aspirin on arrival in hospital.

29. e. Left bundle branch block can be the presenting ECG finding of myocardial infarction, in which case it is often associated with a high mortality. If a patient with left bundle branch block gives a good history of ischaemic-type chest pain within the past 12 h, consistent with a myocardial infarction, thrombolysis is indicated. Patients with recent evidence of bleeding or recent surgery may be at higher risk of bleeding following thrombolysis, which may offset any beneficial effect. Such patients may still be considered appropriate for primary percutaneous coronary intervention.

30. d. Patients with secondary hyperparathyroidism
are **hypo**calcaemic: the low level of serum calcium
causes increased pathyroid hormone production by
the pituitary gland; after a prolonged period this
may lead to a rise in the serum calcium, termed
tertiary hyperparathyroidism. Primary
hyperparathyroidism is a common cause of
hypercalcaemia; this results from excessive secretion
of parathyroid hormone from the pituitary gland,
often due to an adenoma. Sarcoidosis, myeloma
and bronchial carcinoma (with or without bony
metastases) should all be considered in the
differential diagnosis of a patient with
hypercalcaemia.

EMQs answers

1
1. b
2. h
3. f
4. e

2
1. d
2. a
3. c
4. f
5. g
6. b

3
1. f
2. h
3. a
4. d
5. e
6. g
7. c

4
1. c
2. b
3. e
4. d
5. g

5
1. f
2. a
3. b
4. d

6
1. c
2. a
3. f
4. b
5. d

7
1. a
2. g
3. c
4. h
5. e
6. d
7. i

8
1. b
2. c
3. a
4. d

9
1. i
2. b
3. c
4. j
5. e

10
1. c
2. d
3. g
4. a
5. b

Acute Medicine: Clinical Cases Uncovered. By C. Roseveare.
Published 2009 by Blackwell Publishing, ISBN: 978-1-4051-6883-0

SAQs answers

1

a. On the basis of the symptoms and ECG findings, the likely diagnosis is anterior ST elevation myocardial infarction (STEMI).

b. The patient should be prescribed high-flow oxygen, intravenous opiate analgesia (e.g. morphine sulphate) along with an antiemetic (e.g. cyclizine 50 mg intravenously). In addition he should be given aspirin 300 mg orally provided there is no prior history of severe aspirin allergy.

Given that the likely diagnosis is STEMI, thrombolytic drug therapy or primary percutaneous coronary intervention is likely to be necessary. Further history should establish whether there are any risk factors or contraindications for thrombolysis and the precise timing of onset of symptoms.

c. Early complications include arrhythmias (especially ventricular arrhythmias, including ventricular tachycardia and ventricular fibrillation); cardiogenic shock; left ventricular failure; myocardial or valvular rupture. The patient should be connected to a cardiac monitor for at least 24 hours after admission and undergo regular monitoring of pulse, blood pressure, respiratory rate and oxygen saturation.

2

a. The description of the stool colour, consistency and pungent aroma suggests that she has experienced bleeding from the upper gastrointestinal tract. The most likely cause in a patient of this age would be peptic ulcer disease.

b. The combination of tachycardia, postural hypotension and syncope is suggestive of a significant volume of blood loss; this increases the mortality from this condition and suggests that she is likely to require fluid resuscitation and urgent investigation into the cause.

c. At least one (and preferably two) large-bore cannulae should be sited and intravenous fluid resuscitation should be commenced using colloid (e.g. gelofusine 500 mL over 30 min) or crystalloid (e.g. 1 L 0.9% saline over 1 h). Oxygen should also be administered by mask.

d. Further history should be directed at trying to elicit the likely underlying cause of the bleeding. This should include enquiry into previous symptoms suggestive of peptic ulceration, prior use of aspirin or non-steroidal anti-inflammatory drugs, previous documented peptic ulcer disease. A history of previous chronic liver disease or variceal bleeding should raise the possibility of varices as the cause, and a history of weight loss and early satiety may suggest an upper gastrointestinal malignancy. A history of bleeding disorders or anticoagulant use should also be established.

Blood should be sent for full blood count, urea and electrolytes, liver function tests, group and save and blood-clotting studies. Endoscopy should be undertaken within 12 h of admission where possible, or sooner if the patient remains haemodynamically unstable despite fluid resuscitation.

3

a. The combination of tachypnoea (>25 breaths/min), tachycardia (≥110 beats/min) and inability to speak in full sentences indicates that the patient has *acute severe asthma*.

b. She should be prescribed nebulised salbutamol (5 mg) with oxygen as the driving gas, combined with ipratropium bromide 500 µg. An intravenous cannula should be sited and 2 g magnesium sulphate should be administered by infusion over 20 min.

Acute Medicine: Clinical Cases Uncovered. By C. Roseveare.
Published 2009 by Blackwell Publishing, ISBN: 978-1-4051-6883-0

High-flow oxygen should be continued after completion of the nebuliser and her condition should be reassessed.

c. If her condition fails to improve following this treatment, she should be given further nebulised salbutamol ('back-to-back' nebulisers), with consideration of administration of intravenous salbutamol or aminophylline. Referral to the intensive care unit for intubation and mechanical ventilation should be made if there is further deterioration or if she appears to be tiring despite these measures.

4

a. It is important to obtain a history of recent or prior illnesses, particularly previous similar episodes. It is also important to establish whether the onset of confusion is truly 'acute' or whether there has been a more gradual decline in his cognitive state. A detailed drug history should also be obtained, along with a history of any drug allergies, which may influence his treatment (particularly antibiotic allergies). A history of alcohol excess and any recent head injury or falls should also be obtained. Potential sources of history should include the patient's general practitioner, hospital records, ambulance crew, family members or other carers and neighbours.

b. The presence of fever and tachycardia is suggestive of infection as a cause for the confusion; the recent chest symptoms and bibasal respiratory crackles are suggestive of a lower respiratory tract infection. Other sources of infection, particularly in the urinary tract, should also be considered. Cerebral infections (meningitis, encephalitis or cerebral abscess) are less common but should be considered in the presence of severe confusion or if there is evidence of focal neurology or meningism on examination. The symptoms may be exacerbated by dehydration and renal impairment, and drug toxicity should also be considered. Subdural haematoma or a cerebrovascular event should also be listed in the differential for any elderly patient admitted with unexplained confusion. In this case his irregular tachycardia may imply that he is in atrial fibrillation which is a risk factor for ischaemic stroke, but may also imply treatment with digoxin (consider toxicity) and anticoagulant drugs (increasing the risk of

intracranial bleeding). Thyrotoxicosis may present with fast atrial fibrillation and confusion in elderly patients.

c. Initial investigations should include full blood count, urea and electrolytes, liver function tests, C-reactive protein, thyroid function, blood culture, chest radiograph, urine culture and an ECG. If the patient is thought to be taking anticoagulants or digoxin his clotting and digoxin level should also be measured. CT brain scan should be undertaken if there is no clear explanation for the symptoms following these test results, if his conscious level deteriorates or if there is a history of possible head injury or falls.

5

a. Pinpoint pupils and reduced respiratory rate should always raise suspicion of ingestion of opiate drugs (e.g. codeine, morphine, etc.). These may be found in combination with paracetamol in some over-the-counter or prescribed analgesic agents (e.g. co-dydramol, solpadeine, etc.); alternatively this may have been taken separately. In some cases the recreational use of opiates (e.g. heroin) may have preceded a suicide attempt. Effects of opiate use can be reversed using naloxone, so that recognition of these features can enable specific treatment to be given.

b. Administration of naloxone (initially 0.4 mg intravenously) may result in reversal of the impact of the opiate ingestion and will improve his respiratory rate and conscious level. Measurement of paracetamol level 4 h after the time of ingestion will enable the doctor to establish whether he requires treatment with N-acetyl cysteine. Measurement of blood alcohol level may also be helpful, along with the salicylate level, in case he has taken aspirin in combination with the paracetamol. If the paracetamol level is above the 'treatment line' he will require treatment with N-acetyl cysteine.

c. The combination of a suicide note and his apparent recent depression indicates that he may be at high risk of further self-harm following treatment of this episode. It is essential that a formal psychiatric risk assessment is undertaken prior to discharge from hospital and that further follow-up is arranged to manage this problem, via either his general practitioner or community psychiatric team. It is possible that the psychiatric team will want to admit him for further assessment and treatment if he is deemed to be at high risk, and it is essential that he is not permitted to leave the hospital until this risk has been clearly documented. It may be necessary to detain him in the ward under Section 5(2) of the Mental Health Act, pending psychiatric assessment.

6

a. Given the sudden onset of headache, subarachnoid haemorrhage (SAH) should be considered the most likely diagnosis until this can be ruled out. Although the normal CT scan makes this less likely, this does not rule out the diagnosis. Differential diagnoses include 'thunderclap' migraine, pain referred from the neck (cervical radiculopathy) and cerebral venous sinus thrombosis.

b. Lumbar puncture (LP) is required as the next investigation. This should be delayed for around 12 hours from the onset of symptoms as this will enable blood pigments (especially bilirubin) to appear in the cerebrospinal fluid (CSF) following SAH. Red blood cell count may be helpful if the fluid is completely clear; however, if red blood cells are present in the fluid this may simply imply contamination at the time of lumbar puncture ('traumatic tap'). Provided the LP has been delayed for 12 h the absence of bilirubin from the sample is highly sensitive for exclusion of SAH; conversely if bilirubin is present in the sample this is very suggestive of SAH. Measurement of the CSF pressure should be undertaken at the time of LP. If CSF pressure is elevated in the absence of SAH this should raise the suspicion of venous sinus thrombosis as the cause of headache. If SAH is suggested by the results of LP, magnetic resonance arteriography or cerebral angiography should be considered as the next investigations of choice, following neurosurgical referral.

7

a. The likely diagnosis is an acute exacerbation ('flare-up') of his ulcerative colitis.

b. The severity of the problem may be assessed clinically by the stool frequency, haemodynamic effects and presence of pyrexia/abdominal pain. The severity can also be assessed by review of an abdominal radiograph, or by sigmoidoscopic grading of the severity of colitis. Elevation of the white cell count and inflammatory markers (e.g. C-reactive protein) combined with a low albumin are also suggestive of a more severe exacerbation.

c. He should be commenced on intravenous fluid, and will almost certainly require potassium supplementation. He should be given intravenous corticosteroid treatment (e.g. hydrocortisone 100 mg qds) and oral mesalazine (800 mg tds) combined with a hydrocortisone rectal drip (100 mg bid).

8

a. The likely diagnosis is diabetic ketoacidosis (DKA); this should be confirmed by measurement of arterial or venous blood gases and blood glucose.

b. Given the history of diarrhoea and sickness, it is likely that he has acute gastroenteritis as the underlying cause. Acute pancreatitis should also be considered. Breathlessness may indicate a respiratory infection, but is more likely to reflect 'Kussmaul' respiration due to metabolic acidosis. Some patients will, incorrectly, reduce or discontinue their insulin treatment when they start vomiting because of fears regarding hypoglycaemia. It is important to clarify if he has done this, in which case re-education will be required. Paradoxically, patients' insulin requirements often increase during an acute illness, even in the prescence of vomiting – discontinuation of insulin in Type 1 diabetes will frequently result in DKA. Patients should be advised to continue with their normal insulin treatment and to increase the frequency of monitoring in this situation.

c. The mainstay of treatment is intravenous fluid and intravenous insulin. He should start with 1 L of normal saline over 30–60 min along with 6 units of insulin per hour by intravenous infusion. Blood glucose should be recorded hourly and potassium will need to be measured repeatedly as this will fall with administration of intravenous insulin. Cardiac and fluid balance monitoring are essential, as is measurement of the patient's conscious level. Fluid and insulin requirements should be titrated according to the patient's response.

9

a. She is exhibiting the features of *shock*. The most likely cause for this is sepsis, given the pyrexia and recent febrile illness. The source of infection may be urinary, given the renal angle tenderness, although respiratory infection should also be considered; the ejection systolic murmur is probably a 'flow' murmur, resulting from the high cardiac output in septic shock, although infective endocarditis should also be considered. Intracranial infection and meningococcal infection should also be considered given the reduced conscious level and speed of deterioration in her condition.

Other causes of shock should be considered in the differential diagnosis: hypovolaemia (due to poor oral intake and continued diuretic use), cardiogenic shock (past history of myocardial ischaemia increases the likelihood of this); the vasodilatory effects of ramipril may have exacerbated the hypotension.

b. High-flow oxygen should be administered by mask and at least one large-bore intravenous cannula inserted. A fluid challenge should be given (e.g. 500 mL of normal saline over 30 min). She should be connected to a cardiac monitor and undergo continuous pulse oximetry and regular blood pressure measurement (every 10–15 min) to assess response to fluid. Further fluid should be prescribed according to the initial response. Broad-spectrum intravenous antibiotics should be administered after obtaining blood cultures.

Insertion of a urinary catheter for monitoring of urine output is advisable, and a central venous cannula should be considered if her blood pressure fails to respond to initial fluid resuscitation.

c. Initial investigations should include full blood count, urea and electrolytes, liver function tests, clotting, blood cultures, urine culture, chest radiograph and ECG.

10

a. The blood gases show Type 2 respiratory failure (hypoxia combined with hypercapnia) and compensated respiratory alkalosis (normal pH with raised pCO_2 and raised bicarbonate/base excess). The severity of hypoxia is likely to require correction by administration of oxygen; however, overzealous administration of oxygen is likely to result in a further rise in pCO_2 in this situation. Controlled administration of oxygen with regular measurement of arterial blood gases is therefore necessary.

b. The patient should be started on 28% oxygen via a Venturi mask; nebulised salbutamol and ipratropium bromide should be administered, using air as the driving gas (with supplemental oxygen via nasal cannulae if required). His antibiotic and steroid should be continued, with consideration of the addition of a macrolide antibiotic (e.g. erythromycin) or tetracycline (e.g. doxycycline) to cover atypical organisms. Arterial blood gases (ABG) should be repeated 30 min after commencing 28% oxygen; if the pO_2 remains below 8 kPa and the pCO_2 has not risen significantly, the inhaled oxygen concentration may be increased to 35% with further repeat of ABG after 30 min.

c. If the pCO_2 rises significantly with oxygen administration, mechanical ventilatory support is likely to be necessary (assuming reversible causes such as bronchospasm and sputum plugging have been adequately treated). Initially this will take the form of non-invasive ventilation, such as biphasic positive airway pressure (BiPAP). Intubation and mechanical ventilation are sometimes required.

Appendix: Normal ranges, units and common abbreviations for blood tests

Test	Abbreviation	Normal range*	Units
Sodium	Na	135–145	mmol/L
Potassium	K	3.5–5	mmol/L
Urea	Ur	2.9–7.1	mmol/L
Creatinine	Cr	53–97	μmol/L
Total protein	Prot	61–79	g/L
Albumin	Alb	35–48	g/L
Bilirubin	Bil	0–20	μmol/L
Alkaline phosphatase	ALP	42–161	IU/L
Alanine transaminase	ALT	10–40	IU/L
C-reactive protein	CRP	0–7.5	mg/L
Calcium	Ca	2.15–2.65	mmol/L
Magnesium	Mg	0.74–1.03	mmol/L
Phosphate	Phos	0.78–1.53	mmol/L
Creatinine kinase	CK	<171	IU/L
Amylase	Amy	36–128	IU/L
Thyroid-stimulating hormone	TSH	0.35–5.6	mu/L
Thyroxine	T4	7.5–21.1	pmol/L
Haemoglobin	Hb	130–170	g/L
White cell count	WCC	4–11	$\times 10^9$/L
Neutrophil count	Neut	2–7.5	$\times 10^9$/L
Platelet count	Plat	140–400	$\times 10^9$/L
Mean corpuscular volume	MCV	80–100	fL
Mean corpuscular haemoglobin	MCH	27–32	pg
Erythrocyte sedimentation rate	ESR	<35	mm in first hour
International normalised ratio	INR	0.8–1.2	Not applicable

*Note that reference ranges can vary between different laboratories, depending on the method of assay. Always refer to your local laboratory for confirmation of the normal range, particularly in the case of amylase and ALP measurement.

Index of cases by diagnosis

Index

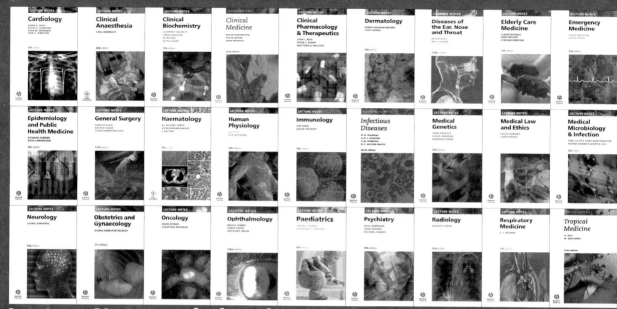
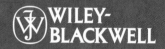
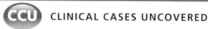
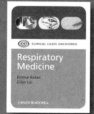
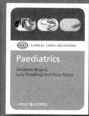
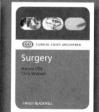
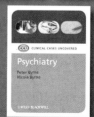
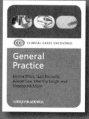
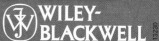